Lyme Borreliosis

Current Problems in Dermatology

Vol. 37

Series Editor

P. Itin Basel

Lyme Borreliosis

Biological and Clinical Aspects

Volume Editors

Dan Lipsker Strasbourg
Benoît Jaulhac Strasbourg

13 figures, 8 in color, and 11 tables, 2009

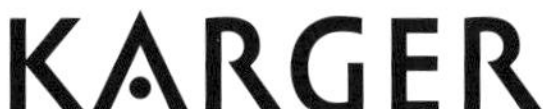

Basel · Freiburg · Paris · London · New York ·
Bangalore · Bangkok · Singapore · Tokyo · Sydney

Current Problems in Dermatology

Dan Lipsker
Clinique Dermatologique
1 Place de l'Hôpital
FR-67091 Strasbourg/France

Benoît Jaulhac
Laboratoire associé au Centre National de Référence des Borrelia
3, rue Koeberlé
FR-67000 Strasbourg/France

Library of Congress Cataloging-in-Publication Data

Lyme borreliosis : biological and clinical aspects / volume editors, Dan Lipsker, Benoît Jaulhac .
p. ; cm. -- (Current problems in dermatology ; v. 37)
Includes bibliographical references and index.
ISBN 978-3-8055-9114-0 (hard cover : alk. paper)
1. Lyme disease. I. Lipsker, Dan. II. Jaulhac, Benoît. III. Series: Current problems in dermatology ; v. 37.
[DNLM: 1. Lyme Disease. W1 CU804L v.37 2009 / WC 406 L98531 2009]
RC155.5.L933 2009
616.9'246--dc22
2009010643

Bibliographic Indices. This publication is listed in bibliographic services, including Pub Med/MEDLINE.

www.karger.com
Printed in Switzerland on acid-free and non-aging paper (ISO 9706) by Reinhardt Druck, Basel
ISSN 1421–5721
ISBN 978–3–8055–9114–0
e-ISBN 978–3–8055–9115–7

Contents

Preface

'Lyme disease', so called since Steere et al. [1, 2] inquired into an arthritis epidemic among young children in the community of Old Lyme, Conn., USA, in the late 1970s, has a very long European history. Its cutaneous manifestations, the most frequent signs of the disease, had already been described at the end of the 19th century and the beginning of the 20th century by physicians like Buchwald, Pick, Herxheimer, Hartman, Afzelius and Lipschütz [3–5]. Additionally, two French physicians in a landmark paper published in 1922, Garin and Bujadoux [6], reported a patient who developed erythema chronicum migrans followed by painful meningoradiculitis. Shortly before the symptoms began, this patient was bitten by a tick and he had a positive Bordet-Wasserman test, which was used at this time to diagnose syphilis. They stated, however, that although this test was positive, this patient did not have syphilis, and concluded that this patient had a tick-borne disease that induced cutaneous and neurological manifestations caused by a spirochete different from *Treponema pallidum*. It was not until the early 1980s that their prediction proved to be correct, when Burgdorfer et al. [7] were able to isolate a bacterium belonging to the family of Spirochaetaceae, first from ticks and then from humans. Interestingly, the first North American observation of Lyme disease, a patient with erythema migrans, was only published in 1970 [8].

In the years after the isolation of the causative bacterium, it was quickly shown that there were significant differences in disease expression between North America and Europe. Furthermore, it could be shown that there was 1 predominant species of *Borrelia* in North America, while there were at least 4 different pathogenic species in Europe [9, 10].

Thus, this disease has a long European history, and therefore to us it seemed necessary to specifically address 'Lyme disease' in Europe (or should we call it 'European borreliosis'?).

We have the great privilege in this volume of *Current Problems in Dermatology* to coordinate a special overview of Lyme disease. The texts were written by some of the top European experts in this field. Though this volume is published in a dermatological book series, all the aspects of Lyme disease are addressed. Microbiologists, infectious disease specialists, neurologists, rheumatologists, internists and dermatologists all contributed to this volume. Indeed, our main goal was to cover a broad range of the characteristics of the disease and to provide current state-of-the-art guidelines on epidemiology, diagnosis, treatment, bacteriology and serology, rather than focus exclusively on the skin disease.

In the last part of this volume, some important topics are addressed in the form of questions. This part of the books deals with questions that are often asked of experts, including 'What should one do in case of a tick bite?', 'When is the best time to order a Western blot and how should it be interpreted?', 'Is serological follow-up useful for patients with cutaneous Lyme borreliosis?', 'How do I manage tick bites and Lyme borreliosis in pregnant women?', 'What should be done in case of persistent symptoms after adequate antibiotic treatment for Lyme disease?' and 'What are the indications for lumbar puncture in patients with Lyme disease?'.

We sincerely hope that this book will be of help and interest to all physicians involved in the diagnosis and care of patients with Lyme borreliosis.

Dan Lipsker
Benoît Jaulhac

References

1 Steere AC, Malawista SE, Snydman DR, Shope RE, Andiman WA, Ross MR, Steele FM: Lyme arthritis: an epidemic of oligoarticular arthritis in children and adults in three Connecticut communities. Arthritis Rheum 1977;20:7–17.
2 Steere AC, Boderick TF, Malawista SE: Erythema chronicum migrans and Lyme arthritis: epidemiologic evidence for a tick vector. Am J Epidemiol 1978;108:312–321.
3 Lipschütz B: Über eine seltene Erythemform (erythema chronicum migrans). Arch Dermatol Syph 1913;118:349–356.
4 Herxheimer K, Hartman K: Über acrodermatitis chronica atrophicans. Arch Dermatol (Berlin) 1902;61:57–76.
5 Marchionini A: A propos de l'étiologie de l'acrodermatite chronique atrophiante de Pick-Herxheimer. Ann Dermatol Venereol 1956;83:601–611.
6 Garin C, Bujadoux D: Paralysie par les tiques. J Med (Lyon) 1922;77:765–767.
7 Burgdorfer W, Barbour AG, Hayes SF, Benach JL, Grunwaldt E, Davis JP: Lyme disease: a tick-borne spirochetosis? Science 1982;216:1317–1319.
8 Scrimenti RJ: Erythema chronicum migrans. Arch Dermatol 1970;102:104–105.
9 Welsh J, Pretzman C, Postic D, Saint Girons I, Baranton G, McClelland M: Genomic fingerprinting by arbitrarily primed polymerase chain reaction resolves *Borrelia burgdorferi* into three distinct phyletic groups. Int J Syst Bacteriol 1992;42:370–377.
10 Richter D, Postic D, Sertour N, Livey I, Matuschka FR, Baranton G: Delineation of *Borrelia burgdorferi* sensu lato species by multilocus sequence analysis and confirmation of the delineation of *Borrelia spielmanii* sp. nov. Int J Syst Evol Microbiol 2006;56:873–881.

Lipsker D, Jaulhac B (eds): Lyme Borreliosis.
Curr Probl Dermatol. Basel, Karger, 2009, vol 37, pp 1–17

Borrelia burgdorferi sensu lato Diversity and Its Influence on Pathogenicity in Humans

Guy Baranton[a] · Sylvie J. De Martino[b]

[a]Centre National de Référence Borrelia, Institut Pasteur, Paris, et [b]Laboratoire associé au CNR Borrelia, Strasbourg, France

Abstract

Among the Spirochaetes, the *Borrelia burgdorferi* sensu lato complex is responsible for Lyme borreliosis. This complex comprises more than 13 *Borrelia* species. Four of them are clearly pathogenic for humans: *B. burgdorferi* sensu stricto, *B. afzelii*, *B. garinii* and *B. spielmanii*. They can generate erythema migrans, an initial skin lesion, and can then spread deeply into the host to invade distant tissues, especially the nervous system, the joints or the skin. In humans, *Borrelia* pathogenicity seems to be linked with taxonomic position, but in vitro studies show the role of plasmids in *B. burgdorferi* s.l. pathogenesis. The inter- and intraspecies genetic diversity of *B. burgdorferi* s.l. evidences a clonal evolution of the chromosome, while plasmid genes are quite variable, suggesting their major role in *Borrelia* adaptability. The plasmid-encoded adhesins and *vlse*, *crasps* and *osp* genes determine invasiveness and host immune evasion of *B. burgdorferi* s.l., and select the bacterial host spectrum. The geographic distribution of *B. burgdorferi* s.l. is closely related to its vectors and competent hosts, and its development within these influences its diversity, taxonomy and pathogenesis, primarily via genetic lateral transfer.

Introduction

Borrelia *Species and Speciation*

The Spirochaetes phylum comprises several genera, but only 4 of them *(Leptospira, Treponema, Brachyspira* and *Borrelia)* contain human pathogens. *Borrelia* genus representatives are characterized by both their strict parasitic way of life and a biphasic cycle involving arthropod vectors and vertebrate hosts. Two distinct groups constitute the *Borrelia* genus: the relapsing fever *Borrelia* group and the *Borrelia burgdorferi* sensu lato complex; the latter is responsible for Lyme borreliosis. When it was discovered, *B. burgdorferi* was first considered to be a unique species responsible for Lyme arthritis. Indeed the 12 isolates first studied (11 from the USA, 1 from Switzerland) belonged to a single species [1], later named *Borrelia burgdorferi* sensu stricto [2]. It appeared that at least 3 pathogenic species could be delineated [2]. Finally, several nonpathogenic species were discovered [3]. Up to now, 13 *Borrelia* species and 2 genospecies have been identified as belonging to this *B. b*urgdorferi s.l. complex [4]. Genospecies usually only differ from named species by a very small number of available isolates [4].

Ecological features associated with formal species (and speciation) are probably diverse, complex and poorly understood; these are: the expansion area, host(s) spectrum, nature of vector(s) species and symptomatology of the disease in man (if this exists).

For instance, *B. burgdorferi* s.s. is mostly present in North America and Europe, and is transmitted by *Ixodes scapularis, I. pacificus* and *I. ricinus* to birds and multiple mammals. In humans, it causes erythema migrans (EM) and arthritis, but also polyneuritis and in particular acrodermatitis chronica atrophicans (ACA) [3]. It coexists with *B. andersonii*, which is restricted to the eastern part of the USA, nonpathogenic for man and transmitted by a single vector *(I. dentatus)* to a single host (cotton tailed rabbit) [5]. Therefore, conditions of speciation in *Borrelia* remain largely due to chance: some sympatric species are narrowly specialized, while others are broadly generalist. Similarly, in Europe, a single vector, *I. ricinus*, is competent for the 6 *Borrelia* species present, including *B. burgdorferi* s.s. Therefore, in North America, 2 vectors are both able to transmit *B. burgdorferi* s.s., the only pathogenic species in the USA.

It is noteworthy that another species, *Borrelia lonestari*, was identified as a causative agent of the southern tick-associated rash illness (STARI), an erythema migrans-like rash observed in the southern USA [6]. However, its sequence analysis showed that this species belongs to the relapsing fever group [7, 8]. The vector of *B. lonestari* is the *Amblyomma americanum* tick, the lone star tick, distributed throughout the southeast USA from central Oklahoma and Texas to the coast and northward into Maine. However, *B. lonestari* has also been isolated in *I. scapularis* ticks, found from the southeastern United States into both Massachusetts and New York [9]. Nevertheless, in patients from Missouri, recent studies could implicate neither *B. burgdorferi* nor *B. lonestari* as the causative agent of STARI [10, 11].

Methods to Evaluate the Genetic Diversity of B. burgdorferi *s.l.*

Since 1987, whole DNA/DNA hybridization (WDDH) was considered as the gold standard in bacterial taxonomy [12], and for 30 years no cultivable bacterial species could be defined without WDDH data. It had been the case for *Borrelia* species up to 2006, when *B. spielmanii* became the first cultivable bacterial species to be delineated without being hybridized [13]. Multilocus sequencing analysis was accepted as an alternative to WDDH by the editors of the leading journal in bacterial taxonomy, the *International Journal of Systematic and Evolutionary Microbiology.*

However, many simpler methods allow an approach to the inter- and intraspecies genetic diversity of bacteria: ribotyping, restriction fragment length polymorphism analysis, multilocus enzyme electrophoresis and pulsed-field gel electrophoresis. Other methods based on polymerase chain reaction (PCR) are usually faster, and therefore frequently used: arbitrarily primed PCR, random amplification of polymorphic DNA, variable number tandem repeat analysis, etc. More recently, PCR and sequencing became popular because of their ease and sensitivity. Analysis of spacers between ribosomal genes are particularly appreciated since the primers, hybridizing on conserved sequences, allow amplification of as many bacteria as wished for, whereas the highly variable amplicons give a deep appreciation of species diversity. In the case of *Borrelia*, the unusual topology of ribosomal genes (*rrl* and *rrf* genes tandemly repeated) allows a quite *B. burgdorferi* s.l.-specific amplification of the *rrl-rrf* spacer leading to simultaneous detection, identification and typing [14]. One must be careful when using sequencing of a single gene to identify species or subspecies because of lateral transfer. Considering *B. burgdorferi* s.l., for instance, genes coding outer membrane proteins or virulence factors which are quite variable and plasmid encoded (e.g. *ospC, dbpAB* genes) are often subjected to such lateral transfer. Conversely, the chromosomally encoded genes are stable and present a clonal evolution. These are conserved too much to be useful as markers of genetic diversity (intergenic spacers excepted).

Multilocus sequences typing (MLST) is a method of studying the genetic diversity in a bacterial group. A very early paper showed that the *Borrelia* chromosome clonally evolves [15]. Three MLST studies have been used to elucidate the *Borrelia* population structure [16–18]. They demonstrated a strong linkage between the multilocus sequence genotypes, and a strong linkage between MLST allelic groups and the major alleles of the *ospC* gene in spite of the high recombination rate in this gene. This suggests a balancing selection of *ospC* as a dominant force to maintain diversity in local populations of *Borrelia.* A similar conclusion had already been reached, showing that OspC local diversity was equivalent to the global one [19]. However, except for *ospC*, sequence variation at plasmid-borne loci exhibits inconsistency with phylogeny, suggesting plasmid transfers between isolates [17], and *ospC* phylogeny consistency in spite of its high polymorphism suggests that *ospC* plays a major role in adaptive differentiation of *B. burgdorferi* [18].

Borrelia *Pathogenicity*

Pathogenicity stricto sensu and virulence of *Borrelia* comprise at least 2 phenomena that are not independent of each other.

Borrelia *Pathogenic Potential Seems to Be Linked to Taxonomic Position*

Of course, since *Borrelia* are strict parasites, all species are able to invade a host. However, the host spectrum as well as the clinical expression differ greatly [20]. When considering, by medical pragmatism, human sensitivity to *Borrelia*, the complex of 15 species is divided into 3 groups:

- 4 clearly pathogenic species: *B. burgdorferi* s.s., *B. afzelii, B. garinii* and *B. spielmanii;*
- 3 rarely, if at all, pathogenic species: *B. bissettii, B. lusitaniae* and *B. valaisiana;*
- 6 species (and 2 genospecies) that have never been isolated in humans.

In the Borrelia *Model, Virulence Is Not Associated with Taxonomic Position*

In nature, an obvious permanent selective pressure eliminates such avirulent variants that are not able to colonize their natural host. Loss of some plasmids, such as lp25 and lp28-1, is involved in a decrease in virulence [21]. Similarly the plasmid (lp25)-encoded *PncA* gene (nicotinamidase) has been shown to be strongly associated with virulence in *Borrelia* [22].

Nevertheless, virulence is an artifact only observed during in vitro experimental conditions and has not been studied further. However, theoretically it is possible that in nature the ticks may be able to diffuse avirulent *Borrelia* isolates by cofeeding [23].

Genes or Products of Potentially Pathogenic Genes

All the genes mentioned in this section, but 2 – P66 and BgP – are plasmid encoded. Several genes have been suggested to be involved in pathogenesis. Potential adhesins, able to attach to diverse mammalian cell surface components, promote the bacterial colonization of the mammalian host.

Adhesins. BgP and P66 are able to bind to platelets and integrins [24]. BbK32 (encoded on lp36) is a fibronectin adhesin [25]. DbpA and B (lp49) are decorin-binding proteins [26]. Decorin-binding proteins and BBK32 (lp36) also bind to glycosaminoglycans [27].

Other Candidate Genes for Pathogenicity. VlsE could be involved in escape from immune response by antigenic variation [28]. Complement regulator-acquiring surface factors (CRASP) are able to inhibit complement activity by combining with factor H or other similar substances of the host [29]. CRASP-1 is located on lp54, CRASP-2 on lp28-3 and CRASP 3–5 are Erp proteins encoded by the cp32 gene family [29]. CRASP from different *Borrelia* species, by binding with factor H of a given host, confer a corresponding serum resistance. This phenomenon could explain the host spectrum of each *Borrelia* species [30].

OspA (lp54), an outer surface lipoprotein, is an adhesin only expressed in vector, and is responsible for attachment to *Ixodes* midgut mucosa [31]. However, exceptionally, in some cases of chronic arthritis due to *Borrelia*, antibodies to OspA have been detected. It has been shown that an OspA motif is quite similar to human leukocyte function-associated antigen-1, which suggests it could be responsible for resistance to treatment Lyme arthritis [32]. OspA has also been involved in plasmin fixation [33].

OspC, another outer surface lipoprotein, is only expressed after the blood meal in vectors and mainly in vertebrate hosts. The *ospC* gene is on cp26, a very stable plasmid comprising metabolic genes [34]. In pathogenicity, *ospC* is a highly variable gene and plays an important role. Its expression is necessary to initiate the host colonization [35]. It has been noticed that only a limited number of *ospC* alleles could allow *Borrelia* to reach deep organs in humans after blood dissemination [36]. It has also been shown that distinct alleles of OspC bind with different affinity to plasminogen [37]. This suggests that only particular *ospC* alleles allow corresponding *Borrelia* to cross the capillary membrane of a given host species to invade its deep organs using host plasminogen. Such isolates, whose *ospC* allelic type is able to bind human plasminogen, are called 'invasive'. OspC has also another indirect role. It has been discovered that salp 15, a tick saliva component, was overexpressed during the blood meal. OspC is able to bind to this and block CD4 T cell activation, leading to an increase in the Spirochaete load due to immunosuppression [38].

OspA and OspC are immunodominant outer-membrane proteins and both elicit bactericidal antibodies in hosts that are quite challenging for the strictly parasitical behavior of *Borrelia*. However, OspA is expressed in ticks only, and OspC local diversity represents a 'repertoire' that allows recontamination of a given host by a new and unrecognized ospC variant [39].

In conclusion, most of the genes that up to now have been identified as involved in pathogenicity are plasmid encoded and upregulated within the host, except the *ospA* gene.

Moreover, autoimmunity and the general interaction of *B. burgdorferi* s.l. with the immune system has also been proposed as a mechanism of pathogenicity in human Lyme borreliosis [40, 41].

B. burgdorferi s.l. Diversity

Borrelia *Species Pathogenic for Humans*

B. burgdorferi *s.s.*

B. burgdorferi s.s. is a highly generalist species: several vectors, such as *I. scapularis, I. pacificus* and *I. ricinus,* are able to transmit it, as are minor ones, such as *I. trianguliceps* and *I. hexagonus* [42]. Both vector cycles and seasonal fluctuations shape the transmission potential of *Borrelia.* As a result, the prevalence of the disease may be drastically different between places close to each other [43]. Similarly, the expansion zone of *B. burgdorferi* s.s. is quite large in the northern hemisphere. In North America, *B. burgdorferi* s.s. has spread over the West Coast and the eastern half of the USA (mainly in the northeast), but also some southern areas such as Florida and Texas. In the Mid-West, some contaminated spots have been recorded. In Canada, the threat exists in the southeast of the country. In Europe, *B. burgdorferi* s.s. is present, but its density is lower than those of the 2 other main pathogenic species: *B. garinii* and *B. afzelii*. In Africa, ticks harboring *B. burgdorferi s.s.* have been reported in Morocco [44]. Currently, it may be abundant, as is the case in the western part of France. Towards the east, *B. burgdorferi* s.s. is considered to be absent from Asia. Indeed, in the borderline area between Asia and Europe, where both *I. ricinus* and *I. persulcatus* coexist, *B. burgdorferi* s.s. was identified only in *I. ricinus* [45]. *B. burgdorferi* s.s. has been isolated in South Central China, but restricted to a hare, *Caprolagus sinensis*, whose associated tick is *Haemaphysalis bispinosa* [46]. *B. burgdorferi* s.s. is also present in Taiwan, but both *ospC* and *ospA* genes from several sequenced Taiwanese isolates are almost identical. It mirrors a strictly clonal population in spite of the different hosts harboring the isolates [47, 48]. Similarly, European *B. burgdorferi* s.s. also represent a subset of the North American population of *B. burgdorferi* s.s., which is largely more diverse intraspecifically. Such genetic bottlenecks are called a 'founder's event', and suggest that some North American clones of *B. burgdorferi* s.s. have been subsequently imported into Europe and then into Taiwan [4, 19, 49].

B. burgdorferi s.s. hosts are still characterized by their diversity in the USA: *Peromyscus leucopus, Tamias striatus, Blarina brevicauda, Sciurus carolinensis and Sciurus griseus,* and also passerine birds, blackbirds, robins, pheasants and veeries [42, 50]. Each distinct host harbors different *B. burgdorferi* s.s. genotypes at different frequencies, shaping the *Borrelia* population into distinct enzootic niches [43, 50]. However, in Europe the range of *B. burgdorferi* s.s. hosts are less well known, and include red squirrels and hedgehogs [42].

Concerning its pathogenicity, *B. burgdorferi* s.s. – like any other pathogenic *B. burgdorferi* s.l. species – is able to provoke EM. It has been shown that lesions correspond to the intradermic inflammatory response fighting the centrifugal migration of bacteria from the inoculation point [51]. The physiology of multiple EM is quite different: it reflects the ability of some *Borrelia* to penetrate the blood vessels and migrate via this route into different parts of the body, including the skin. This necessarily supposes these bacteria to be invasive ones.

Further, Lyme borreliosis may be inconstantly characterized by secondary lesions distant from the inoculation point, sometimes in deep organs. Septicemia is the way that the *Borrelia* invade the whole organism at this late stage. Each pathogenic *Borrelia* species exhibits a preferential organotropism [20]. *B. burgdorferi* s.s. have been associated with arthritis. For instance in the USA, where *B. burgdorferi* s.s. is the only pathogenic *B. burgdorferi* s.l. species present, arthritis is the most reported late clinical presentation (33%) [52]. However, this organotropism is elective since *B. burgdorferi* s.s., still in the USA, also causes neurological problems (5%) [52]. In western Europe, too, *B. burgdorferi* s.s. has been reported as the species prominently isolated from arthritic forms [53], but in eastern areas where *B. garinii* is highly represented, such as Germany, the etiology of arthritis is more diverse [54].

Although some European *B. burgdorferi* s.s. isolates are very close to North American ones, whatever the method used, polymorphism of *B. burgdorferi* s.s. is much larger in North America than in Europe, and only few alleles are endemic in Europe [55, 56]. These features characterize a founder's event, suggesting a recent importation of *B. burgdorferi* s.s. from North America to Europe. This hypothesis is strengthened by the fact that, although in Europe a significant part of the polymorphism of *ospC* gene is due to lateral transfer from other *B. burgdorferi* s.l. species (mainly *B. afzelii* and *B. garinii*), no sequence of this type has been found in the USA, suggesting that migration from Europe towards the USA is unlikely [49, 56].

The pathogenic potential of *B. burgdorferi* s.s. isolates is variable. In the New York area, 21 groups have been delineated by sequence analysis of the *ospC* gene. Among them, only 4 groups exhibited an invasive potential in the USA [36]. On a global scale, a single 5th 'invasive' group specific to Europe was defined later on [57].

B. garinii

B. garinii is a very complex species. It has spread all over Europe and Asia (from Turkey to Siberia, to northern and eastern China and Japan) [58] and even into North Africa [42, 59]. In Europe and North Africa, it is transmitted by *I. ricinus*. In Asia, the main vector is *I. persulcatus* and, much more rarely, *I. trianguliceps*.

However, a second cycle involving seabirds and their associated ticks *(I. uriae)* maintains *B. garinii* in many worldwide bird colonies, including those in the southern hemisphere and boreal part of North America [60, 61]. Although the seabird or *I. uriae*-associated *Borrelia* isolates do not differ genetically from other *B. garinii* (20047 group), this cycle seems to be enzootic and not to play an important role in the dissemination of Lyme disease. Within *B. garinii*, 2 subspecies (both pathogenic for humans) are genetically delineated [45, 58]:

- The 20047 group that is spread in both Asia, where it is transmitted by *I. persulcatus,* and Europe, where *I. ricinus* is the main vector. The usual hosts of the 20047 group are birds in Europe [62], but rodents and birds in Asia [58].
- The NT29 (or Ip89) group [45, 58], which is restricted to Asia (vector *I. persulcatus*). Rodents and not birds are reservoirs for NT29 group which has never been found in *I. ricinus*.

A high diversity within these 2 subspecies, genetically delineated, has been observed by monoclonal antibody typing. This allows us to define 6 serotypes [63], whereas for other pathogenic *Borrelia*, a serotype corresponds to 1 species only. The *B. garinii* diversity is seen in the CSF of patients presenting with neuroborreliosis [64]. In addition, rodents instead of birds are the reservoir host for serotype 4 isolates [65]. Serotype 4 also corresponds to both ospA and ospC genotypes [39, 64].

Concerning organotropism of *B. garinii*, the neural apparatus is the main target organ: symptoms reflect meningitis and inflammatory lesions of the peripheral nervous system [3, 20, 64, 66]. Less frequently, *B. garinii* has been detected in joints [48], and in exceptional cases it causes ACA [67].

B. afzelii

B. afzelii [68] is present in both Europe and Asia (from Turkey to Siberia, to northern and eastern China and Japan) [58]. It is particularly frequent in eastern and northern Europe. The only known vectors of *B. afzelii* are *I. ricinus* in Europe and *I. persulcatus* in Asia. *I. ricinus* is the most permissive *Ixodes* vector for *Borrelia* since it is able to transmit *B. burgdorferi* s.s., *B. garinii, B. afzelii, B. valaisiana, B. lusitaniae* and *B. spielmanii*, while *I. persulcatus* only transmits *B. garinii* and *B. afzelii.*

In humans, *B. afzelii* seems to have an organotropism for the skin, since it preferentially causes lymphadenosis benigna cutis [69] and is the etiological agent of ACA [3, 20]. However, *B. afzelii* have sometimes been isolated from either joints or CSF [54]. ACA has never been observed in American citizens who have never left the USA, confirming the suspicion that endemic *B. burgdorferi* s.s. are not able to induce this cutaneous lesion. By contrast, in Europe *B. burgdorferi* s.s. isolates have occasionally been isolated from ACA biopsies [70].

B. spielmanii

B. spielmanii is the last pathogenic Borrelia species to have been discovered [13, 71]. It is very rarely isolated, although strains have been observed in different European countries: The Netherlands, the Czech Republic, France, Poland and Russia, among others (but neither in Asia, nor in North America). It is transmitted by *I. ricinus*, but the reason for the scarcity of isolates is due to its unique reservoir: dormice *(Eliomys quercinus)*. It is unambiguously a pathogenic species since about one half of the available isolates have been isolated from human skin biopsies. Up to now, only EM has been associated with *B. spielmanii,* and it is not known whether or not this species comprises potentially invasive isolates.

Borrelia *Species Rarely if At All Pathogenic for Humans*

B. bissettii

B. bissettii is a large and diverse species. It is mainly isolated in California, where 4 ticks usually harbor *B. bissettii: I. spinipalpis, I. neotomae, I. jellisonii* and *I. pacificus. B. bissettii* has been observed in other US states, like Colorado and Florida, and rarely in Wisconsin and New York (in both areas 1 strain from *I. scapularis* has been isolated). Known hosts are *Neotoma fuscipes, Dipodomys californiensis* and *Odocoileus hemionus* in California, *Peromyscus difficilis, P. maniculatus* and *N. mexicana* and *Microtus ochrogaster* in Colorado, and *P. gossypinus* and *Sigmodon hispidus* in Florida [4, 72].

In the USA, *B. bissettii* has never been isolated from humans, and therefore is not considered as a pathogenic species. In Europe, *B. bissettii* has never been isolated from ticks nor hosts, except in Slovenia from 9 patients with EM [73]. However, these isolations are very controversial since they were characterized in the USA and are no longer available in Slovenia. Moreover, none of them have been made available to the scientific community, suggesting a technical mistake.

B. valaisiana

B. valaisiana [74] has spread all over Eurasia. Its vectors are *I. ricinus* in Europe and *I. granulatus* in Asia (China, Japan and Korea). It is associated with birds, *Turdus* spp., passerines and pheasants, as a *B. garinii* European subgroup (20047). Additionally, in cases of mixed infection in ticks, B. *valaisiana* and B. *garinii* are frequently associated, underlining their bird relationships [45]. On some occasions, *B. valaisiana* has been identified by PCR in human skin [75] and once in the CSF [76], but has never been isolated from patients. One hypothesis for this rarely observed pathogenic potential is the lateral transfer of a gene involved in pathogenesis from a pathogenic species to *B. valaisiana*. The *ospC* gene, whose lateral transfer has been documented, is such a candidate gene [56, 77].

B. lusitaniae

B. lusitaniae [78] is present in both Europe and North Africa, but this distribution is heterogeneous; it is quite frequent and highly polymorphic in Portugal, and also frequent in North Africa, but this time it is monomorphic [59, 79]. In other places in Europe, *B. lusitaniae* is very scarce. This heterogeneity in distribution and diversity could be due to the original reservoir of *B. lusitaniae*: lizards [80].

Although usually isolated only from *I. ricinus* ticks, *B. lusitaniae* has been isolated recently from skin lesions of a Portuguese patient [81].

Nonpathogenic Borrelia

B. japonica

B. japonica [82] is restricted to Japan [58], and has only been isolated from *I. ovatus*. It has never been associated with human infection.

B. tanukii

B. tanukii [83] has only been isolated from *I. tanuki* (raccoon tick in Asia) in both Japan and Nepal [58]. No human infection has been reported.

B. turdi

B. turdi [83] is associated with *I. turdus*, a Japanese tick found on Turdidae birds. This species is restricted to Japan, and no human infection due to this species has been observed.

B. sinica

B. sinica has recently been delineated [84], and has been found in *I. ovatus* in both China and Nepal [58]. It has never been observed in humans.

B. andersonii

B. andersonii [5] is characterized by both a specific vector *(I. dentatus)* and a specific host (cottontail rabbit; *Oryctolagus cuniculus*). Restricted to the eastern part of the USA, this species has never been associated with disease in humans.

B. californiensis

B. californiensis [4] is a rather homogeneous species, up to now restricted to California. It is associated with a major host, the kangaroo rat *D. californicus,* which was previously identified as a reservoir for *B. burgdorferi* s.l. [85], and more rarely associated with *O. hemionus* (commonly referred to as the mule deer). Identified vectors are *I. jellisonii, I. spinipalpis* and *I. pacificus.*

Genospecies 1 and 2

At the moment, each of these genospecies comprise only 2 strains, which all have been isolated from *I. pacificus.* They have been found only in California [4].

Considerations about Diversity, Taxonomy and Pathogenicity of *B. burgdorferi* s.l.

Geographic Distribution of Borrelia *Species*

The *B. burgdorferi* s.l. complex is mainly spread across the northern hemisphere. Furthermore, we have noticed that 12 out of the 15 known species have been reported in 1 of 2 areas located at the same latitude (30–40° N) on each side of the Pacific Ocean: California on one side (*B. burgdorferi* s.s., *B. bissettii, B. californiensis*, genospecies 1 and 2) and Japan, Korea and western China on the other side (*B. afzelii, B. garinii, B. valaisiana, B. tanukii, B. japonica, B. turdi, B. sinica* and even *B. burgdorferi* s.s.). Indeed, each of these 2 sets of species usually constitutes a monophyletic clade in phylogenetic trees drawn with highly conserved genes or by multilocus sequencing analysis: the 'Californian' clade including European *B. burgdorferi s.s.* isolates [4]. Conversely, *B. garinii* and *B. afzelii* associated with both *I. ricinus* and *I. persulcatus* and with an open range of reservoirs – birds and rodents, respectively – have a large expansion area. Concerning *B. burgdorferi* s.s., it is noteworthy that the maximum intraspecies diversity is observed in California [55, 72], just as if it had evolved locally long enough in *I. pacificus* before some clones adapted to *I. scapularis* and progressed towards the east coast and finally got transported overseas to Europe [4, 49, 55], where they could adapt to *I. ricinus,* and then move onwards to Taiwan.

The 3 *Borrelia* species absent from both California and north-western Asia are characterized by their narrow and unusual reservoirs (lizards for *B. lusitaniae*, cottontail rabbit for *B. andersonii* and dormice for *B. spielmanii*). The 2 first ones usually constitute their own deep and peripheral branch in phylogenetic trees, although *B. spielmanii* is close to *B. afzelii.*

Schematically, there are 2 kinds of *Borrelia* species:

- Those associated with a vector characterized by both a broad spectrum of hosts *(I. ricinus, I. persulcatus* or *I. scapularis)* and by a huge expansion area. These species have large populations of individuals and a variety of different vertebrate hosts which do not fully characterize the concerned *Borrelia* species. These species are genetically quite diverse and usually pathogenic or potentially pathogenic (*B. burgdorferi* s.s., *B. garinii, B. afzelii, B. valaisiana, B. lusitaniae,* etc.). The best example of such a species is *B. garinii*: highly diverse genetically with distinct groups differing both genetically and ecologically, but still in the species frame (see '*B. garinii*').
- In contrast, there is a second kind of species associated with either a unique reservoir and a unique specialized vector *(B. andersonii, B.turdi, B. tanukii)*, or an unspecialized vector but still a unique reservoir *(B. spielmanii)*.

The genome of *B. burgdorferi* s.l. is quite unusual for a bacterium since it comprises many (15–22) replicons, both linear and circular [86]. The plasmids represent almost 40% of the genome. The linear chromosome is quite stable and clonally evolving by genetic drift (no genetic lateral transfer reported) [15]. In contrast, most of the plasmid replicons are submitted to duplications and lateral transfers (either complete plasmid transfers or more often simple transfers of plasmid segments or genes) leading to redundancy and pseudogenes [86].

Most of the genes involved in fitness of *Borrelia* with either tick or host reservoirs are plasmid encoded. Those which play a role in host invasion or persistence are probably also involved in pathogenicity in humans. The numerous rearrangements among plasmid and plasmidic genes allow the reassortment of genes to define new combinations optimal for a particular subset of hosts or vectors. The successful combinations are positively selected, leading to particular fitness between a clone on the one hand and a given spectrum of hosts or vectors on the other hand. Although many plasmidic genes vary, most of the genome (mainly the chromosome) remains unchanged. Heterogeneity in the frequency of a given clone according to the host species has indeed been recorded [50] within a *Borrelia* species. It seems that the main species are *B. burgdorferi* s.s., *B. garinii* and *B. afzelii* in this case. The best example is *B. garinii* (high genetic and phenotypic diversity): European (20047) and Asian (NT29) groups have different hosts, similarly for serotype 4 of the European group, even the seabird-associated cycle coexists with the main one within *B. garinii*.

It is well known that speciation occurs when a small population becomes isolated either spatially or by a particular behavior. Once built by fast plasmidic fluidity, a successful new genetic combination, reflecting the fitness between clones and hosts, leads to intraspecific diversity. If a unique clone with a unique host relationship is maintained long enough and stabilized, for instance in a place where the considered host is highly predominant, a situation of isolation is created which would allow a slow genetic drift of both the chromosome and the newly specialized plasmids. These local conditions allow the development of a new *Borrelia* species. *B. spielmanii,* specifically adapted to a single rare rodent species (dormice), could have been individualized this way from another *I. ricinus*-transmitted *Borrelia* (probably *B. afzelii,* the closest species to *B. spielmanii* and whose reservoirs also are rodents species). This mechanism of rapid plasmidic changes may also lead a clone to adapt to a new vector. If the new vector has a unique host, the clone would easily become a new species *(B. andersonii?).* However, when the vector has a broad spectrum of hosts it could only increase the intraspecific diversity (*B. burgdorferi* s.s. in Europe).

Taxonomic Lateral Transfer and Pathogenicity

Pathogenic Potential of B. valaisiana *and* B. lusitaniae

Pathogenicity of *Borrelia* for humans appears to be linked to taxonomy with very few exceptions. Up to now, these exceptions only concerned Europe, where both *B. valaisiana* (associated with birds) and *B. lusitaniae* (associated with lizards) have occasionally been detected in human tissues [76, 81]. In Europe, 4 pathogenic *Borrelia* species coexist; moreover, the 4 pathogenic and the 2 nonpathogenic species are transmitted by a single vector, *I. ricinus,* which implies frequent mixed infection of the vector [45]. This promiscuous presence of 2 or more *Borrelia* populations in the midgut of ticks provides an opportunity for plasmid or plasmidic gene exchanges. Among the exchangeable loci, some of them allow the colonization of a given host species. They could be either a specific adhesin or CRASP, which confer resistance to the complement of a given species (the affinity of different CRASP alleles for the Factor H of distinct potential hosts has been shown to be variable [30]). However, concerning CRASP, it has been recently shown that the mechanism of host selection is probably more complex [87].

Invasiveness

Several authors have shown that within a pathogenic species, the population is heterogeneous at the pathogenicity level [36, 88]. When MLST studies are performed to define the population structure, the leading role of the *ospC* gene is usually highlighted [16, 18]. Indeed, Seinost et al. [36] first showed that a restricted number of ospC groups were responsible for most of the late symptoms of Lyme disease. This suggests that only isolates belonging to these *ospC* groups are able to invade blood vessels and to migrate into deep organs or distant from the inoculation point [36, 39, 57]. A possible mechanism could be the ability of OspC protein from the so-called invasive groups to bind with high affinity to human plasminogen which, once activated in plasmin, allows the concerned isolates to cross the vascular endothelium and other tissue membranes [37].

Another striking feature of the *ospC* gene is the high level of recombination it exhibits: OspC protein sequences look like mosaics of fragments from different origins and species [15, 49]. On other occasions, the whole gene or a very large fragment is laterally transferred within or between species. Such large transfers have been observed, even with a pathogenic species as donor and a nonpathogenic one as receiver. Such recombinations could explain how *B. valaisiana* isolates have been involved in neuroborreliosis [76]. Indeed, a *B. valaisiana* isolate (M7) bearing an OspC protein quite similar to typically *B. afzelii* invasive genotypes isolated from ACA (ACA1) has been found in nature [56].

Taxonomy, Organotropism and Lateral Transfer

All the pathogenic species, when infecting humans, are able to provoke EM at the inoculation point. Some isolates of pathogenic species can provoke multiple EM after blood dissemination. Later on, when the infection persists, each species exhibits a particular organotropism (unclear for the rare species *B. spielmanii*, which up to now has only been isolated from EM). Schematically, *B. burgdorferi* s.s. is responsible for arthritis, *B. garinii* for neuroborreliosis and *B. afzelii* for ACA and lymphadenosis benigna cutis [3, 20]. However, there is usually no strict association: *B. burgdorferi* s.s. is also involved in neuroborreliosis [3] and *B. garinii* is sometimes isolated from synovial tissues [53]. In contrast, there are very few exceptions to the unique *B. afzelii* etiology of ACA [75]. For instance, in the USA the rare ACA recordings were always found in patients who had travelled abroad; no locally acquired ACA have been reported [89]. This would mean that *B. burgdorferi* s.s. per se is unable to provoke ACA. By contrast, in Europe on a few occasions *Borrelia* other than *B. afzelii* have been identified (PCR with chromosomal stable loci) in ACA skin lesions [67, 75]. However, a Danish *B. burgdorferi* s.s. isolate, DK7 (invasive isolate), was once isolated from ACA skin [90]. The absence of indigenous ACA patients in the USA is obviously due to the absence of *B. afzelii*. The reason why *B. burgdorferi* s.s. may be involved in ACA in Europe and not in the USA is less clear. Again, a lateral transfer of certain plasmidic loci from *B. afzelii*, the usual agent of this pathology, is a convincing hypothesis.

References

1 Johnson RC, Schmid GP, Hyde FW, Steigerwalt AG, Brenner DJ: *Borrelia burgdorferi* sp. nov.: etiologic agent of Lyme disease. Int J Syst Bacteriol 1984;34:496–497.

2 Baranton G, Postic D, Saint Girons I, Boerlin P, Piffaretti JC, Assous M, Grimont PA: Delineation of *Borrelia burgdorferi* sensu stricto, *Borrelia garinii* sp. nov., and group VS461 associated with Lyme borreliosis. Int J Syst Bacteriol 1992;42:378–383.

3 Wang G, van Dam AP, Schwartz I, Dankert J: Molecular typing of *Borreli burgdorferi* sensu lato: taxonomic, epidemiological, and clinical implications. Clin Microbiol Rev 1999;12:633–653.

4 Postic D, Garnier M, Baranton G: Multilocus sequence analysis of atypical *Borrelia burgdorferi* sensu lato isolates – description of *Borrelia californiensis* sp. nov. and genomospecies 1 and 2. Int J Med Microbiol 2007;297:253–271.

5 Marconi RT, Liveris D, Schwartz I: Identification of novel insertion elements, restriction fragment length polymorphism patterns, and discontinuous 23S rRNA in Lyme disease spirochetes: phylogenetic analyses of rRNA genes and their intergenic spacers in *Borrelia japonica* sp. nov. and genomic group 21038 (*Borrelia andersonii* sp. nov.) isolates. J Clin Microbiol 1995;33:2427–2434.

6 James AM, Liveris D, Wormser GP, Schwartz I, Montecalvo MA, Johnson BJ: *Borrelia lonestari* infection after a bite by an *Amblyomma americanum* tick. J Infect Dis 2001;183:1810–1814.

7 Armstrong PM, Rich SM, Smith RD, Hartl DL, Spielman A, Telford SR 3rd: A new *Borrelia* infecting Lone Star ticks. Lancet 1996;347:67–68.

8 Barbour AG, Maupin GO, Teltow GJ, Carter CJ, Piesman J: Identification of an uncultivable *Borrelia* species in the hard tick *Amblyomma americanum*: possible agent of a Lyme disease-like illness. J Infect Dis 1996;173:403–409.

9 Taft SC, Miller MK, Wright SM: Distribution of borreliae among ticks collected from eastern states. Vector Borne Zoonotic Dis 2005;5:383–389.

10 Philipp MT, Masters E, Wormser GP, Hogrefe W, Martin D: Serologic evaluation of patients from Missouri with erythema migrans-like skin lesions with the C6 Lyme test. Clin Vaccine Immunol 2006; 13:1170–1171.

11 Wormser GP, Masters E, Liveris D, Nowakowski J, Nadelman RB, Holmgren D, Bittker S, Cooper D, Wang G, Schwartz I: Microbiologic evaluation of patients from Missouri with erythema migrans. Clin Infect Dis 2005;40:423–428.

12 Wayne LG: International Committee on Systematic Bacteriology: announcement of the report of the ad hoc Committee on Reconciliation of Approaches to Bacterial Systematics. Zentralbl Bakteriol Mikrobiol 1988;268:433–434.

13 Richter D, Postic D, Sertour N, Livey I, Matuschka FR, Baranton G: Delineation of *Borrelia burgdorferi* sensu lato species by multilocus sequence analysis and confirmation of the delineation of *Borrelia spielmanii* sp. nov. Int J Syst Evol Microbiol 2006; 56:873–881.

14 Postic D, Assous MV, Grimont PA, Baranton G: Diversity of *Borrelia burgdorferi* sensu lato evidenced by restriction fragment length polymorphism of *rrf* (5S)-*rrl* (23S) intergenic spacer amplicons. Int J Syst Bacteriol 1994;44:743–752.

15 Dykhuizen DE, Polin DS, Dunn JJ, Wilske B, Preac-Mursic V, Dattwyler RJ, Luft BJ: *Borrelia burgdorferi* is clonal: implications for taxonomy and vaccine development. Proc Natl Acad Sci USA 1993;90: 10163–10167.

16 Bunikis J, Garpmo U, Tsao J, Berglund J, Fish D, Barbour AG: Sequence typing reveals extensive strain diversity of the Lyme borreliosis agents *Borrelia burgdorferi* in North America and *Borrelia afzelii* in Europe. Microbiology 2004;150:1741–1755.

17 Qiu WG, Schutzer SE, Bruno JF, Attie O, Xu Y, Dunn JJ, Fraser CM, Casjens SR, Luft BJ: Genetic exchange and plasmid transfers in *Borrelia burgdorferi* sensu stricto revealed by three-way genome comparisons and multilocus sequence typing. Proc Natl Acad Sci USA 2004;101:14150–14155.

18 Attie O, Bruno JF, Xu Y, Qiu D, Luft BJ, Qiu WG: Co-evolution of the outer surface protein C gene (*ospC*) and intraspecific lineages of *Borrelia burgdorferi* sensu stricto in the northeastern United States. Infect Genet Evol 2007;7:1–12.

19 Wang IN, Dykhuizen DE, Qiu W, Dunn JJ, Bosler EM, Luft BJ: Genetic diversity of *ospC* in a local population of *Borrelia burgdorferi* sensu stricto. Genetics 1999;151:15–30.

20 Assous MV, Postic D, Paul G, Nevot P, Baranton G: Western blot analysis of sera from Lyme borreliosis patients according to the genomic species of the *Borrelia* strains used as antigens. Eur J Clin Microbiol Infect Dis 1993;12:261–268.

21 Labandeira-Rey M, Seshu J, Skare JT: The absence of linear plasmid 25 or 28-1 of *Borrelia burgdorferi* dramatically alters the kinetics of experimental infection via distinct mechanisms. Infect Immun 2003;71:4608–4613.

22 Purser JE, Lawrenz MB, Caimano MJ, Howell JK, Radolf JD, Norris SJ: A plasmid-encoded nicotinamidase (PncA) is essential for infectivity of *Borrelia burgdorferi* in a mammalian host. Mol Microbiol 2003;48:753–764.

23 Randolph SE, Gern L, Nuttall PA: Co-feeding ticks: epidemiological significance for tick-borne pathogen transmission. Parasitol Today 1996;112:472–479.

24 Parveen N, Cornell KA, Bono JL, Chamberland C, Rosa P, Leong JM: Bgp, a secreted glycosaminoglycan-binding protein of *Borrelia burgdorferi* strain N40, displays nucleosidase activity and is not essential for infection of immunodeficient mice. Infect Immun 2006;74:3016–3020.

25 Seshu J, Esteve-Gassent MD, Labandeira-Rey M, Kim JH, Trzeciakowski JP, Höök M, Skare JT: Inactivation of the fibronectin-binding adhesin gene *bbk32* significantly attenuates the infectivity potential of *Borrelia burgdorferi*. Mol Microbiol 2006; 59:1591–1601.

26 Guo BP, Brown EL, Dorward DW, Rosenberg LC, Höök M: Decorin-binding adhesins from *Borrelia burgdorferi*. Mol Microbiol 1998;30:711–723.

27 Fischer JR, LeBlanc KT, Leong JM: Fibronectin binding protein BBK32 of the Lyme disease spirochete promotes bacterial attachment to glycosaminoglycans. Infect Immun 2006;74:435–441.

28 Zhang JR, Hardham JM, Barbour AG, Norris SJ: Antigenic variation in Lyme disease borreliae by promiscuous recombination of VMP-like sequence cassettes. Cell 1997;89:275–285.

29 von Lackum K, Miller JC, Bykowski T, Riley SP, Woodman ME, Brade V, Kraiczy P, Stevenson B, Wallich R: *Borrelia burgdorferi* regulates expression of complement regulator-acquiring surface protein 1 during the mammal-tick infection cycle. Infect Immun 2005;73:7398–7405.

30 Stevenson B, El-Hage N, Hines MA, Miller JC, Babb K: Differential binding of host complement inhibitor factor H by *Borrelia burgdorferi* Erp surface proteins: a possible mechanism underlying the expansive host range of Lyme disease spirochetes. Infect Immun 2002;70:491–497.
31 Pal U, de Silva AM, Montgomery RR, et al: Attachment of *Borrelia burgdorferi* within *Ixodes scapularis* mediated by outer surface protein A. J Clin Invest 2000;106:561–569.
32 Gross DM, Forsthuber T, Tary-Lehmann M, Etling C, Ito K, Nagy ZA, Field JA, Steere AC, Huber BT: Identification of LFA-1 as a candidate autoantigen in treatment-resistant Lyme arthritis. Science 1998; 281:703–706.
33 Fuchs H, Wallich R, Simon MM, Kramer MD: The outer surface protein A of the spirochete *Borrelia burgdorferi* is a plasmin(ogen) receptor. Proc Natl Acad Sci USA 1994;91:12594–12598.
34 Byram R, Stewart PE, Rosa P: The essential nature of the ubiquitous 26-kilobase circular replicon of *Borrelia burgdorferi*. J Bacteriol 2004;186:3561–3569.
35 Grimm D, Tilly K, Byram R, et al: Outer-surface protein C of the Lyme disease spirochete: a protein induced in ticks for infection of mammals. Proc Natl Acad Sci USA 2004;101:3142–3147.
36 Seinost G, Dykhuizen DE, Dattwyler RJ, Golde WT, Dunn JJ, Wang IN, Wormser GP, Schriefer ME, Luft BJ: Four clones of *Borrelia burgdorferi* sensu stricto cause invasive infection in humans. Infect Immun 1999;67:3518–3524.
37 Lagal V, Portnoi D, Faure G, Postic D, Baranton G: *Borrelia burgdorferi* sensu stricto invasiveness is correlated with OspC-plasminogen affinity. Microbes Infect 2006;8:645–652.
38 Ramamoorthi N, Narasimhan S, Pal U, Bao F, Yang XF, Fish D, Anguita J, Norgard MV, Kantor FS, Anderson JF, Koski RA, Fikrig E: The Lyme disease agent exploits a tick protein to infect the mammalian host. Nature 2005;436:573–577.
39 Baranton G, Seinost G, Theodore G, Postic D, Dykhuizen D: Distinct levels of genetic diversity of *Borrelia burgdorferi* are associated with different aspects of pathogenicity. Res Microbiol 2001;152: 149–156.
40 Steere AC, Klitz W, Drouin EE, Falk BA, Kwok WW, Nepom GT, Baxter-Lowe LA: Antibiotic-refractory Lyme arthritis is associated with HLA-DR molecules that bind a *Borrelia burgdorferi* peptide. J Exp Med 2006;203:961–971.
41 Soulas P, Woods A, Jaulhac B, et al: Autoantigen, innate immunity, and T cells cooperate to break B cell tolerance during bacterial infection. J Clin Invest 2005;115:2257–2267.
42 Humair P, Gern L: The wild hidden face of Lyme borreliosis in Europe. Microbes Infect 2000;2:915–922.
43 Kurtenbach K, Hanincova K, Tsao JI, Margos G, Fish D, Ogden NH: Fundamental processes in the evolutionary ecology of Lyme borreliosis. Nat Rev Microbiol 2006;4:660–669.
44 Sarih M, Jouda F, Gern L, Postic D: First isolation of *Borrelia burgdorferi* sensu lato from *Ixodes ricinus* ticks in Morocco. Vector Borne Zoonotic Dis 2003;3:133–139.
45 Postic D, Korenberg E, Gorelova N, Kovalevski YV, Bellenger E, Baranton G: *Borrelia burgdorferi* sensu lato in Russia and neighbouring countries: high incidence of mixed isolates. Res Microbiol 1997;148: 691–702.
46 Zhang Z, Xiu L: Personal communication 1996.
47 Shih CM, Chao LL: An *OspA*-based genospecies identification of Lyme disease spirochetes (*Borrelia burgdorferi*) isolated in Taiwan. Am J Trop Med Hyg 2002;66:611–615.
48 Shih CM, Chao LL: Genetic analysis of the outer surface protein C gene of Lyme disease Spirochaetes (*Borrelia burgdorferi* sensu lato) isolated from rodents in Taiwan. J Med Microbiol 2002;51:318–325.
49 Marti Ras N, Postic D, Foretz M, Baranton G: *Borrelia burgdorferi* sensu stricto, a bacterial species 'made in the USA'? Int J Syst Bacteriol 1997;47: 1112–1117.
50 Brisson D, Dykhuizen DE: *ospC* diversity in *Borrelia burgdorferi*: different hosts are different niches. Genetics 2004;168:713–722.
51 Berger BW, Johnson RC, Kodner C, Coleman L: Cultivation of *Borrelia burgdorferi* from erythema migrans lesions and perilesional skin. J Clin Microbiol 1992;30:359–361.
52 http://www.cdc.gov/ncidod/dvbid/lyme/ld_humandisease_symptoms.htm.
53 Jaulhac B, Heller R, Limbach FX, et al: Direct molecular typing of *Borrelia burgdorferi* sensu lato species in synovial samples from patients with Lyme arthritis. J Clin Microbiol 2000;38:1895–1900.
54 Vasiliu V, Herzer P, Rossler D, Lehnert G, Wilske B: Heterogeneity of *Borrelia burgdorferi* sensu lato demonstrated by an ospA-type-specific PCR in synovial fluid from patients with Lyme arthritis. Med Microbiol Immunol 1998;187:97–102.
55 Foretz M, Postic D, Baranton G: Phylogenetic analysis of *Borrelia burgdorferi* sensu stricto by arbitrarily primed PCR and pulsed-field gel electrophoresis. Int J Syst Bacteriol 1997;47:11–18.
56 Dykhuizen DE, Baranton G: The implications of a low rate of horizontal transfer in *Borrelia*. Trends Microbiol 2001;9:344–350.

57 Lagal V, Postic D, Ruzic-Sabljic E, Baranton G: Genetic diversity among *Borrelia* strains determined by single-strand conformation polymorphism analysis of the *ospC* gene and its association with invasiveness. J Clin Microbiol 2003;41:5059–5065.

58 Masuzawa T: Terrestrial distribution of the Lyme borreliosis agent *Borrelia burgdorferi* sensu lato in East Asia. Jpn J Infect Dis 2004;57:229–235.

59 Younsi H, Postic D, Baranton G, Bouattour A: High prevalence of *Borrelia lusitaniae* in *Ixodes ricinus* ticks in Tunisia. Eur J Epidemiol 2001;17:53–56.

60 Olsen B, Duffy DC, Jaenson TG, Gylfe A, Bonnedahl J, Bergstrom S: Transhemispheric exchange of Lyme disease spirochetes by seabirds. J Clin Microbiol 1995;33:3270–3274.

61 Smith RP Jr, Muzaffar SB, Lavers J, Lacombe EH, Cahill BK, Lubelczyk CB, Kinsler A, Mathers AJ, Rand PW: *Borrelia garinii* in seabird ticks (Ixodes uriae), Atlantic Coast, North America. Emerg Infect Dis 2006;12:1909–1912.

62 Comstedt P, Bergstrom S, Olsen B, Garpmo U, Marjavaara L, Mejlon H, Barbour AG, Bunikis J: Migratory passerine birds as reservoirs of Lyme borreliosis in Europe. Emerg Infect Dis 2006;12: 1087–1095.

63 Wilske B, Jauris-Heipke S, Lobentanzer R, Pradel I, Preac-Mursic V, Rössler D, Soutschek E, Johnson RC: Phenotypic analysis of outer surface protein C (OspC) of *Borrelia burgdorferi* sensu lato by monoclonal antibodies: relationship to genospecies and OspA serotype. J Clin Microbiol 1995;33:103–109.

64 Wilske B, Busch U, Eiffert H, et al: Diversity of OspA and OspC among cerebrospinal fluid isolates of *Borrelia burgdorferi* sensu lato from patients with neuroborreliosis in Germany. Med Microbiol Immunol 1996;184:195–201.

65 Huegli D, Hu CM, Humair PF, Wilske B, Gern L: Apodemus species mice are reservoir hosts of *Borrelia garinii* OspA serotype 4 in Switzerland. J Clin Microbiol 2002;40:4735–4737.

66 Jaulhac B, Nicolini P, Piemont Y, Monteil H: Detection of *Borrelia burgdorferi* in cerebrospinal fluid of patients with Lyme borreliosis. N Engl J Med 1991; 324:1440.

67 Picken RN, Strle F, Picken MM, Ruzic-Sabljic E, Maraspin V, Lotric-Furlan S, Cimperman J: Identification of three species of *Borrelia burgdorferi* sensu lato (*B. burgdorferi* sensu stricto, *B. garinii*, and *B. afzelii*) among isolates from acrodermatitis chronica atrophicans lesions. J Invest Dermatol 1998;110:211–214.

68 Canica MM, Nato F, du Merle L, Mazie JC, Baranton G, Postic D: Monoclonal antibodies for identification of *Borrelia afzelii* sp. nov. associated with late cutaneous manifestations of Lyme borreliosis. Scand J Infect Dis 1993;25:441–448.

69 Grange F, Wechsler J, Guillaume JC, Tortel J, Tortel MC, Audhuy B, Jaulhac B, Cerroni L: *Borrelia burgdorferi*-associated lymphocytoma cutis simulating a primary cutaneous large B-cell lymphoma. J Am Acad Dermatol 2002;47:530–534.

70 Rijpkema SG, Tazelaar DJ, Molkenboer MJ, Noordhoek GT, Plantinga G, Schouls LM, Schellekens JF: Detection of *Borrelia afzelii*, *Borrelia burgdorferi* sensu stricto, *Borrelia garinii* and group VS116 by PCR in skin biopsies of patients with erythema migrans and acrodermatitis chronica atrophicans. Clin Microbiol Infect 1997;3:109–116.

71 Richter D, Schlee DB, Allgower R, Matuschka FR: Relationships of a novel Lyme disease spirochete, *Borrelia spielmani* sp. nov., with its hosts in Central Europe. Appl Environ Microbiol 2004;70:6414–6419.

72 Postic D, Ras NM, Lane RS, Hendson M, Baranton G: Expanded diversity among Californian *Borrelia* isolates and description of *Borrelia bissettii* sp. nov. (formerly *Borrelia* group DN127). J Clin Microbiol 1998;36:3497–3504.

73 Strle F, Picken RN, Cheng Y, Cimperman J, Maraspin V, Lotric-Furlan S, Ruzic-Sabljic E, Picken MM: Clinical findings for patients with Lyme borreliosis caused by *Borrelia burgdorferi* sensu lato with genotypic and phenotypic similarities to strain 25015. Clin Infect Dis 1997;25:273–280.

74 Wang G, van Dam AP, Le Fleche A, Postic D, Peter O, Baranton G, de Boer R, Spanjaard L, Dankert J: Genetic and phenotypic analysis of *Borrelia valaisiana* sp. nov. (*Borrelia* genomic groups VS116 and M19). Int J Syst Bacteriol 1997;47:926–932.

75 Rijpkema SG, Molkenboer MJ, Schouls LM, Jongejan F, Schellekens JF: Simultaneous detection and genotyping of three genomic groups of *Borrelia burgdorferi* sensu lato in Dutch *Ixodes ricinus* ticks by characterization of the amplified intergenic spacer region between 5S and 23S rRNA genes. J Clin Microbiol 1995;33:3091–3095.

76 Diza E, Papa A, Vezyri E, Tsounis S, Milonas I, Antoniadis A: *Borrelia valaisiana* in cerebrospinal fluid. Emerg Infect Dis 2004;10:1692–1693.

77 Wang G, van Dam AP, Dankert J: Evidence for frequent OspC gene transfer between *Borrelia valaisiana* sp. nov. and other Lyme disease spirochetes. FEMS Microbiol Lett 1999;177:289–296.

78 Le Fleche A, Postic D, Girardet K, Peter O, Baranton G: Characterization of *Borrelia lusitaniae* sp. nov. by 16S ribosomal DNA sequence analysis. Int J Syst Bacteriol 1997;47:921–925.

79 Younsi H, Sarih M, Jouda F, Godfroid E, Gern L, Bouattour A, Baranton G, Postic D: Characterization of *Borrelia lusitaniae* isolates collected in Tunisia and Morocco. J Clin Microbiol 2005;43:1587–1593.

80 Dsouli N, Younsi-Kabachii H, Postic D, Nouira S, Gern L, Bouattour A: Reservoir role of lizard *Psammodromus algirus* in transmission cycle of *Borrelia burgdorferi* sensu lato (Spirochaetaceae) in Tunisia. J Med Entomol 2006;43:737–742.
81 Collares-Pereira M, Couceiro S, Franca I, Kurtenbach K, Schäfer SM, Vitorino L, Gonçalves L, Baptista S, Vieira ML, Cunha C: First isolation of *Borrelia lusitaniae* from a human patient. J Clin Microbiol 2004;42:1316–1318.
82 Kawabata H, Masuzawa T, Yanagihara Y: Genomic analysis of *Borrelia japonica* sp. nov. isolated from *Ixodes ovatus* in Japan. Microbiol Immunol 1993; 37:843–848.
83 Fukunaga M, Hamase A, Okada K, Nakao M: *Borrelia tanukii* sp. nov. and *Borrelia turdae* sp. nov. found from *Ixodid* ticks in Japan: rapid species identification by 16S rRNA gene-targeted PCR analysis. Microbiol Immunol 1996;40:877–881.
84 Masuzawa T, Takada N, Kudeken M, Fukui T, Yano Y, Ishiguro F, Kawamura Y, Imai Y, Ezaki T: *Borrelia sinica* sp. nov., a Lyme disease-related *Borrelia* species isolated in China. Int J Syst Evol Microbiol 2001;51:1817–1824.
85 Brown RN, Lane RS: Reservoir competence of four chaparral-dwelling rodents for *Borrelia burgdorferi* in California. Am J Trop Med Hyg 1996;54:84–91.
86 Casjens S, Palmer N, van Vugt R, Huang WM, Stevenson B, Rosa P, Lathigra R, Sutton G, Peterson J, Dodson RJ, Haft D, Hickey E, Gwinn M, White O, Fraser CM: A bacterial genome in flux: the twelve linear and nine circular extrachromosomal DNAs in an infectious isolate of the Lyme disease spirochete *Borrelia burgdorferi*. Mol Microbiol 2000;35: 490–516.
87 Woodman ME, Cooley AE, Miller J: *Borrelia burgdorferi* binding of host complement regulator factor H is not required for efficient mammalian infection. Infect Immun 2007;75:3131–3139.
88 Wang G, Ojaimi C, Wu H, Saksenberg V, Iyer R, Liveris D, McClain SA, Wormser GP, Schwartz I: Disease severity in a murine model of Lyme borreliosis is associated with the genotype of the infecting *Borrelia burgdorferi* sensu stricto strain. J Infect Dis 2002;186:782–791.
89 DiCaudo DJ, Su WP, Marshall WF, Malawista SE, Barthold S, Persing DH: Acrodermatitis chronica atrophicans in the United States: clinical and histopathologic features of six cases. Cutis 1994;54:81–84.
90 Theisen M, Borre M, Mathiesen MJ, Mikkelsen B, Lebech AM, Hansen K: Evolution of the *Borrelia burgdorferi* outer surface protein OspC. J Bacteriol 1995;177:3036–3044.

Sylvie De Martino
Laboratoire de Bactériologie, CNR Borrelia Laboratoire associé, CHU de Strasbourg
3, rue Koeberlé
FR–67000 Strasbourg (France)
Tel. +33 3 90 24 38 05, Fax +33 3 90 24 38 08, E-Mail sylvie.demartino@medecine.u-strasbg.fr

Lipsker D, Jaulhac B (eds): Lyme Borreliosis.
Curr Probl Dermatol. Basel, Karger, 2009, vol 37, pp 18–30

Life Cycle of *Borrelia burgdorferi* sensu lato and Transmission to Humans

Lise Gern

Institute of Biology, University of Neuchâtel, Neuchâtel, Switzerland

Abstract

Lyme borreliosis is a zoonosis: its causative agent, *Borrelia burgdorferi* sensu lato, circulates between *Ixodes ricinus* ticks and a large variety of vertebrates. *I. ricinus* has a wide geographical distribution throughout Europe within the latitudes of 65° and 39° and from Portugal into Russia. Enzootic cycles in Europe involve at least 7 *Borrelia* species. Apparently, associations exist in nature between *Borrelia* species and hosts. *B. afzelii* and *B. burgdorferi* sensu stricto are associated with rodents, and *B. garinii* and *B. valaisiana* with birds. *B. lusitaniae* may be transmitted to ticks by some lizard species and birds. *B. spielmanii* appears to be associated with dormice and hedgehogs. Less strict associations also exist. Transmission of *Borrelia* infection by *I. ricinus* to their hosts, including humans, does not occur immediately when ticks attach to host skin. A delay is observed, which may depend on the *Borrelia* species infecting the tick. *B. afzelii* can be transmitted during the first 24 h, whereas *B. burgdorferi* needs 48 h of tick attachment before its transmission begins. Nothing is known about the other *Borrelia* species; however, success of transmission always increases with tick attachment duration. Therefore, careful visual examinations of the body for at least 2 successive days are recommended after visiting an endemic area.

Among diseases due to vector-borne pathogens in Europe, Lyme borreliosis, which is transmitted by the tick *Ixodes ricinus*, is the most widespread and has a big impact on human health. Lyme borreliosis is a zoonosis: its causative agent, *Borrelia burgdorferi* sensu lato (s.l.), circulates between ticks and a large variety of vertebrates that act as hosts for ticks. By acquiring the infection through infected tick bites and by developing clinical manifestations of Lyme borreliosis, humans reveal the presence of the microorganism in various geographical areas. Humans are not involved in the transmission cycle of *B. burgdorferi* s.l. in nature. They act as dead-end hosts.

Biology of *I. ricinus*

I. ricinus has a very wide geographical distribution throughout Europe. It has been found within the latitudes of 65° and 39° and from Portugal into Russia, and also in North Africa (Tunisia, Algeria and Morocco) [1]. In continental Europe, *I. ricinus* is mainly present in deciduous woodlands and mixed forests. Ticks colonize biotopes offering a high relative humidity. In fact, *I. ricinus* only survives where the relative humidity in its microhabitat does not fall under 80%. The duration of its life cycle can vary regionally and from one habitat to another, and can be affected by climatic factors and host density. The large geographical distribution of *I. ricinus* implies that this tick has to survive under various environmental conditions, i.e. throughout this large geographical area, temperatures vary considerably. Since temperature is known to have an effect on tick questing activity and on tick development rates, it is an important parameter in the dynamic of seasonal activity. Several papers described that the seasonal activity of questing *I. ricinus* presents different patterns under different climatic conditions. This seasonal activity pattern may be unimodal with a major peak of tick activity in spring or in winter, or may be bimodal with 2 peaks of tick activity, one in spring and another one in autumn [2]. This is important information because seasonal questing activity of *I. ricinus* influences the risk of being bitten by ticks, geographically and temporally.

The vertical distribution limit of *I. ricinus* differs throughout Europe according to geographical position. However, recently many studies reported a shift in this limit to higher altitudes, most probably due to the increase in temperature observed during these last decades [2]. Interestingly, due to the vertical distribution limit observed in tick distribution, it is frequently believed that the higher the altitude, the less ticks. This should not be considered as a rule; various reports have recently shown that in some habitats the opposite has been observed: the higher the altitude, the more ticks. However, it is important to note that the tick densities described at the highest altitudes were usually rather low.

In many aspects, ticks differ from insects. One way is that each of their developmental stages (larvae, nymphs and adult females) feeds once on a host, and this lasts for several consecutive days (fig. 1). Each blood meal is followed by a developmental phase, except for the females that will lay eggs after their blood meal and then die. Male ticks may take up a very small quantity of blood, but they never take large blood meals. The total duration of blood meals of *I. ricinus* is short, and does not last more than 12–20 days. Larvae feed for 2 to 4 days, nymphs for 4 to 6 days and females for 6 to 10 days. Ticks can survive for years in their biotopes; however, they spend only a small part of their life in a parasitic phase. Most of the *I. ricinus* lifetime is spent outside of the hosts, either on the ground or in vegetation. To find a host, *I. ricinus* climbs onto low vegetation and waits at the tip where they quest for a host for time-limited periods. During these periods of questing, *I. ricinus* ticks stay mainly immobile at the tip of the vegetation. When ticks are questing, they respond to mechanical and chem-

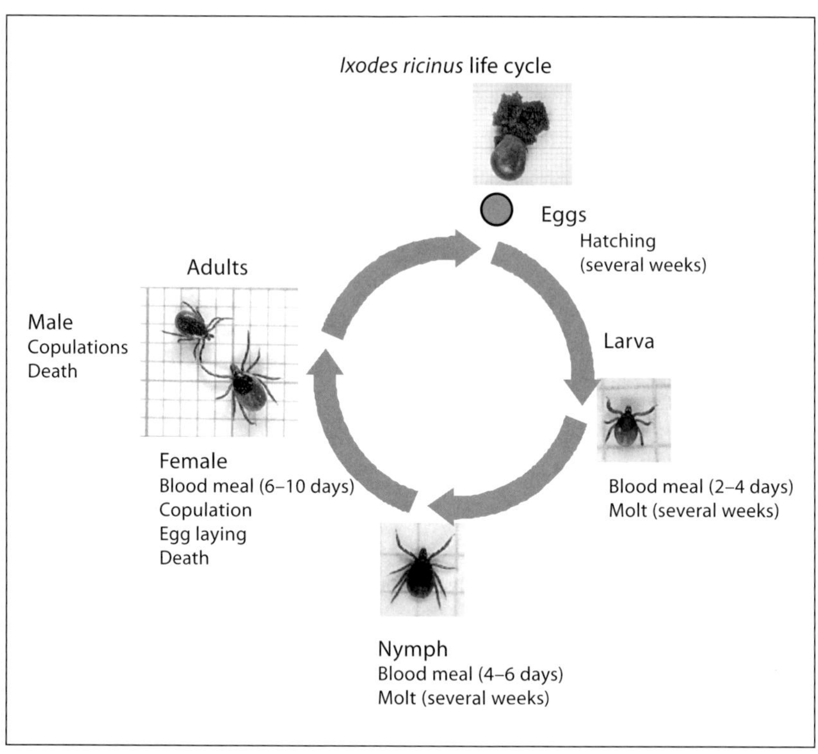

Fig. 1. Complete life cycle of the *I. ricinus* tick.

ical stimuli produced by hosts, including humans. When hosts pass close enough, questing ticks grab their hosts. This behaviour of *I. ricinus* is important since it implies that hosts, including humans, take some active part in the tick-host encounter.

During questing periods, *I. ricinus* often experiences desiccating conditions. As already mentioned, *I. ricinus* ticks are susceptible to desiccation when questing for hosts on vegetation, and high humidity is a prerequisite for tick survival. The atmosphere is often unsaturated, and this represents a net water loss for the ticks. Therefore, questing ticks have to rehydrate, and to do so they regularly leave their questing place and move to the litter zone. There, to maintain their water balance, ticks actively absorb water from the subsaturated atmosphere. High humidity is found at the base of vegetation, where ticks uptake atmospheric water. One aspect of the life cycle of ticks is that they do not have unlimited time to find their hosts. Indeed, their survival is limited by the amount of energy they gain with blood meals and by their ability to maintain their water content in a desiccating atmosphere. For example, if highly desiccating conditions develop, ticks reduce their questing duration and move more often to the soil to rehydrate; eventually, their energy reserves will run out before they find a host and they will die. In nature, abrupt declines in questing tick populations have been reported to coincide with abrupt increases in saturation deficit (measurement of the drying power of the air that includes relative humidity and temperature) [3–5]. Long-lasting high saturation deficit may influence the evolution of seasonal questing tick density, and also impair tick population maintenance in some areas [2, 6]. If highly desiccating conditions are lasting and they coincide with tick questing activity period, tick populations may greatly suffer from this moisture stress and may be dramatically reduced. It was observed that under warmer episodes in spring and summer, when synchrony of weather conditions with the tick life cycle occurred – e.g. in spring, when many ticks quest and long-lasting highly desiccating conditions are present – questing duration was reduced and tick mortality was increased, leading to a lower questing tick population [4, 5].

Life Cycle of *B. burgdorferi* s.l.

At the time of its discovery in the beginning of the 1980s, the causative agent of Lyme borreliosis, *B. burgdorferi,* was thought to be a uniform organism. Currently, 12 *Borrelia* species are included in the complex *B. burgdorferi* s.l., and 7 of them have been reported in *I. ricinus* in Europe: *B. burgdorferi* sensu stricto (s.s.), *B. garinii, B. afzelii, B. valaisiana, B. lusitaniae, B. bissettii* and *B. spielmanii* [7, 8]. *B. bissettii* has been reported only once in *I. ricinus* ticks in Europe. This was in a report from Slovakia, where 1 tick was found to be reactive with probes specific for *B. bissettii* [9]; this tick was also reactive with probes for 2 other species of *B. burgdorferi,* which complicated the specific identification of the spirochetes present in this tick, and, as a result, the presence of *B. bissettii* in *I. ricinus* has to be confirmed by additional reports.

In Europe, *B. burgdorferi* s.l. has been reported from Italy to Iceland and from Portugal to Russia [7]. The reported mean rates of *B. burgdorferi* in *I. ricinus* are 1.9% for larvae, 10.8% for nymphs and 17.4% for adults [10]. Occasionally, higher infection rates have been reported, mainly using PCR, as for example in Portugal where *B. burgdorferi* DNA in *I. ricinus* ticks reached 75% [7]. Local and temporal variations in the infection prevalences of *Borrelia* in ticks have been recorded.

B. garinii and *B. afzelii* are the most frequent and most widely distributed species, whereas *B. burgdorferi* s.s. and *B. valaisiana* are less common [7]. *B. lusitaniae* presents an interesting geographical distribution. In fact, *B. lusitaniae,* first isolated from *I. ricinus* ticks in Portugal, has been reported in various European countries, for example Bulgaria, Portugal, Slovakia, Switzerland, the Czech Republic, Moldavia, Ukraine, Poland and Spain [1, 7]. Its presence has also been described in North Africa [11]. Interestingly, *B. lusitaniae* is very common and greatly exceeds the other species in *I. ricinus* ticks in Portugal and North Africa, whereas this *Borrelia* species is only sporadically reported in ticks from the other areas. Rauter and Hartung [7] in their meta-analysis give a detailed distribution of the main *Borrelia* species in different parts of Europe. However, it is important to repeat here that the distribution of the various species of *B. burgdorferi* s.l. and their frequency vary in endemic areas

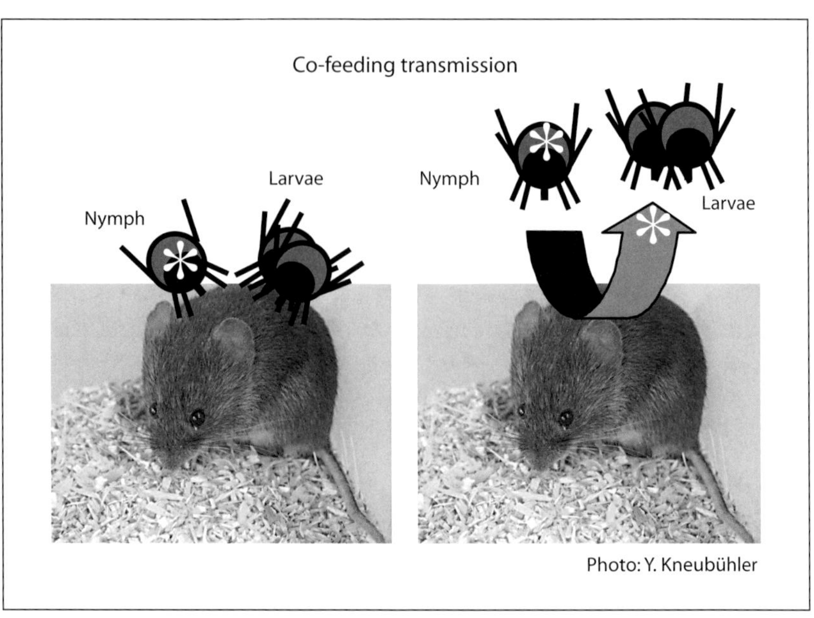

Fig. 2. Co-feeding transmission.

over time. For example, *B. afzelii* may alternatively dominate in an area with *B. garinii*. The recently described species, *B. spielmanii,* has been reported in *I. ricinus* from The Netherlands, Denmark, Hungary, Slovenia, Germany and France [8]. The reported geographical distribution of the different *Borrelia* species and their frequency, and especially of those which are less frequently reported, may greatly change in the future due to the implementation of more molecular analysis techniques.

Since, in some endemic areas in Europe, at least 6 *Borrelia* species may circulate, mixed infection with more than 1 species in ticks can be observed. Infections by multiple *B. burgdorferi* s.l. species have been observed in ticks in many parts of Europe [7]. Different combinations of mixed infections with 2 or 3 species have been detected in *I. ricinus. B. garinii* and *B. valaisiana* constitute the majority of mixed infections, followed by mixed infections with *B. garinii* and *B. afzelii.* Such mixed infections are reported less frequently than single infections, and are often detected by PCR methods. Rauter and Hartung [7], in their analysis of data collected throughout Europe, reported 13% mixed infections in *I. ricinus* ticks. These multiple infections may result from the feeding of ticks on a host infected by more than 1 *Borrelia* species or from infected ticks feeding simultaneously with uninfected ticks on a host and exchanging the *Borrelia* species through co-feeding transmission from infected to uninfected ticks (fig. 2) [12]. Moreover, ticks may acquire various *Borrelia* species through their successive blood meals on various hosts, and maintain the infection to the subsequent stage via transstadial transmission. Transovarial transmission of *Borrelia* from infected *I. ricinus* females to their progeny is also possible, but it represents a rare phenomenon [1]. Nevertheless, transovarially transmitted spirochetes may also contribute to mixed infections in ticks.

The efficient persistence of the borreliae in endemic areas requires the involvement of reservoir hosts. Potential hosts for ticks are numerous, and more than 300 vertebrate species have been identified as hosts for *I. ricinus,* including small mammals, birds, larger mammals and reptiles. Among these hosts, some act as blood meal sources and as reservoir hosts for pathogens, others as blood meal sources only. Natural hosts do not seem to develop clinical manifestations of the disease, although it is difficult to evaluate the impact of *Borrelia* infection on their health, and minor clinical manifestations may escape our attention.

Only a few dozen of the hosts for ticks have been currently identified as reservoir hosts for *B. burgdorferi* s.l. in Europe. Globally, little information is available on the real significance of most animal hosts as sources for infecting ticks with *B. burgdorferi* s.l. At present, several species of mice, voles, rats and shrews are recognized as reservoirs of *B. burgdorferi* s.l. in Europe [1]. In particular, it was evidenced that the mice *Apodemus flavicollis*, *A. sylvaticus*, *A. agrarius* and the vole, *Clethrionomys glareolus*, play key roles in the ecology of Lyme borreliosis as reservoirs for *B. burgdorferi* s.l. in many European countries. Once infected by an infectious tick bite, some reservoir hosts, like *Apodemus* mice, have been shown to persistently remain infectious for ticks. Small rodents are frequently parasitized by larval and nymphal *I. ricinus,* and this also contributes to their importance as reservoirs. Less information has been obtained on the roles of other small mammal species in the maintenance cycles of *Borrelia* in nature. Nevertheless, another species of vole *(Microtus agrestis)* in Sweden, and black rats *(Rattus rattus)* and Norway rats *(R. norvegicus)* in urbanized environments in Germany and in Madeira, may serve as sources of infection for *I. ricinus* ticks. Similarly, only few data have been collected on *B. burgdorferi* s.l. in shrews *(Sorex minutus* and *S. araneus* and *Neomys fodiens)* or in ticks attached on them. Observations in endemic areas of Germany and France showed that edible dormice *(Glis glis)* and garden dormice *(Eliomys quercinus)* are reservoir hosts for *Borrelia*. Other rodent species, like grey squirrels *(Sciurus carolinensis)* in the UK and red squirrels *(S. vulgaris)* in Switzerland, also contribute to the amplification of *Borrelia* in the tick population. Red and grey squirrels are usually very heavily infested with ticks, and 1 study reported a high prevalence of infection (69%) in ticks feeding on red squirrels. In other investigations in Ireland, Germany and Switzerland, it was reported that the European hedgehog *(Erinaceus europaeus)* also perpetuates *B. burgdorferi* s.l. [7]. In Switzerland, an enzootic transmission cycle of *B. burgdorferi* s.l. involving hedgehogs and another tick vector, *I. hexagonus*, has been observed in an urban environment. This shows that gardens can also represent zones at risk of Lyme borreliosis as further discussed below. Examination of the role of lagomorphs *(Lepus europaeus, L. timidus,* and *Oryctolagus cuniculus)* in the support of the enzootic cycle of *B. burgdorferi* s.l. has also elucidated their roles as reservoirs [1].

When attention was first directed at the role of birds in the ecology of Lyme borreliosis, their role was minimized. However, at the beginning of the 1990s, the reservoir role of birds was clarified in Europe, and now it is unanimously accepted that some bird species are reservoirs for *B. burgdorferi* s.l. In 1998, 2 studies clearly defined the reservoir role of birds, one on a passerine bird, the blackbird *(Turdus merula)*, the other one on a gallinaceous bird species, the pheasant *(Phasianus colchicus)* [1]. Both studies examined the reservoir role of these bird species using xenodiagnosis. Tick xenodiagnosis consists of infecting uninfected ticks – usually larvae – during feeding on the animal suspected to be reservoir host. These results and others have evidenced the contribution of birds to the circulation of *Borrelia* in endemic areas. Interestingly, a transmission cycle of *B. burgdorferi* s.l. was discovered in environmental settings other than the biotopes where *I. ricinus* usually live. In fact, it was demonstrated, on a Swedish island, that *B. burgdorferi* spirochetes could be maintained in seabird colonies among razorbills *(Alca torda)* by an associated tick species, *I. uriae*. Of course, interest in birds was also focused on the potential role of migrating birds in transporting infected ticks. This approach turned out to be justified, and spirochetes were reported in ticks collected from migratory birds in various studies. The involvement of seabirds and *I. uriae* (in the marine environment) in the transport of infected *Borrelia* between the northern and the southern hemispheres was described. In this context, it is interesting to mention that in a laboratory study, reactivation of latent *Borrelia* infection could be induced in passerines experimentally submitted to stressful conditions simulating migration. This implies that during their migration, birds can infect ticks all along their migration route. Bird migration also allows the transfer and establishment of particular *Borrelia* species, as described for *B. lusitaniae*. In fact, birds migrating between south-west Europe/North Africa to north-western Europe have been suggested to be responsible for the transfer of *B. lusitaniae* from North Africa and south-west Europe, where this *Borrelia* species clearly dominates, to north-west Europe where it is much less frequent [13].

Assessment of the reservoir competency of large mammals is clearly a difficult task. It necessitates, if xenodiagnosis is applied, capture of the animals and maintenance in a laboratory structure. The consequence of this is that the role of medium-sized and large mammalian species has been studied less and is not yet clearly understood. Red foxes seem to be implicated in the maintenance of *Borrelia* in nature, as described in Germany. However, these animals do not appear to be very potent reservoirs, since spirochetes were poorly transmitted to ticks feeding on them. According to various reports, ruminants appear to act primarily as sources of blood for ticks. Controversy long surrounded the exact role of large animals, particularly cervids, in the maintenance cycle of *Borrelia* in endemic areas. Currently, most studies seem to indicate that they do not play a role as reservoirs. In fact, studies undertaken in Sweden and in the UK on roe deer *(Capreolus capreolus)*, moose *(Alces alces)*, red deer *(Cervus elaphus)* and fallow deer *(Dama dama)* suggested that these species do not infect feeding ticks with *B. burgdorferi* s.l. However, according to some recent developments, the possibility exists that they may act as supports for co-feeding transmission of *Borrelia* between infected and uninfected ticks, and therefore may represent amplifying hosts.

As previously mentioned, in Europe, at least 6 *Borrelia* species may circulate between vertebrate hosts and ticks. This raises a fundamental question: how do the different *Borrelia* species interact with the different host species in endemic areas? The first findings showing an association between a *Borrelia* species and some host species date back to the middle of the 1990s. At that time, it was shown that *Borrelia* species isolated from *Apodemus* spp. captured in 2 sites in Switzerland all belonged to *B. afzelii*, whereas *Borrelia* species diversity in ticks collected by flagging vegetation in these sites displayed heterogeneity. Later, it was shown that small rodents of the genus *Apodemus* and of the genus *Clethrionomys* as well as red *(Sciurus vulgaris)* and grey squirrels *(S. carolinensis)* were usually infected by *B. afzelii* and less frequently by *B. burgdorferi* s.s. and that they transmitted these 2 *Borrelia* species to ticks feeding on them. On the other hand, at the same time, *B. garinii* was shown to be associated with migratory birds, and *B. garinii* and *B. valaisiana* with blackbirds and pheasants. *B. garinii* was also described as the *Borrelia* species involved in marine environments – in seabird colonies and in the tick *I. uriae* – located in both the northern and southern hemispheres.

As far as less common *Borrelia* species are concerned, like *B. lusitaniae* and *B. spielmanii*, recent works identified associations with some vertebrate hosts as well. Thus, Dsouli et al. [11] demonstrated the reservoir role of the lizard *Psammodromus algirus* for *B. lusitaniae* in North Africa (Tunisia), Richter and Matuschka [14] the roles of the common wall lizard *Podarcis muralis* and sand lizard *Lacerta agilis* in Germany, and, finally, Amore et al. [15] reported that *P. muralis* was a reservoir for this *Borrelia* species in Italy. Poupon et al. [13] observed *B. lusitaniae* in *I. ricinus* larvae collected from birds that were migrating between southwest Europe/North Africa and northwestern Europe. These authors strongly suspected the role of migratory birds in the dispersal of *B. lusitaniae.* Concerning *B. spielmanii*, the garden dormouse, *E. quercinus* [16], and the hedgehog *E. europaeus* [17] have been described as contributing the majority of *B. spielmanii*-infected ticks in areas endemic for this *Borrelia* species.

At this point, one might justifiably ask: What element is behind this host-specificity of *B. burgdorferi* s.l.? Explanation for this observation came from studies showing that determinants for the described phenomenon were linked to the host complement system [18]. It was demonstrated in vitro that *B. burgdorferi* s.s., *B. garinii, B. valaisiana* and *B. afzelii* showed different patterns of resistance or sensitivity to serum according to host species, corresponding to the host specificity observed in nature [18]. The main disadvantage of this in vitro system is that a great heterogeneity is present among *Borrelia* strains in nature, and therefore a very large number of various *Borrelia* strains have to be tested in relation to a very large number of host sera to be able to mimic situations encountered in nature. An illustration of this is

B. lusitaniae. Kurtenbach et al. [18] reported that *B. lusitaniae* is sensitive to the complement of some bird and lizard species, and hence is destroyed by these host sera. However, as reported before, *B. lusitaniae* has been found to be associated with some lizard and bird species in nature. Further research in this field is required to better understand all subtleties governing these interactions. This is particularly important because besides these strict associations between *Borrelia* and vertebrate hosts, loose associations between *Borrelia* and hosts have also been described in the natural environment. *B. garinii* has occasionally been described as associated with rodents, and *B. afzelii* has been detected in xenodiagnostic ticks that fed on birds. The existence of such loose associations between hosts and *Borrelia* was confirmed recently in studies using less classical methods to identify host reservoirs. In fact, the use of molecular tools upon field-collected ticks – that allow the identification of host DNA remaining in the tick midgut from the previous blood meal, along with the detection of *Borrelia* – tended to show that in parallel to the strict associations between *Borrelia* species and hosts, less strict associations also exist [19]. All this goes to show that in nature strict and loose associations probably occur between *Borrelia* species and host species. Additional studies are required to really understand the relationships between the various *Borrelia* species and strains and their hosts in nature.

It is striking that among the 300 vertebrate species serving as hosts for ticks, only a few have been identified as reservoir hosts. We have already touched on the difficulties in assessing the reservoir competency of vertebrates, particularly large mammals. This can be mainly attributed to the fact that, as a gold standard, reservoir identification implies tick xenodiagnosis. This necessitates animal trappings and temporary maintenance of these animals in captivity. It is obvious that most tick hosts are difficult to capture and to maintain in a laboratory. That is one of the reasons why researchers have recently developed molecular tools allowing identification of hosts that have fed the field-collected ticks in their previous developmental stages. This method coupled with the simultaneous detection of pathogens in ticks, mainly in nymphs, has been developed and applied in the field. Two main host genes have been targeted in these studies, the nuclear 18S rRNA gene [20] and the 12S rDNA mitochondrial gene [21]. The method based on the nuclear 18S rRNA gene appears to be less sensitive, in the sense that it allows the discrimination of only major groups of vertebrate hosts [20]. The other method, based on the 12S rDNA mitochondrial gene, has the advantage of allowing identification of host DNA to the species level, narrowing down host identification [21]. The use of these molecular tools may help to elucidate the maintenance and the circulation of *B. burgdorferi* s.l. among their different hosts throughout the large geographical distribution of *I. ricinus* ticks in Europe and North Africa.

Transmission of *B. burgdorferi* to Humans

Let us first remember here that the encounter between ticks and their hosts, including humans, comprises a tick that is immobile on vegetation waiting for a host that is moving; this means that the encounter between these 2 elements of the eco-epidemiological chain is based mainly on the active part of the host. Once the encounter has taken place, the tick will move on its host to look for an adequate place to introduce its mouthparts into the skin of its host. In humans, it may take a few minutes to hours before the tick attaches to the skin. The duration of attachment of the tick *I. ricinus* to its hosts, as we mentioned before, can vary between 3 and 10 days depending on the developmental stage. *B. burgdorferi* s.l. spirochetes are transmitted to their hosts orally while ticks are taking their blood meal. It took a few years after the discovery of *B. burgdorferi* in ticks in North America in the 1980s for the mechanism of how the spirochetes were transmitted to the host to be elucidated. This was mainly due to the fact that before blood meal, in unfed ticks, spirochetes are located in the tick midgut. Thus, for some years, regurgitation of midgut content was considered as the mode of transmission of *B. burgdorferi* s.l., before the transmission route was elucidated. Currently, it is well established that *B. burgdorferi* s.l. is transmitted to the host via infected saliva during the blood meal. Very few studies have investigated the transmission dynamic of *B. burgdorferi* s.l. by *I. ricinus*; however, these studies showed that, in the majority of infected *I. ricinus* ticks, spirochetes (that are present in the midgut of ticks before blood meal begins) migrate during blood feeding to the salivary glands, from which they are transmitted to the host via saliva. Furthermore, microscopic examination of unfed nymphal and adult *I. ricinus* ticks collected in endemic areas demonstrated that spirochetes may also be present in the salivary glands of ticks even before any blood uptake [22].

When unfed *I. ricinus* attaches to a vertebrate host, *Borrelia* transmission does not occur at the beginning of the blood uptake but later on, and transmission efficiency increases with the duration of the blood meal [23, 24]. The uptake of blood seems to trigger spirochetes to migrate from tick midgut to the salivary glands. The delay in transmission observed during the first hours of the blood meal might be due to this phenomenon, the migration of the spirochetes. In a laboratory study, an early transmission of borreliae with high efficiency was described for *I. ricinus*. In fact, Kahl et al. [23] reported that 50% of laboratory animals were infected by *B. burgdorferi* s.l. after only 16.7 h of tick attachment. The observations of high infection rates in salivary glands of unfed *I. ricinus* suggest that systemically infected ticks may transmit *Borrelia* early after attachment to hosts [22], and this might be a factor that might reduce the delay in transmission after attachment of the ticks to the hosts. Crippa et al. [24], comparing transmission dynamic of spirochetes by *B. burgdorferi* s.s.- and *B. afzelii*-infected ticks, reported that this delay might also be influenced by the *Borrelia* species infecting the ticks. In fact, earlier transmission by *I. ricinus* occurred when ticks were infected by *B. afzelii* rather than by *B. burgdorferi* s.s. These authors reported that during the first 48 h of attachment to the host, *B. burgdorferi* s.s.-infected ticks did not infect the 18 exposed mice, whereas *B. afzelii*-infected ticks transmitted infection to 33% of the mice [24]. This study not only showed that *I. ricinus* transmits *B. afzelii* earlier than *B. burgdorferi* s.s., but also that *I. ricinus* is a more efficient vector for *B. afzelii* than for *B. burgdorferi* s.s. Unfortunately, nothing is known on the transmission delay for other pathogenic *Borrelia* species infecting *I. ricinus*, such as *B. garinii*, *B. valaisiana* and the recently described species *B. spielmanii*. All this indicates that ticks should be removed as soon as they are found attached to the skin.

The migration of *Borrelia* from the midgut to the salivary glands during tick feeding is associated with variable protein expression. From studies mainly on the North American tick vector, *I. scapularis*, but also on *I. ricinus*, it is known that in unfed ticks, before the beginning of blood uptake, spirochetes located in the midgut express outer surface protein A (OspA). On its surface, OspA possesses a receptor for plasminogen of the host organism. After tick feeding starts on the host, plasminogen changes into plasmin, which facilitates migration through the midgut wall to the salivary glands. During blood feeding, OspA synthesis is repressed and OspC synthesis is induced. In *I. ricinus*, very few studies addressed this point. Leuba-Garcia et al. [22] observed that *B. afzelii* spirochetes expressing OspA and OspC were present in the midgut of unfed ticks, and that spirochetes expressing OspA were not detected in ticks attached to the host for more than 24 h. In salivary glands of engorged ticks, *B. afzelii* spirochetes expressed OspC. This study also reported that in the skin of mice infected by *B. afzelii*-infected nymphs, spirochetes expressed OspC. Later, Fingerle et al. [25], using different *B. afzelii* and *B. garinii* strains, demonstrated that in capillary-infected *I. ricinus* ticks, OspA was expressed in the tick midgut and that the proportion of OspC-positive borreliae was usually greater when the borreliae reached the salivary glands. In this study, a *B. afzelii* strain unable to produce OspC was unable to disseminate and to induce infection in salivary glands, showing the role of OspC in *Borrelia* dissemination in *I. ricinus*. The degree of strain specificity on the dynamics of Osp expression and the dissemination of spirochetes in the vector is an interesting topic. The interactions of the various *Borrelia* species and strains with *I. ricinus* are clearly extremely complex and insufficiently studied.

We cannot end this chapter without adding some words on another tick species, the hedgehog tick *(I. hexagonus)*, that may transmit *Borrelia* infection to humans. Its vector competence has been demonstrated under laboratory conditions, and confirmed under field conditions. This tick species is one of the most widespread tick species in Europe. *I. hexagonus* is a nidicolous species, which means that this tick lives in the nest, burrow or cave of its hosts. Hosts for this tick species are mainly recorded among carnivores. In view of its habitats, *I. hexagonus* rarely comes in contact with humans. However, hedgehogs are also frequent hosts for *I. hexagonus,* and since hedgehogs are frequent hosts in our gardens, humans can come into contact with this tick (particularly when they handle nests of hedgehogs, which have surface nests, when gardening). *I. hexagonus* bites humans, although less frequently than *I. ricinus*, and may transmit *Borrelia* infection to them. In addition to *I. ricinus* and *I. hexagonus*, other tick species and even insect species have been found to be infected by *B. burgdorferi* s.l., but without evidence of vector competence. A list of these insect and tick species can be found in a report by Gern and Humair [1].

We have seen that once on their host, *I. ricinus* ticks do not attach immediately to the skin, but look for a suitable place. We have also reported that the risk of transmission of *Borrelia* by feeding ticks increases with attachment duration. Both these elements are important in the prevention of Lyme borreliosis. It means that careful visual examinations of body may prevent tick bites as well as *Borrelia* infection. Body examination is recommended not only during and immediately after stays in tick biotopes, but also during the following days.

References

1 Gern L, Humair PF: Ecology of *Borrelia burgdorferi* sensu lato in Europe; in Gray JS, Kahl O, Lane RS, Stanek G (eds): Lyme Borreliosis: Biology, Epidemiology and Control. Wallingford, CAB International, 2002, pp 149–174.

2 Morán Cadenas F, Rais O, Jouda F, Douet V, Humair PF, Moret J, Gern L: Phenology of *Ixodes ricinus* and infection with *Borrelia burgdorferi* sensu lato along a north- and south-facing altitudinal gradient on Chaumont Mountain, Switzerland. J Med Entomol 2007;44:683–693.

3 Randolph SE, Storey K: Impact of microclimate on immature tick-rodent host interactions (Acari: Ixodidae): implications for parasite transmission. J Med Entomol 1999;36:741–748.

4 Perret JL, Guigoz E, Rais O, Gern L: Influence of saturation deficit and temperature on *Ixodes ricinus* tick questing activity in a Lyme borreliosis endemic area (Switzerland). Parasitol Res 2000;86:554–557.

5 Perret JL, Rais O, Gern L: Influence of climate on the proportion of *Ixodes ricinus* nymphs and adults questing in a tick population. J Med Entomol 2004;41:361–365.

6 Burri C, Morán Cadenas F, Douet V, Moret J, Gern L: *Ixodes ricinus* density and infection prevalence of *Borrelia burgdorferi* sensu lato along a north facing altitudinal gradient in the Rhône Valley (Switzerland). Vector Borne Zoonotic Dis 2007;7:50–58.

7 Rauter C, Hartung T: Prevalence of *Borrelia burgdorferi* sensu lato species in *Ixodes ricinus* ticks in Europe: a metaanalysis. Appl Environ Microbiol 2005;71:7203–7216.

8 Richter D, Postic D, Sertour N, Livey I, Matuschka FR, Baranton G: Delineation of *Borrelia burgdorferi* sensu lato species by multilocus sequence analysis and confirmation of the delineation of *Borrelia spielmanii* sp. nov. Int J Syst Evol Microbiol 2006;56:873–881.

9 Hanincová K, Taragelová V, Koci J, Schäfer SM, Hails R, Ullmann AJ, Piesman J, Labuda M, Kurtenbach K: Association of *Borrelia garinii* and *B. valaisiana* with songbirds in Slovakia. Appl Environ Microbiol 2003;69:2825–2830.

10 Hubálek Z, Halouzka J: Prevalence rates of *Borrelia burgdorferi* sensu lato in host-seeking *Ixodes ricinus* ticks in Europe. Parasit Res 1998;84:167–172.

11 Dsouli N, Younsi-Kabachii H, Postic D, Nouira S, Gern L, Bouattour A: Reservoir role of the lizard, *Psammodromus algirus*, in the transmission cycle of *Borrelia burgdorferi* sensu lato (Spirochaetacea) in Tunisia. J Med Entomol 2006;43:737–742.

12 Gern L, Rais O: Efficient transmission of *Borrelia burgdorferi* between cofeeding *Ixodes ricinus* ticks (Acari: Ixodidae). J Med Entomol 1996;33:189–192.

13 Poupon MA, Lommano E, Humair PF, Douet V, Rais O, Schaad M, Jenni L, Gern L: Prevalence of *Borrelia burgdorferi* sensu lato in ticks collected from migratory birds in Switzerland. Appl Environ Microbiol 2006;72:976–979.

14 Richter D, Matuschka FR: Perpetuation of the Lyme disease spirochete *Borrelia lusitaniae* by lizards. Appl Environm Microbiol 2006;72:4627–4632.

15 Amore G, Tomassone L, Grego E, Ragagli C, Bertolotti L, Nebbia P, Rosati S, Mannelli A: *Borrelia lusitaniae* in immature *Ixodes ricinus* (Acari: Ixodidae) feeding on common wall lizards in Tuscany, central Italy. J Med Entomol 2007;44:303–307.
16 Richter D, Schlee DB, Allgöver R, Matuschka FR: Relationships of a novel Lyme disease spirochete, *Borrelia spielmani* sp. nov., with its hosts in central Europe. Appl Environ Microbiol 2004;70:6414–6419.
17 Skuballa J, Oehme R, Hartelt K, Petney T, Bücher T, Kimmig P, Taraschewski H: European hedgehogs as hosts for *Borrelia* spp., Germany. J Emerg Dis 2007;13:952–953.
18 Kurtenbach K, Schäfer SM, de Michelis S, Etti S, Sewell HS: *Borrelia burgdorferi* sensu lato in the vertebrate host; in Gray JS, Kahl O, Lane RS, Stanek G (eds): Lyme Borreliosis: Biology, Epidemiology and Control. Wallingford, CAB International, 2002, pp 117–150.
19 Morán Cadenas F, Rais O, Humair PF, Douet V, Moret J, Gern L: Identification of host bloodmeal source and *Borrelia burgdorferi* sensu lato in field-collected *Ixodes ricinus* ticks in Chaumont (Switzerland). J Med Entomol 2007;44:1109–1117.
20 Pichon B, Egan D, Rogers M, Gray JS: Detection and identification of pathogens and host DNA in unfed host-seeking *Ixodes ricinus* L. (Acari: Ixodidae). J Med Entomol 2003;40:723–731.
21 Humair PF, Douet V, Morán Cadenas F, Schouls L, Van De Pol I, Gern L: Molecular identification of blood meal source in *Ixodes ricinus* ticks using 12S rDNA as a genetic marker. J Med Entomol 2007;44: 869–880.
22 Leuba-Garcia S, Martinez R, Gern L: Expression of outer surface proteins A and C of *Borrelia afzelii* in *Ixodes ricinus* ticks and in the skin of mice. Zentlbl Bakt Hyg 1998;287:475–484.
23 Kahl O, Janetzki-Mittmann C, Gray JS, Jonas R, Stein J, de Boer R: Risk of infection with *Borrelia burgdorferi sensu lato* for a host in relation to the duration of nymphal *Ixodes ricinus* feeding and the method of tick removal. Zentlbl Bakt Hyg 1998;287: 41–52.
24 Crippa M, Rais O, Gern L: Investigations on the mode and dynamics of transmission and infectivity of *Borrelia burgdorferi* sensu stricto and *Borrelia afzelii* in *Ixodes ricinus* ticks. Vector Borne Zoonotic Dis 2002;2:3–9.
25 Fingerle V, Goettner G, Gern L, Wilske B, Schulte-Spechtel U: Complementation of a *Borrelia afzelii* OspC mutant highlights the crucial role of OspC for dissemination of *Borrelia afzelii* in *Ixodes ricinus*. Int J Med Microb 2007;297:97–107.

Lise Gern
Institute of Biology
Emile Argand 11, Case postale 158
CH–2009 Neuchâtel (Switzerland)
Tel. +41 32 718 3000, Fax +41 32 718 3001, E-Mail lise.gern@unine.ch

Lipsker D, Jaulhac B (eds): Lyme Borreliosis.
Curr Probl Dermatol. Basel, Karger, 2009, vol 37, pp 31–50

Epidemiology of Lyme Borreliosis

Zdenek Hubálek
Institute of Vertebrate Biology, Academy of Sciences of the Czech Republic, Brno, Czech Republic

Abstract
Lyme borreliosis (LB) is the most frequent ixodid tick-borne human disease in the world, with an estimated 85,500 patients annually (underlying data presented in this review: Europe 65,500, North America 16,500, Asia 3,500, North Africa 10; approximate figures). This chapter summarizes the up-to-date knowledge about facts and factors important in the epidemiology of LB all over the world. Individual sections briefly describe geographic (latitudinal and altitudinal) distribution and incidence rates of LB in individual countries; seasonal distribution of the disease; effects of patients' age, sex, and profession; comparison of urban versus rural settings; weather-related effects on LB incidence; risk factors for LB acquisition by humans; and risk assessment. This chapter finishes by recommending a more thorough epidemiological surveillance for LB, including morbidity notification in some additional countries where it has not yet been fully implemented.

Introduction

Lyme borreliosis (LB), usually called Lyme disease (LD) in North America, is the most abundant ixodid-borne disease of humans in the world, though it only occurs in the northern hemisphere. It is in fact an old disease that was surprisingly only fully recognized at the end of the 20th century.

Several excellent reviews on LB epidemiology have been published previously [1–7]. The purpose of this review is to summarize the up-to-date knowledge on, and discuss briefly all facts and factors important in, the epidemiology of LB over the world.

Geographic Distribution and Incidence Rate

LB occurs in North America (from the Mexican border in the south to the southern Canadian provinces in the north), the whole of Europe, parts of North Africa (Maghreb), and northern Asia (Russian Siberia and the Far East, Sakhalin, Japan,

China, and Korea). In North America, only a few US states do not report LB or even record it (Alaska, Arizona, Montana, Nebraska, New Mexico, and Wyoming). Occasional reports of the occurrence of LB in the southern hemisphere (Central and South America, sub-Saharan Africa, South Asia, Australia) have never been reliably confirmed. The geographic distribution of LB correlates closely with the range of the principal vector, ticks of the *Ixodes ricinus* complex.

Incidence Rates

Incidence rates of LB in different countries are summarized in table 1. However, LB is not a mandatorily notifiable disease in a number of European and North American countries, e.g. Austria, Sweden, Switzerland (in the last decade), France, Belgium, The Netherlands, Ireland, England and Wales, and Canada. Therefore, the incidence data from these countries presented here are qualified estimates, based on several prospective epidemiological studies, usually limited to certain areas (very often those with a high incidence of LB), and incidence rates of comparable neighboring countries. The mean annual numbers of LB cases, as summarized from notified cases and qualified estimates in countries without an obligatory notification system for LB, are 65,467 in Europe; 3,450 in Asia; 16,340 in North America; and 7 in North Africa (Maghreb); the annual world total is 85,264 LB cases. In a previous review, about 85,000 LB cases were estimated in Europe only, with an additional 15,000–20,000 annual cases in the USA [7]. Our estimates are more conservative.

Many experts admit that there is a significant underreporting of LB, and some of them estimate that the real LB incidence rate may be 2–3 times higher than reported. For instance, Campbell et al. [8] calculated an about 2.8-fold real incidence of LB in Westchester county, N.Y., than that notified by the current passive reporting system. A very similar figure was found in north-central Wisconsin, where only 34% of LB cases were reported to the state, i.e. the real incidence was 2.9-fold higher [9]. Overreporting that follows overdiagnosis can also pose problems under certain circumstances (e.g. state of California in the first years of notification implementation). Nevertheless, the reported figures that are presented here form a relatively good basis for the comparison of LB incidence among countries, especially when the more recent periods (1995–2006) are taken into consideration. If the coefficient of 3 is accepted for underreporting, the mean total annual number of LB cases in the world might be as many as 255,000.

Additional problems in LB notification are caused by different definitions of LB cases, and diagnostic pitfalls with LB. A recent review [10] summarizes well most of the problems associated with the clinical diagnosis of erythema migrans (EM) and with various case definitions of LB in both North America and Europe [11, 12]. Moreover, the method used for the serological diagnosis of LB is not unimportant in that different laboratories use various serological kits and tests, and the proportion of

Table 1. Geographic distribution of mean annual incidence of LB (expressed mean annual LB cases per 100,000 of the population)

Country (region)	Incidence (per 100,000)	Range	Years	Annual cases, n	Remarks	Reference number
Europe				(65,467)		
Albania	n.a.			(5)	no data about LB	
Austria	(130)	(50–350)		(4,500)	not notifiable – a rough estimate	2, 3, 13
Belarus	n.a.			(1,200)	not notifiable	65
Belgium	12.58	8.2–16.3	1999–2006	1,297		Ducoffre, G., pers. commun., 2007
Bulgaria	5.44	1.9–13.0	1993–2005	433		Christova, I., pers. commun., 2007
Croatia	5.91	5.2–7.5	1993–2000	264	compulsory LB reporting started in 1991	40
Czechland	31.73	14.0–61.2	1989–2006	3,263	LB reporting since 1990	108
Denmark	1.68	0.3–2.7	1994–2006	89		109
Estonia	31.01	14.3–43.8	1994–2006	424	notifiable	109 and Vasilenko, V., pers. commun., 2007
Finland	18.46	7.8–23.5	1999–2006	962		109
France	8.2		1999–2000	(4,900)		24
Germany	(25)			(18,000)	not notifiable – except for 6 eastern states	13, 49
Eastern 6 states	26.05	17.8–36.5	2002–2006	4,440	notifiable in: Berlin, Brandenburg, Mecklenburg-Vorpommern, Sachsen, Sachsen-Anhalt, Thüringen	47–49, 111
Great Britain						
England and Wales	0.59	0.3–1.1	1997–2005	311	not notifiable; only 0.2% seroprevalence in farmers	110
Scotland	1.72	1.6–1.9	2002–2005	87	notifiable	111
Greece	n.a.			(10)	very low seroprevalence in Navy recruits (ELISA 3.3%, Western blot 0.3%)	112
Hungary	12.79	12.2–14.3	2001–2005	1,288	reportable	58
Iceland	0.56	0.0–1.1	1999–2003	2	seroprevalence 1–2%; *B. garinii* detected in *I. uriae* in seabird colonies	13, 109
Ireland	0.6		1995	25	no reliable data on incidence; not notifiable disease	13 (estimate of Gray, J.)
Italy	0.02	0.001–0.5	2001–2005	11	notifiable since 1991	111
Latvia	21.64	11.7–30.6	1998–2006	507	notifiable	109
Lithuania	42.93	21.7–106.5	1995–2006	1,502	notifiable	109 (data of Asokliene, L.)
Luxembourg	n.a.			(60)		
Moldova	0.73	0.7–0.8	2003–2005	31		Gheorghitsa, S., thesis, 2006
The Netherlands	2.01	1.4–2.7	2001–2005	327	not notifiable; estimates of EM hospital admissions	113
Norway	4.5	2.6–9.8	1992–2006	199	notifiable from 1989 to 1995	109, 111, 114
Poland	9.29	4.8–17.5	2000–2006	3,549		115

Table 1 (continued)

Country (region)	Incidence (per 100,000)	Range	Years	Annual cases, n	Remarks	Reference number
Portugal	0.48	0.2–0.8	1993–2004	49	serologic data on LB cases	116
	0.04	0.01–0.15	1999–2004	4	notified cases; notifiable since 1999	116
Romania	n.a.			(1,500)	LB occurs; seroprevalence: 4.3% (blood donors), 9.3% (forestry workers)	
Russia (European okrug)	4.6	4.0–5.7	1999–2006	4,789	recorded since 1992	Korenberg, E.I., pers. commun., 2007 (all okrug)
North-west	9.24	5.6–15.8	1999–2006	1,314		
Central	3.39	2.1–4.7	1999–2006	1,263		
Volga	6.8	5.8–8.5	1999–2006	2,192		
Southern	0.09	0.04–0.17	1999–2006	20		
Serbia and Montenegro	2.44	1.4–3.3	1988–1994	239		50
Slovakia	12.12	6.3–18.4	1991–2006	650		51 and Bazovska, S., pers. commun.
Slovenia	136.86	72–206	1991–2005	2,724	reported since 1988	20, 21, 111
Spain	9.8			(26)		7
Sweden		55–110		(8,000)	http://www.socialstyrelsen.se	Bennet, L., pers. commun.
Southern Sweden	69	26–160	1992		24% of the population, and 11% of the area of Sweden	28
Northern Sweden	very low				seroprevalence only 1–2%; infection rate of *I. ricinus* only 0–5%	13
Switzerland	25.09	18.9–32.4	1988–1998	1,743	not reportable in the last 10 years	117
Turkey (European part)	0.01		1990–2002	1	<20 cases 1990–2002	118
Ukraine	n.a.			(2,500)	LB occurs	Korenberg, E.I., pers. commun.
North America				(16,340)		
USA[1]	5.78	3.2–8.4	1991–2005	15,840		22 (including states)
California	0.3	0.2–0.5	1993–2005	102		
Connecticut	72.48	37.7–133.8	1991–2005	2,433		
Delaware	24.4	7.8–76.6	1991–2005	189		
Maryland	11.19	3.7–22.0	1991–2005	586		
Massachusetts	11.98	2.5–36.5	1991–2005	847		
Minnesota	8.81	3.1–20.1	1992–2005	429		
New Hampshire	7.81	1.3–20.5	1991–2005	98		
New Jersey	23.51	9.0–38.6	1991–2005	1,951		
New York (incl. NYC)	24.12	15.5–29.2	1991–2005	4,502		
Pennsylvania	22.99	8.9–46.3	1992–2005	2,782		
Rhode Island	47.49	15.6–79.7	1991–2004	459		
Wisconsin	12.35	7.2–26.3	1991–2005	654		
Canada	low			(500)	not notifiable	Ogden, N., pers. commun.
Ontario	0.25	0.2–0.4	1999–2004	29		Public Health Canada

Table 1 (continued)

Country (region)	Incidence (per 100,000)	Range	Years	Annual cases, n	Remarks	Reference number
Asia				(3,450)		
Russia (Asian part) with the Urals	8.26	7.0–10.7	1999–2006	3,200		Korenberg, E.I., pers. commun., 2007 (including okrug)
The Urals Federal okrug	9.81	7.3–13.9	1999–2006	1,226		
Siberian Federal okrug	8.15	6.1–10.4	1999–2006	1,671		
Far Eastern Federal okrug	4.33	3.1–5.8	1999–2006	303		
Sverdlovsk/ Jekaterinbg.	14.7		1994			13
Novosibirsk area	(10)	9–11.5				119
Tomsk region	28		1993–1994			29, 30
Turkey (Asian part)	very low			<1	*B. burgdorferi* s.l. isolated from ixodid ticks	118
Kyrgyzstan	low			(20)	*B. burgdorferi* s.l. isolated from ixodid ticks	Korenberg, E.I., pers. commun., 1993
Kazakhstan	very low			(10)	LB likely to occur	Korenberg, E.I., pers. commun., 1994
Mongolia	n.a.			(5)	no data about LB	
China	low			(200)	no incidence data available; *B. garinii* and *B. afzelii* isolates from *I. persulcatus* and rodents	120, 121
Taiwan	<0.01			0.1	1 case of LB; also isolations of *B. burgdorferi* s.l. from rodents	122
Korea	very low			(5)	no incidence data available; *B. garinii* and *B. afzelii* isolated from *I. persulcatus* and rodents	120, 121
Japan	<0.01		1987–1994	11	notifiable since 1999: 84 LB cases since 1987 (mainly from Hokkaido and Honshu); many *B. burgdorferi* s.l. isolates have been obtained from patients and ixodid ticks	120
Africa				7		
Morocco	<0.01			<1		124
Algeria	<0.01			<1		125
Tunisia	0.06		1992–1996	5	*B. lusitaniae* often isolated from local *I. ricinus*	126, 127
Madeira Island	<0.01			<1	2 cases in 1999–2004; seroprevalence in inhabitants 8.7%; at least 1.3% of nymphal *I. ricinus* ticks infected with *B. burgdorferi* s.l.	116, 123

Incidence data (cases) in parentheses are qualified estimates, based on restricted prospective studies, extrapolation, incidence data from neighboring countries, and population size. The figures without parentheses show the number of notified cases.
n.a. = No data (not available).
[1] The listed states have the highest LB morbidity, except California.

false-positive or false-negative serum samples might be relatively high in particular circumstances [13, 14]. Probably the best serological assays at present are immunoassays (ELISA) for IgM and IgG antibodies, combined with immunoblotting.

Incidence Trends

In many countries, both in Europe and North America, no marked trends in the incidence rate of LB have been recorded (just irregular fluctuations in the morbidity; for references, see table 1), e.g. in Belgium, Switzerland, Czechland (syn. Czech Republic; fig. 1), Slovakia, Hungary, Latvia, Estonia, Lithuania, Croatia, European and Asian Russia, and the US states of Connecticut, Rhode Island and New York, whereas other countries have reported a growing incidence of this disease in the last decade, e.g. The Netherlands, Germany (eastern states), Norway, Finland, Denmark, England, Wales, Poland and Bulgaria, and the US states of Pennsylvania, Wisconsin, Minnesota and Delaware. However, some of these 'increasing' trends might be biased and caused, in fact, by an improved notification system, greater awareness/vigilance, and better diagnostics for LB over the last years in particular countries. For instance, it is of interest that in most US states where LB is followed with great care for years (e.g. New England), no significantly increasing trends of LB incidence have been recorded in the last decade.

LB reveals a distinctly focal pattern of distribution, even within small countries and regions, that is determined by the heterogeneous spatial distribution of vector ticks [15, 16]. The amount and composition of forest habitats (woodland) play a great role, of course. Within the whole geographic range of LB, there are some hyperendemic high-risk areas ('hot spots'), with annual incidences of >100 LB cases per 100,000 of the population. Such districts have been reported in southern Sweden, e.g. Blekinge County on the coastline along the Baltic Sea (mean incidence rate of 465 per 100,000 between 1997 and 2003, and a maximum of 664 in 2000 [17]), the Estonian-owned island Saaremaa [385/100,000; Kutsar, K., pers. commun.], the Åland islands of Finland (approx. 200/100,000 [18]), several Brandenburg counties in Germany (Brieskow-Finkenheerd and Scharmützelsee, with 311 and 298 cases per 100,000, respectively, in 2003 [19]), the whole of Slovenia (>200 per 100,000 in some parts of the country [20, 21]), certain parts of Austria, Connecticut (Old Lyme: up to 1,000 per 100,000), and Massachusetts (Nantucket County, with a morbidity rate between 449 and 1,247 per 100,000 from 1992 to 1999 [22]).

Influence of Latitude

LB occurs between approximately 35 and 60°N in Europe, and between 30 and 55°N in North America. In countries at the southern limits of the LB range, its incidence decreases rapidly along the north-to-south gradient. For instance in Italy, LB is quite

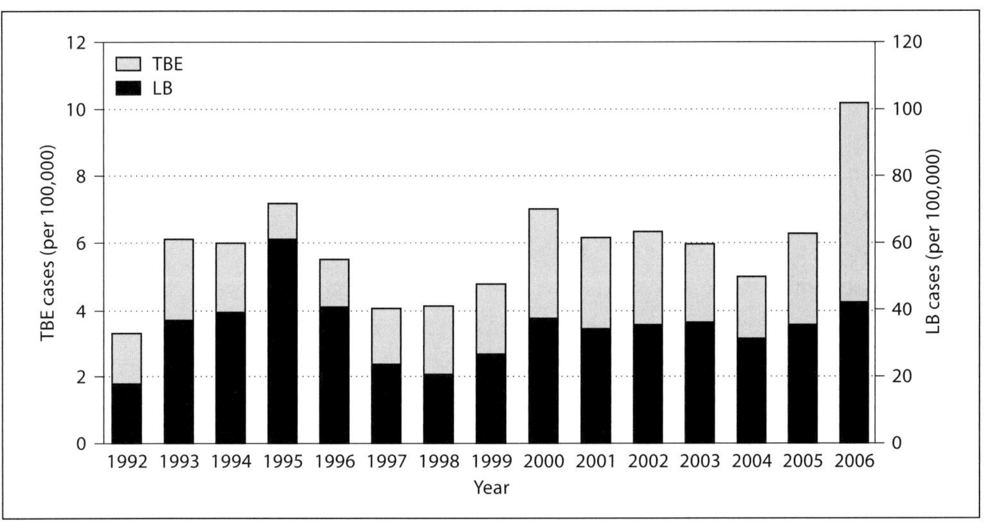

Fig. 1. Incidence rates of LB and tick-borne encephalitis (TBE; transmitted by the same vector species) in Czechland, 1992–2006 [108]. Pearson correlation between the incidence rates is highly significant: $r = 0.718$ ($p < 0.01$).

frequent in northern Italy, whereas it is much less common in central and southern Italy [23]. The situation is similar in France [24], Spain [25], the Balkans (including Bulgaria) [26, 27], and the southern states of the USA [22]. Conversely, at the northern limits of its occurrence, the LB incidence decreases sharply with increasing latitude, i.e. along the south-to-north gradient, e.g. in Scandinavia and European Russia [7, 13, 17, 28–30] or North America [12, 31]. This pattern closely reflects the distribution of ixodid vectors of LB, which is determined by types of climate (mainly temperature and humidity) permissive for the *I. ricinus* tick.

Influence of Altitude

A very low incidence of LB was observed at elevations >1,000 m above sea level (a.s.l.) in Austria [32], although *I. ricinus* ticks infected with borreliae were recently detected in Austrian mountains at 1,350 m a.s.l. [33]. In Czechland, *I. ricinus* has started to occur at higher altitudes, up to 1,100 m a.s.l., compared to elevations of up to only approx. 800 m a.s.l. two decades ago [34, 35]. It has nevertheless been demonstrated that the prevalence rate of *Borrelia burgdorferi* s.l. in *I. ricinus* decreases with altitude, as shown for example in Switzerland along an altitudinal gradient of 750–1,020 m a.s.l. [36]. Already, Aeschlimann et al. [37] have reported individual ticks infected with borreliae in Switzerland found at 1,250 m a.s.l. (Kiental), and their infection rate decreased with the elevation.

Seasonal Distribution of LB

The annual distribution pattern of LB is strongly affected by the seasonal pattern of host-seeking (questing) tick activity, lagged by the incubation period of LB which is usually 1–4 weeks (but up to 2 months in a few cases; median is about 7–12 days) for EM, 3–9 weeks (median 4–6) for early neuroborreliosis, 1.5–8 months (median 2) for arthritis, 6–12 months for late neuroborreliosis, and several to many years for acrodermatitis chronica atrophicans (ACA) [13, 21, 24, 38, 39]. Therefore, LB as a disease in all its forms occurs in all months of the year, although its incidence is (very) low in late autumn, winter, and early spring – usually only chronic manifestations of LB (arthritis, late neuroborreliosis, ACA) are reported in those periods. The peak of annual LB incidence, the curve of which is usually unimodal, occurs from June to July in Austria [32], Belgium [Ducoffre, G., pers. commun.], Bulgaria [27], Croatia [40], Czechland [41, 42], France [43, 44], Germany [38, 45–49], Russia [39], Serbia [50], Slovakia [51], Slovenia [21], southeastern Sweden [17], and the USA [5, 15, 22], indicating that most infections are acquired during late May to late June. In northern countries (Estonia, Sweden), the peak of LB incidence could include August [Kutsar, K., pers. commun; 28], while in Alsace (France), May was reported as the peak [52]. In southern Europe, sometimes a smaller secondary peak in the annual incidence rate of LB occurs in autumn (October to November), when the local weather is warm and permissive for tick and human outdoor activity, e.g. in Slovenia [21].

In most countries, the timing of LB differs according to clinical manifestation. For instance in Austria, the peak occurrence of EM is in July, whereas the peak for neuroborreliosis is in August and September [53]. Similarly, in southern Sweden, most of the EM forms started in August, while the other clinical manifestations of LB peaked in September [28]. This is caused by the different incubation periods for particular clinical forms.

An additional factor affecting the seasonality of LB is human behavior and outdoor activity, i.e. the coincidence of maximum vector tick activity with summer-related leisure behavior of people [49]. For instance, vacation times overlapping with enhanced exposure to vector ticks during hiking and berry/mushroom picking in forests are usually June, July, and August in Europe [1].

Patient Characteristics

Lyme borreliosis could affect persons of all age categories, but the age distribution of the disease is usually bimodal in most countries, with the first (lower) maximum occurring in children 5–9 (14) years old, and the second (higher) maximum in adults aged (45) 50–64 (69) years. A marked depression in LB morbidity appears among young people between (15) 20 and 24 years of age. Such a pattern has been reported in Belgium [Ducoffre, G., pers. commun.], Bulgaria [54], Croatia [40], Czechland [41, 42,

55], England and Wales [56], Germany [38, 45–49], Hungary [57, 58], Serbia [50], Slovakia [51], Slovenia [21], southeastern Sweden [17, 59], and the USA [5, 15, 22]. Interestingly, a serological survey in Sweden also showed the bimodal pattern according to the age groups: the antibodies against *B. burgdorferi* s.l. were most prevalent in children and young persons below 20 years of age and in persons older than 50 years, while they were much less frequent in persons aged 21–50 years, with an absolute minimum at the 21- to 30-year-old group [60]. Explanation of the striking differences between age groups could be related to the different outdoor activity and leisure-time behavior patterns among these population strata [49]. However, some of these figures might be biased in that most of them are not recalculated as specific incidence rates, i.e. cases per number of inhabitants of a particular age category in the corresponding area.

Lymphocytoma manifestation occurs much more often or almost exclusively in children under 16 years, whereas ACA is predominant in elderly persons [2, 11, 28, 38, 45, 57]. Also, neuroborreliosis and arthritis cases can be more frequent in children than in adults [45]. Berglund et al. [28] reported the neuroborreliosis form of LB in 28% of children, but only 14% of adult patients in southern Sweden.

Bites of vector ticks vary in their localization on the human body between age groups: in children they predominate on ears, head, and neck region (49% of bites vs. 2% in adults in Sweden, 23 vs. 1% in adults in Germany, 23 vs. 2% in adults in Bulgaria), while in adults the predilection sites for ticks are the lower limbs: 62, 60, and 63.5% of bites in Sweden, Germany, and Bulgaria, respectively [28, 45, 54].

Sex

Results of gender-related analyses differ among countries. In the USA, males (51.9%) slightly outnumbered females in 1992–1998, especially among children and adolescents aged 5–19 years, but also in the category of adults aged ≥60 years [5, 15]. On the other hand, a slight female preponderance (usual range of 54–60% females among recorded LB patients) is reported in most European countries, e.g. Austria [53], Czechland [41, 61], Germany [45, 49], Slovakia [51], Slovenia [21], and Switzerland [37]. In southeastern Sweden, among 3,443 EM cases reported in 1997–2003, 54.5% were females, and the predominance of females was especially marked in the age group 50–74 years (60.1%) [59]. In Italy, females are infected more often than males [23], while only 49.9% of the 1,175 LB patients in Hungary were female [57]. However, some of these figures might be biased in that most of them are not recalculated as specific incidence rates, i.e. per number of inhabitants of particular gender category in the corresponding area.

Females are affected more often than males by ACA, the late chronic cutaneous manifestation of LB [2, 37, 38]. Reinfection with borreliae was reported 6 times more frequently for females than for males in southern Sweden, and nearly all reinfected women were older than 40 years and postmenopausal. Interestingly, Swedish females also attract more tick bites than males, though they spend approximately 30% less time outdoors than men [59].

Bites of vector ticks vary in their localization on the human body between gender: the predilection sites for ticks are the lower limbs and breast region in females, and the lower limbs and genital region in males [28].

Occupation

Examples of population groups at risk are forestry workers, military field personnel, farmers, deer handlers, gamekeepers, hunters, rangers, and outdoor workers in general. For instance, LB seropositivity is high among forestry workers in most countries tested: France 22% (while only 4% in normal population [62]), Austria 14–18% [2], Bulgaria 18% [26] and Italy up to 27% [23]. Farmers also often have a higher seropositivity rate, e.g. 15% in Bulgaria [26].

However, in most European countries, occupational exposure generally constitutes only 2% of LB cases [63]; it is typically a recreation time disease, contracted during holidays and leisure time exposure [24, 58, 63], including sport in forested areas. In Switzerland, 8.1% of 558 orienteers seroconverted over 1 season, but only 0.8% of them revealed clinical symptoms of LB – the ratio of apparent to inapparent infection was therefore 1:9 [64].

Urban versus Rural Inhabitants

There is a low or no significant difference in LB incidence rates between urban and rural populations [24], or the LB incidence among urban inhabitants is even higher, e.g. in Finland where the mean morbidity (per 100,000 population) is 13 in Helsinki but only 6.6 in rural areas [18], or in Russia where 84% of LB cases are among urban residents [30, 65], and Bulgaria [54]. In addition, infected ticks also occur in urban parks [66].

Weather-Related Effects on LB Incidence

In southeast Sweden and Scotland, LB incidence increased following mild winters (i.e. number of days in preceding winter with mean temperature >0°C) and during warm humid summers (i.e. the mean monthly summer temperatures combined with the number of summer days with relative air humidity >86%), but higher mean monthly precipitation (excess summer rainfall) had a depressing effect on LB morbidity [17, 67]. The authors have concluded that the main mechanism of these weather factors is either increasing/decreasing precipitation, which also has an impact upon human outdoor activity (and subsequently the rate of human exposure to ticks) that is the leading cause of LB morbidity. However, the tick activity should also be taken into consideration. In 7 northeastern US states, the June moisture index (Palmer Hydrological Drought Index) 2 years previously correlated well with the current LB incidence, most probably by enhancing the nymphal *I. scapularis* survival during the more humid conditions; further, a warmer winter, lagged 1.5 years, increased LB incidence, probably due to the higher survival and activity of the white-footed mouse, the principal local vertebrate amplifying host of borreliae [68]. Precipitation during May and June, not temperature, stimulated LB incidence in the northeastern USA in the period 1992–2002 [69]. Ashley and Meentemeyer [70] found that LB incidence is affected by meteorological variables prevalent during April to June, and more by moisture (total soil moisture surplus, total precipitation) than by mean air temperature, which could be used for LB risk assessment. In general, summer temperature and rainfall affect tick populations [71]. The effects of weather (and climate) on vector ticks are quite complicated and simple solutions of the interrelationships are usually not the best ones.

Risk Factors for LB Acquisition by Humans and Risk Assessment

LB risk is clearly a product of 2 principal factors: the abundance (density) of infectious vector ticks and the intensity of human exposure to the vector (degree of human-tick contact).

Vector Tick Stage

The only competent vectors of pathogenic borreliae to humans are ticks of the *I. ricinus* complex: *I. ricinus, I. persulcatus, I. scapularis,* and *I. pacificus.* Most of the LB patients are infected by nymphal rather than female *Ixodes* ticks, both in North America and Europe [1, 63, 72–78]. Nymphs are more numerous in the field and, because of their smaller size, more difficult to be detected (at that moment and later) on the human body than adult female ticks. In Connecticut 1989–1996, Westchester county (New York state) 1991–1996 and South Moravia (Czechland) 1991–2001, 3 independent teams found that the local annual incidence of human LB correlated significantly (R^2 = 58–69%) with the abundance of nymphal, but not female, vector ticks [74, 75, 79].

Transmission Risk

The risk of developing LB symptoms after a vector tick bite is estimated to be 2–4% [63], or sometimes even ≤1% in Europe [4]. However, in a LB-endemic area of Poland,

4.7% of 426 forestry workers bitten by a tick contracted clinical disease [80], and similarly in Russia, LB transmission was reported in 4–5% persons with attached ticks [30]. Nahimana et al. [78] followed 376 persons after a tick bite in Switzerland: EM developed in 2.1% of the probands. In Germany, 2.6% of 730 persons with tick bites developed LB [81]. In Sweden, 4.6% of persons with attached ticks seroconverted, but not all of them revealed clinical symptoms of LB [82]. A seroconversion without LB symptoms is quite common in Europe and results in a high seropositivity rate in the European population [78]. In New England, the risk of LB after tick bites has been reported to be 1.2% [83], 3.7% [84], and 3.2% [85].

Duration of Tick Attachment (Transmission Timing)

There is a difference between North America and Europe in the duration of tick attachment required for transmission of borreliae into the human host. The US (Centers for Disease Control and Prevention) paradigm is that borreliae are only present in the midgut of infected unfed (host-seeking) ticks, and during the blood feeding on a host they migrate through the tick's hemocele to salivary glands after 24–48 h, and only then can the tick infect the host with saliva. In accordance with that, most North American epidemiological studies state that transmission of borreliae to humans can occur only 48 h after attachment [86]. This is obviously not correct for Europe, where significant transmission of borreliae to the human host may occur within the first 24 h of attachment [63]. For instance, G. Stanek [pers. commun.] observed several LB patients in Vienna who contracted LB following a tick attachment of no longer than 8 h.

Importantly, generalized infection with borreliae (including the salivary glands) has repeatedly been observed in some host-seeking unfed *I. ricinus* ticks, e.g. in Switzerland [87–89]. These cases of systemic infection are probably most common with the ticks containing large numbers of borreliae in their midguts – in some individual ticks thousands of borreliae have been observed. The proportion of unfed ticks with >100 borreliae were found to be 5.0% in 2,380 female and 1.7% in 3,546 nymphal *I. ricinus* examined in Czechland [90]; it is noteworthy that the prevalence rate of the *B. burgdorferi* s.l. highly loaded nymphs (and females) closely matches the proportion of tick bites giving rise to LB in humans (1–5%, see 'Transmission Risk'). Ticks with such a high spirochetal load can transfer them to the host much faster than ticks with a low burden of borreliae [90, 91]. This difference between the American and European experiences could probably be explained by the quicker transmission rate of *B. afzelii* and/or *B. garinii* than that of *B. burgdorferi* s.s. [92]. Kahl et al. [93] found that half of experimental Mongolian gerbils *(Meriones unguiculatus)* were already infected by spirochete-carrying *I. ricinus* nymphs 17 h after attachment.

Piesman et al. [72] proposed as a standard risk measure the number of infected ticks per unit sampling effort (area, time). Ginsberg [94] formulated a simple transmission risk index, the number of tick bites per person. Hubálek et al. [95] quantified the LB risk exposure as the mean time necessary to encounter the first (heavily) infected tick, measured by flagging. For risk assessment, Nicholson and Mather [31] suggested using the abundance of nymphal ticks and prevalence of borrelial infection in ticks, and combine these with geographic information system analysis. An ecological risk index [96] has been proposed to identify risk areas for LB transmission; it is composed of 5 components: habitat suitability, habitat amount, habitat accessibility, tick abundance, and the tick infection rate (all classified on a scale of 1–5). However, this is not a very useful predictor of LB incidence without taking into account the data on human behavior [97].

Risk ecosystems and habitats are deciduous or mixed forest ecosystems or woodlands matching the distribution of the principal vector (ticks of the *I. ricinus* complex), along with city parks and urban gardens [45–48, 66], especially gardens within 200 m of forests [98]. In the Würzburg region in Germany, many cases of LB were reported in the northwestern wooded area, but few cases in the southern, predominantly agricultural area [45]. Similarly in Brandenburg State, Germany, the majority of LB cases were acquired in localities close to humid forests, while very low morbidity has been reported in areas with extended agroecosystems [48]. Brandenburg, steadily reporting about half of all LB cases from 6 eastern German states, is very rich in forests and water habitats compared to the 5 other states [48].

There is a higher risk of contracting LB in the ecotones between forests and fields/meadows, although higher densities of infected vector ticks are within forests; this is an effect of frequent human presence along the edges of these habitats [99]. Also, forest fragmentation in suburban areas (Connecticut, USA) theoretically poses a greater risk (higher entomological risk) due to an enhanced proportion of ecotones [100, 101]. However, in 1 study, the LB incidence was surprisingly lower in fragmented habitats, and human behavior played a more significant role in the LB risk [102]. Prusinski et al. [103] studied the effect of forest habitat structure on LB risk, and found that understory vegetation structure and coverage dictates vector density. On the other hand, Nicholson and Mather [31] did not find plant communities as predictive in LB risk assessment in a geographic information system-based analysis.

Ecological risk factors involve a number of variables. For instance, reforestation usually causes an increased population not only of forest rodents, but also of deer, the principal host of adult vector ticks. Growing deer populations (principal hosts of adult vector ticks in woodland, but not competent hosts for borreliae) increase LB morbidity [104]. In central Bohemia, Zeman and Januška [105] found that LB risk correlated with overall population density of game (red deer, roe deer, mouflon, wild boar) regardless of mouse abundance. Nevertheless, in general, increased populations of competent hosts (forest rodents) usually stimulate the LB incidence. Increased acorn production favors populations of forest rodents and deer, and results in an increase in vector ticks [106].

Age and Sex

As shown previously, children and elderly people are at higher risk than middle-aged persons. Bennet et al. [59] found that in southeast Sweden women ≥40 years old had a 48% higher risk of attracting tick bites than men of this age group, a 42% higher risk than women younger than 40 years, and a 96% higher risk than men younger than 40 years.

Occupation

Outdoor employment and work (forestry workers, military personnel in the field, farmers, gardeners, gamekeepers, hunters, rangers) are at risk.

Permanent residence in endemic areas with a high density of infectious ticks (e.g. forested suburban localities in the US states of Connecticut, New Jersey, and New York) is a serious risk factor for LB.

Risk Behavior

All activities that increase human contact with ticks present risks, especially: recreational (leisure time) activities in forested areas, such as camping (including children's holiday camps), picnicking, walking and hiking, sitting on logs or on leaves, jogging, orienteering, and berry/mushroom picking [107]; seasonal or occasional living by urban residents in country cottages ('dachas') in endemic areas with a high density of infectious ticks [26]; mowing and clearing of brush around the home in forested areas and gardening, especially when the garden is within 200 m from a forest [98], even in urban gardens [16, 45]. In Scotland, the 2001 foot-and-mouth disease outbreak led to countryside access restrictions, decreasing the visitor numbers during summer months, which resulted in reductions in tick exposure and LB incidence [67]. Ownership of pet dogs and cats could also present a relative risk in cases where the pets are frequently parasitized by ticks and the owner removes the ticks [98].

Epidemiological Surveillance

Epidemiological surveillance for LB is a paramount task for Europe, and this effort should be coordinated by the European Centre for Disease Prevention and Control, based in Sweden. It should include such things as improved awareness and recognition of the disease at national and continental levels, but first of all mandatory reporting of LB in all European countries where the disease occurs (and it occurs virtually in all of them). Under certain circumstances, serosurveys among people, domestic animals (dogs), and wild vertebrates might also bring useful results. Better surveillance systems for LB should also be installed in some Asian, North African (Maghreb) and North American (Canada) countries.

Acknowledgments

I am very much obliged to a number of experts who supplied the LB incidence data for particular countries, or significantly assisted in obtaining these data (listed alphabetically): Loreta Asokliene (Centre for Communicable Diseases Prevention and Control, Lithuania); Sylvia Bazovská (Komenský University, Faculty of Medicine, Department of Epidemiology, Slovakia); Louise Bennet (University Hospital of Malmö, Sweden); Iva Christova (National Centre of Infectious and Parasitic Diseases, National Reference Laboratory for LB and Leptospirosis, Sofia, Bulgaria); Geneviève Ducoffre (National Institute of Public Health, LB Reference Laboratory, Belgium); Lise Gern (University of Neuchâtel, Switzerland); Johan Giesecke (ECDC Stockholm, Sweden); Jeremy Gray (School of Biology and Environmental Science, University College, Dublin, Ireland); Agnetha Hofhuis (RIVM – Epidemiology and Surveillance, Bilthoven, The Netherlands); Eduard I. Korenberg (Gamaleya Institute of Epidemiology and Microbiology, LB Reference Laboratory, Moscow, Russia); Andras Lakos (Centre for Tick-Borne Diseases, Budapest, Hungary); Laurent Letrilliart (University of Lyon, Department of General Practice, France); Catherine Linard (University of Louvaine, Belgium); Elisabet Lindgren (CTM, Stockholm University, Sweden); Nicholas Ogden (University of Montreal, Canada); Agostino Pugliese (University of Torino, Italy); and Veera Vasilenko (National Institute of Health Development, Tallinn, Estonia).

This review was partially funded by the EU grant GOCE-2003-010284 EDEN; it is catalogued by the EDEN Steering Committee as EDEN0063 (http://www.eden-fp6project.net). The contents of this publication are the responsibility of the author and do not necessarily reflect the views of the European Commission.

References

1 Jaenson TGT: The epidemiology of Lyme borreliosis. Parasitol Today 1991;7:39–45.
2 Stanek G, Satz N, Strle F, Wilske B: Epidemiology of Lyme borreliosis; in Weber K, Burgdorfer W (eds): Aspects of Lyme Borreliosis. Berlin, Springer, 1993, pp 358–370.
3 O'Connell S, Granström M, Gray JS, Stanek G: Epidemiology of European Lyme borreliosis. Zentralbl Bakteriol 1998;287:229–240.
4 Gern L, Falco RC: Lyme disease. Rev Sci Tech 2000; 19:121–135.
5 Dennis DT, Hayes EB: Epidemiology of Lyme disease; in Gray J, Kahl O, Lane RS, Stanek G (eds): Lyme Borreliosis: Biology, Epidemiology and Control. Wallingford, CABI, 2002, pp 251–280.
6 Piesman J, Gern L: Lyme borreliosis in Europe and North America. Parasitology 2004;129(suppl):191–220.
7 Lindgren E, Jaenson TGT: Lyme borreliosis in Europe: influences of climate and climate change, epidemiology and adaptation measures; in Menne B, Ebi KL (eds): Climate Change and Adaptation Strategies for Human Health. Darmstadt, Steinkopff, 2006, pp 157–188.

8 Campbell GL, Fritz CL, Fish D, Nowakowski J, Nadelman RB, Wormser GP: Estimation of the incidence of Lyme disease. Am J Epidemiol 1998;148: 1018–1026.

9 Naleway AL, Belongia EA, Kazmierczak JJ, Greenlee RT, Davis JP: Lyme disease incidence in Wisconsin: a comparison of state-reported rates and rates from a population-based cohort. Am J Epidemiol 2002;155:1120–1127.

10 Tibbles CD, Edlow JA: Does this patient have erythema migrans? JAMA 2007;297:2617–2627.

11 Stanek G, O'Connell S, Cimmino M, Aberer E, Kristoferitsch W, Granström M, Guy E, Gray J: European Union Concerted Action on Risk Assessment in Lyme borreliosis: clinical case definitions for Lyme borreliosis. Wien Klin Wochenschr 1996; 108:741–747.

12 Centers for Disease Control and Prevention: Case definitions for infectious conditions under public health surveillance. MMWR Recomm Rep 1997;46: 1–55.

13 World Health Organization: Report of WHO workshop on Lyme borreliosis diagnosis and surveillance (who/cds/vph/95141-1). Warsaw, 20–22 June 1995, pp 1–220.

14 Hunfeld KP, Stanek G, Straube E, Hagedorn HJ, Schörner C, Mühlschlegel F, Brade V: Quality of Lyme disease serology. Wien Klin Wochenschr 2002;114:591–600.

15 Orloski KA, Hayes EB, Campbell GL, Dennis DT: Surveillance for Lyme disease – United States, 1992–1998. MMWR CDC Surveill Summ 2000; 49:1–11.

16 Robert Koch-Institut: Risikofaktoren für Lyme-Borreliose: Ergebnisse einer Studie in einem Brandenburger Landkreis. Epidemiol Bull 2001;21:147–149.

17 Bennet L, Halling A, Berglund J: Increased incidence of Lyme borreliosis in southern Sweden following mild winters and during warm, humid summers. Eur J Clin Microbiol Infect Dis 2006;25: 426–432.

18 Junttila J, Peltomaa M, Soini H, Marjamäki M, Viljanen MK: Prevalence of *Borrelia burgdorferi* in *Ixodes ricinus* ticks in urban recreational areas of Helsinki. J Clin Microbiol 1999;37:1361–1365.

19 Robert Koch-Institut: Zur Lyme-Borreliose im Land Brandenburg. Epidemiol Bull 2005;20:173–178.

20 Strle F: Lyme borreliosis in Slovenia. Zentralbl Bakteriol 1999;289:643–652.

21 Strle F, Videčnik J, Zorman P, Cimperman J, Lotrič-Furlan S, Maraspin V: Clinical and epidemiological findings for patients with erythema migrans – comparison of cohorts from the years 1993 and 2000. Wien Klin Wochenschr 2002;31:493–497.

22 Centers for Disease Control and Prevention: Reports with statistics on Lyme disease cases. Morb Mort Week Rep, continuously up to August 2007.

23 Ciceroni L, Ciarrocchi S: Lyme disease in Italy, 1983–1996. New Microbiol 1998;21:407–418.

24 Letrilliart L, Ragon B, Hanslik T, Flahault A: Lyme disease in France: a primary care-based study. Epidemiol Infect 2005;133:935–942.

25 Estrada-Peña A, Oteo JA, Estrada-Peña R, Gortázar C, Osácar JJ, Moreno JA, Castellá J: *Borrelia burgdorferi* sensu lato in ticks (Acari: Ixodidae) from two different foci in Spain. Exp Appl Acarol 1995; 19:173–180.

26 Angelov L, Aeschlimann A, Korenberg E, Gern L, Shchereva C, Marinova R, Kalinin M: Data on the epidemiology of Lyme disease in Bulgaria (in Russian). Med Parazitol Parazit Bol 1990;4:13–14.

27 Angelov L, Arnaudov D, Rakadjieva T, Lipchev G, Kostova E: Lyme borreliosis in Bulgaria. Report WHO Workshop Lyme Borreliosis Diagn Surveill, Warsaw, 20–22 June 1995, pp 41–52.

28 Berglund J, Eitrem R, Ornstein K, Lindberg A, Ringner A, Elmrud H, Carlsson M, Runehagen A, Svanborg C, Norrby R: An epidemiological study of Lyme disease in southern Sweden. N Engl J Med 1995;333:1319–1324.

29 Korenberg EI: Ixodid tick-borne borrelioses (ITBBs), infections of the Lyme borreliosis group, in Russia. Report WHO Workshop Lyme Borreliosis Diagn Surveill, Warsaw, 20–22 June 1995, pp 128–136.

30 Korenberg EI: Infections of the Lyme borreliosis group – ixodid tick-borne borrelioses in Russia (in Russian). Med Parazitol Parazit Bolez 1996;3:14–18.

31 Nicholson MC, Mather TN: Methods for evaluating Lyme disease risk using geographic information systems and geospatial analysis. J Med Entomol 1996;33:711–720.

32 Stanek G, Flamm H, Groh V, Hirschl A, Kristoferitsch W, Neumann R, Schmutzhard E, Wewalka G: Epidemiology of *Borrelia* infections in Austria. Zentralbl Bakteriol Mikrobiol Hyg [A] 1986;263: 442–449.

33 Stünzner D, Hubálek Z, Halouzka J, Wendelin I, Sixl W, Marth E: Prevalence of *Borrelia burgdorferi* sensu lato in the tick *Ixodes ricinus* in the Styrian mountains of Austria. Wien Klin Wochenschr 2006;118:682–685.

34 Daniel M, Danielová V, Kříž B, Jirsa A, Nožička J: Shift of the tick *Ixodes ricinus* and tick-borne encephalitis to higher altitudes in Central Europe. Eur J Clin Microbiol Infect Dis 2003;22:327–328.

35 Zeman P, Beneš Č: A tick-borne encephalitis ceiling in Central Europe has moved upwards during the last 30 years: possible impact of global warming? Int J Med Microbiol 2004;293(suppl 37):48–54.

36 Burri C, Cadenas FM, Douet V, Moret J, Gern L: *Ixodes ricinus* density and infection prevalence of *Borrelia burgdorferi* sensu lato along a north-facing altitudinal gradient in the Rhône Valley (Switzerland). Vector Borne Zoon Dis 2007;7:50–58.

37 Aeschlimann A, Chamot E, Gigon F, Jeanneret JP, Kesseler D, Walther C: *Borrelia burgdorferi* in Switzerland. Zentralbl Bakteriol Mikrobiol Hyg [A] 1986;263:450–458.

38 Wilske B, Steinhuber R, Bergmeister H, Fingerle V, Schierz G, Preac-Mursic V, Vanek E, Lorbeer B: Lyme borreliosis in South Germany. Epidemiologic data on the incidence of cases and on the epidemiology of ticks (Ixodes ricinus) carrying *Borrelia burgdorferi* (in German). Dtsch Med Wochenschr 1987; 112:1730–1736.

39 Korenberg EI, Kuznetsova RI, Kovalevskij JV, Vasilenko ZE, Mebel BD: Basic epidemiological patterns of Lyme borreliosis in the north-west of the USSR (in Russian). Med Parazitol Parazit Bolez 1991;3:14–17.

40 Borčić B, Kaić B, Kralj V: Some epidemiological data on TBE and Lyme borreliosis in Croatia. Zentralbl Bakteriol 1999;289:540–547.

41 Janovská D, Hálková B, Ranná M: Surveillance of Lyme borreliosis in the Czech Republic. Abstracts 3rd Czech Days on Lyme Borreliosis, Prague, 27–29 Aug 1997.

42 Kříž B, Beneš Č: Lyme Borreliosis (in Czech). Prague, National Institute of Public Health, 2007. http://www.szu.cz/cem.

43 Dournon E, Villeminot S, Hubert B: Le maladie de Lyme en France: enquête réalisée auprès d'un réseau sentinelle de médecins généralistes. Bull Épidém Hebd 1989;45:185–186.

44 Degeilh B, Pichot J, Gilot B, Allen S, Doche B, Guiguen C: Dynamique annuelle des cas de primoinfestation humaine de borreliose de Lyme (erythème chronique migrant) en France et phenologie des populations de tiques vectrices (*Ixodes ricinus* Linné, 1758): essai de correlation. Acarologia 1996;37:7–17.

45 Huppertz HI, Böhme M, Standaert SM, Karch H, Plotkin SA: Incidence of Lyme borreliosis in the Würzburg region of Germany. Eur J Clin Microbiol Infect Dis 1999;18:697–703.

46 Robert Koch-Institut: Zur Lyme-Borreliose in ausgewählten Bundesländern. Epidemiol Bull 2000;50: 395–398.

47 Robert Koch-Institut: Erkrankungen an Lyme-Borreliose in den sechs östlichen Bundesländern in den Jahren 2002 und 2003. Epidemiol Bull 2004;28: 219–222.

48 Robert Koch-Institut: Neuerkrankungen an Lyme-Borreliose im Jahr 2004. Epidemiol Bull 2005;32: 285–288.

49 Mehnert WH, Krause G: Surveillance of Lyme borreliosis in Germany, 2002 and 2003. Euro Surveill 2005;10:83–85. http://www.eurosurveillance.org/ViewArticle.aspx?ArticleId=531.

50 Dmitrovic R: Lyme borreliosis in Yugoslavia 1987–1994. Report WHO Workshop Lyme Borreliosis Diagn Surveill, Warsaw, 20–22 June 1995, pp 182–191.

51 Bazovska S, Machacova E, Spalekova M, Kontrosova S: Reported incidence of Lyme disease in Slovakia and antibodies to *B. burgdorferi* antigens detected in healthy population. Bratisl Lek Listy 2005; 106:270–273.

52 Schmitt M, Encrenaz N, Chubilleau C, Verrier A: Données épidémiologiques sur la maladie de Lyme en Alsace, Limousin et Rhône-Alpes. Bull Épidém Hebd 2006;27–28:202–203.

53 Stanek G, Kristoferitsch W, Hirschl A, Wewalka G: *Borrelia*-Infektionen in Österreich 1984. Mitt Österr Ges Tropenmed Parasitol 1985;7:55–62.

54 Christova I, Komitova R: Clinical and epidemiological features of Lyme borreliosis in Bulgaria. Wien Klin Wochenschr 2004;116:42–46.

55 Hulínská D, Janovská D, Bašta J: Lyme borreliosis – epidemiological survey in the Czech Republic in 1994. Report WHO Workshop Lyme Borreliosis Diagn Surveill, Warsaw, 20–22 June 1995, pp 53–75.

56 Smith R, O'Connell S, Palmer S: Lyme disease surveillance in England and Wales, 1986–1998. Emerg Infect Dis 2000;6:404–407.

57 Lakos A: Lyme borreliosis in Hungary. Report WHO Workshop Lyme Borreliosis Diagn Surveill. Warsaw, 20–22 June 1995, pp 84–102.

58 Epinfo (Epidemiológiai Információs Hetilap): Magyarország 2005. Évi Járványügyi Helyzete 2007;14:46.

59 Bennet L, Sternberg L, Berglund J: Effect of gender on clinical and epidemiologic features of Lyme borreliosis. Vector Borne Zoon Dis 2007;7:34–41.

60 Gustafson R, Svennungson B, Gardulf A, Stiernstedt G, Forsgren M: Prevalence of tick-borne encephalitis and Lyme borreliosis in a defined Swedish population. Scand J Infect Dis 1990;22: 297–306.

61 Pazdiora P, Benešová J, Böhm K, Brejcha O, Kubátová A, Machovská E, Mareš J, Morávková I, Spáčilová M, Turková D, Vodrážková Z: Incidence of Lyme borreliosis in the West Bohemian Region, 1988–1992 (in Czech). Epidemiol Mikrobiol Immunol 1994;43:71–74.

62 Doby JM, Couatarmanac'h A, Fages J, Chevrier S: Les spirochétoses à tiques chez les professionnels de la forêt. Arch Mal Profess 1989;50:751–757.

63 Gray J: Risk assessment in Lyme borreliosis. Wien Klin Wochenschr 1999;111:990–993.

64 Fahrer H, van der Linden SM, Sauvain MJ, Gern L, Zhioua E, Aeschlimann A: The prevalence and incidence of clinical and asymptomatic Lyme borreliosis in a population at risk. J Infect Dis 1991;163: 305–310.

65 Korenberg EI: Comparative ecology and epidemiology of Lyme disease and tick-borne encephalitis in the former Soviet Union. Parasitol Today 1994; 10:157–160.

66 Hubálek Z, Halouzka J, Juřicová Z: Prevalence of borreliae in *Ixodes ricinus* ticks from urban parks. Folia Parasitol 1993;40:236.

67 Joss AWL, Mavin S, Ho-Yen DO: Increased incidence of Lyme borreliosis following mild winters and during warm, humid summers. Eur J Clin Microbiol Infect Dis 2007;26:79.

68 Subak S: Effects of climate on variability in Lyme disease incidence in the northeastern United States. Am J Epidemiol 2003;157:531–538.

69 McCabe GJ, Bunnell JE: Precipitation and the occurrence of Lyme disease in the northeastern United States. Vector Borne Zoon Dis 2004;4:143–148.

70 Ashley ST, Meentemeyer V: Climatic analysis of Lyme disease in the United States. Clim Res 2004; 27:177–187.

71 Estrada-Peña A, Venzal JM: Changes in habitat suitability for the tick *Ixodes ricinus* (Acari: Ixodidae) in Europe (1900–1999). Ecohealth 2006;3:154–162.

72 Piesman J, Mather TN, Dammin GJ, Telford SR, Lastavica CC, Spielman A: Seasonal variation of transmission risk of Lyme disease and human babesiosis. Am J Epidemiol 1987;126:1187–1189.

73 Hubálek Z, Halouzka J, Juřicová Z: A comparison of the occurrence of borreliae in nymphal and adult *Ixodes ricinus* ticks. Zentralbl Bakteriol 1991;276: 133–137.

74 Hubálek Z, Halouzka J Juřicová Z: Longitudinal surveillance of the tick *Ixodes ricinus* for borreliae. Med Vet Entomol 2003;17:46–51.

75 Hubálek Z, Halouzka J, Juřicová Z: Borreliae in *Ixodes ricinus* ticks feeding on humans. Med Vet Entomol 2004;18:228–231.

76 Falco RC, McKenna DF, Daniels TJ, Nadelman RB, Nowakowski J, Fish D, Wormser GP: Temporal relation between *Ixodes scapularis* abundance and risk for Lyme disease associated with erythema migrans. Am J Epidemiol 1999;149:771–776.

77 Dorn W, Flügel C, Grübner I: Data on human-biting *Ixodes ricinus* ticks in a region of Thuringia (Germany). Int J Med Microbiol 2002;291(suppl 33):219.

78 Nahimana I, Gern L, Blanc DS, Praz G, Francioli P, Péter O: Risk of *Borrelia burgdorferi* infection in western Switzerland following a tick bite. Eur J Clin Microbiol Infect Dis 2004;23:603–608.

79 Stafford KC, Cartter ML, Magnarelli LA, Ertel SH, Mshar PA: Temporal correlations between tick abundance and prevalence of ticks infected with *Borrelia burgdorferi* and increasing incidence of Lyme disease. J Clin Microbiol 1998;36:1240–1244.

80 Bialowas K, Jablonowski Z: Frequency of contact with ticks and pathogenic effects of such contacts in forestry workers of north-eastern Poland. Int J Med Microbiol 2002;291(suppl 33):214.

81 Maiwald M, Oehme R, March O, Petney TN, Kimmig P, Naser K, Zappe HA, Hassler D, von Knebel Doeberitz M: Transmission risk of *Borrelia burgdorferi* sensu lato from *Ixodes ricinus* ticks to humans in southwest Germany. Epidemiol Infect 1998;121:103–108.

82 Gustafson R, Svennungson B, Forsgren M, Gardulf A, Granstrom M: Two-year survey of the incidence of Lyme borreliosis and tick-borne encephalitis in a high-risk population in Sweden. Eur J Clin Microbiol Infect Dis 1992;11:894–900.

83 Shapiro ED, Gerber MA, Holabird NB, Berg AT, Feder HM, Bell GL, Rys PN, Persing DH: A controlled trial of antimicrobial prophylaxis for Lyme disease after deer-tick bites. N Engl J Med 1992;327: 1769–1773.

84 Sood SK, Salzman MB, Johnson BJB, Happ CM, Feig K, Carmody L, Rubin LG, Hilton E, Piesman J: Duration of tick attachment as a predictor of the risk of Lyme disease in an area in which Lyme disease is endemic. J Infect Dis 1997;175:996–999.

85 Nadelman RB, Nowakowski J, Fish D, Falco RC, Freeman K, McKenna D, Welch P, Marcus R, Agüero-Rosenfeld ME, Dennis DT, Wormser GP: Prophylaxis with single-dose doxycycline for the prevention of Lyme disease after an *Ixodes scapularis* tick bite. N Eng J Med 2001;345:79–84.

86 Piesman J, Mather TN, Sinsky RJ, Spielman A: Duration of tick attachment and *Borrelia burgdorferi* transmission. J Clin Microbiol 1987;25:557–558.

87 Lebet N, Gern L: Histological examination of *Borrelia burgdorferi* infection in unfed *Ixodes ricinus* nymphs. Exp Appl Acarol 1994;18:177–183.

88 Leuba-Garcia S, Kramer MD, Wallich R, Gern L: Characterization of *Borrelia burgdorferi* isolated from different organs of *Ixodes ricinus* ticks collected in nature. Zentralbl Bakteriol 1994;280:468–475.

89 Zhu Z: Histological observations on *Borrelia burgdorferi* growth in naturally infected female *Ixodes ricinus*. Acarologia 1998;39:11–22.

90 Hubálek Z, Halouzka J, Juřicová Z: Investigation of haematophagous arthropods for borreliae – summarized data, 1988–1996. Folia Parasitol 1998;45: 67–72.

91 Korenberg EI, Gorban LY, Kovalevskii YV, Frizen VI, Karavanov AS: Risk for human tick-borne encephalitis, borrelioses, and double infection in the pre-Ural region of Russia. Emerg Infect Dis 2001; 7:459–462.
92 Crippa M, Reis O, Gern L: Investigations on the mode and dynamics of transmission and infectivity of *Borrelia burgdorferi* sensu stricto and *B. afzelii* in *Ixodes ricinus* ticks. Vector Borne Zoon Dis 2002;2:3–9.
93 Kahl O, Janetzki-Mittmann C, Gray JS, Jonas R, Stein J, de Boer R: Risk of infection with *Borrelia burgdorferi* sensu lato for a host in relation to the duration of nymphal *Ixodes ricinus* feeding and the method of tick removal. Zentralbl Bakteriol 1998;287:41–52.
94 Ginsberg HS: Transmission risk of Lyme disease and implications for tick management. Am J Epidemiol 1993;138:65–73.
95 Hubálek Z, Halouzka J, Juřicová Z: A simple method of transmission risk assessment in enzootic foci of Lyme borreliosis. Eur J Epidemiol 1996;12:331–333.
96 Schulze TL, Taylor RC, Taylor GC, Bosler EM: Lyme disease: a proposed ecological index to assess areas of risk in the northeastern United States. Am J Publ Health 1991;81:714–718.
97 Connally NP, Ginsbergh HS, Mather TN: Assessing peridomestic entomological factors as predictors for Lyme disease. J Vector Ecol 2006;31:364–370.
98 Fitzner J, Ammon A, Baumann I, Talaska T, Schönberg A, Stöbel K, Fingerle V, Wilske B, Petersen L: Risk factors in Lyme borreliosis: a German case-control study. Int J Med Microbiol 2002;291(suppl 33):220.
99 Horobik V, Keesing F, Ostfeld RS: Abundance and *Borrelia burgdorferi*-infection prevalence of nymphal *Ixodes scapularis* ticks along forest-field edges. Ecohealth 2007;3:262–268.
100 Stafford KC, Magnarelli LA: Spatial and temporal patterns of *Ixodes scapularis* (Acari: Ixodidae) in southeastern Connecticut. J Med Entomol 1993; 30:762–771.
101 Fish D: Environmental risk and prevention of Lyme disease. Am J Med 1995;98(suppl 4A):2–9.
102 Brownstein JS, Skelly DK, Holford TR, Fish D: Forest fragmentation predicts local scale heterogeneity of Lyme disease risk. Oecologia 2005; 146:469–475.
103 Prusinski MA, Chen H, Drobnack JM, Kogut SJ, Means RG, Howard JJ, Oliver J, Lukacik G, Backenson PB, White DJ: Habitat structure associated with *Borrelia burgdorferi* prevalence in small mammals in New York State. Environ Entomol 2006;35:308–319.
104 Steere AC: Lyme disease. N Eng J Med 1989;321: 586–596.
105 Zeman P, Januška J: Epizootiologic background of dissimilar distribution of human cases of Lyme borreliosis and tick-borne encephalitis in a join endemic area. Comp Immunol Microbiol Infect Dis 1999;22:247–260.
106 Ostfeld RS: The ecology of Lyme disease risk. Am Sci 1997;85:338–346.
107 Lane RS, Steinlein DB, Mun J: Human behaviors elevating exposure to *Ixodes pacificus* (Acari: Ixodidae) nymphs and their associated bacterial zoonotic agents in a hardwood forest. J Med Entomol 2004;41:239–248.
108 Epidat: Notification of Infectious Diseases in the Czech Republic National Public Health Institute. Prague, Centre of Epidemiology and Microbiology, 2007. http://www.szu.cz/cema/hpcema.htm.
109 EpiNorth: Data on Lyme borreliosis. 2007. http://www.epinorth.org.
110 Health Protection Agency: UK Data on Lyme borreliosis. 2007. http://www.hpa.org.uk/infections.
111 Smith R, Takkinen J: Lyme borreliosis: Europe-wide coordinated surveillance and action needed? Euro Surveill 2006;11:E0606221.1. http://www.eurosurveillance.org/ViewArticle.aspx?ArticleId=2977.
112 Stamouli M, Totos G, Braun HB, Michel G, Gizaris V: Very low seroprevalence of Lyme borreliosis in young Greek males. Eur J Epidemiol 2000;16: 495–496.
113 Hofhuis A, van der Giessen JWB, Borgsteede FHM, Wielinga PR, Notermans DW, van Pelt W: Lyme borreliosis in the Netherlands: strong increase in GP consultations and hospital admissions in past 10 years. Euro Surveill 2006; 11:E060622.2. http://www.eurosurveillance.org/ViewArticle.aspx?ArticleId=2978.
114 Hasseltvedt V: Cases of Lyme borreliosis notified in Norway, 2000. Euro Surveill 2001;5:010809.2. http://www.eurosurveillance.org/ViewArticle.aspx?ArticleId=1706.
115 Epimeld: Infectious Diseases and Poisonings in Poland. Warsaw, National Research Centre of Public Health, 2007. http://www.pzh.gov.pl.
116 Lopes de Carvalho I, Núncio MS: Laboratory diagnosis of Lyme borreliosis at the Portuguese National Institute of Health (1990–2004). Euro Surveill 2006;11:257–260.
117 Gern L: Lyme borreliosis in Switzerland. Report WHO Workshop Lyme Borreliosis Diagn Surveill. Warsaw, 20–22 June 1995, pp 152–156.
118 Güner ES, Hashimoto N, Takada N, Kaneda K, Imai Y, Masuzawa T: First isolation and characterization of *Borrelia burgdorferi* sensu lato strains from *Ixodes ricinus* ticks in Turkey. J Med Microbiol 2003;52:807–813.

119 Romanova EV, Buchinskaya EA: Peculiarities of clinical manifestations of tick-borne borrelioses based on the data from 1st Novosibirsk City Infectious Diseases Hospital (in Russian); in Matushenko AA (ed): Current Aspects of Diseases with Natural Focality. Omsk, 2001, pp 123–124.
120 Miyamoto K, Masuzawa T: Ecology of *Borrelia burgdorferi* sensu lato in Japan and East Asia; in Gray J, Kahl O, Lane RS, Stanek G: Lyme Borreliosis – Biology, Epidemiology and Control. Wallingford, CABI, 2002, pp 201–222.
121 Masuzawa T: Terrestrial distribution of the Lyme borreliosis agent *Borrelia burgdorferi* sensu lato in East Asia. Jap J Infect Dis 2004;57:229–235.
122 Shih CM, Wang JC, Chao LL, Wu TN: Lyme disease in Taiwan: first human patient with characteristic erythema chronicum migrans skin lesion. J Clin Microbiol 1998;36:807–808.
123 Matuschka FR, Eiffert H, Ohlenbusch A, Richter D, Schein E, Spielman A: Transmission of the agent of Lyme disease on a subtropical island. Trop Med Parasitol 1994;45:39–44.
124 Ouhabi H, Slassi I, El Aloui-Frais M: Paralysie faciale et maladie de Lyme. Arch Inst Pasteur Maroc 1994;9:51–55.
125 Rousselle C, Floret D, Cochat P, Reignier F, Wright C: Encéphalite aige à *Borrelia burgdorferi* (maladie de Lyme) chez un enfant algérien. Pédiatrie 1989; 44:265–269.
126 Aoun K, Kechrid A, Lagha N, Zarrouk A, Bouzouaia N: La maladie de Lyme en Tunisie, résultats d'une étude clinico-sérologique (1992–1996). Cah Santé 1998;8:98–100.
127 Younsi H, Postic D, Baranton G, Bouattour A: High prevalence of *Borrelia lusitaniae* in *Ixodes ricinus* ticks in Tunisia. Eur J Epidem 2001;17:53–56.

Dr. Z. Hubálek
Medical Zoology Laboratory, Institute of Vertebrate Biology, Academy of Sciences
Klasterni 2
CZ–69142 Valtice (Czech Republic)
Tel. +420 519 352 961, Fax +420 519 352 387, E-Mail zhubalek@ivb.cz

Lipsker D, Jaulhac B (eds): Lyme Borreliosis.
Curr Probl Dermatol. Basel, Karger, 2009, vol 37, pp 51–110

Clinical Manifestations and Diagnosis of Lyme Borreliosis

Franc Strle[a] · Gerold Stanek[b]

[a]Department of Infectious Diseases, University Medical Center Ljubljana, Ljubljana, Slovenia;
[b]Medical University of Vienna, Clinical Institute of Hygiene and Medical Microbiology, Vienna, Austria

Abstract

Lyme borrelosis is a multi-systemic disease caused by *Borrelia burgdorferi* sensu lato. A complete presentation of the disease is an extremely unusual oberservation, in which a skin lesion follows a tick bite, the lesion itself is followed by heart and nervous system involvement, and later on by arthritis; late involvement of the eye, nervous system, joints and skin may also occur. Information on the relative frequency of individual clinical manifestations of Lyme borreliosis is limited; however, the skin is most frequently involved and skin manifestations frequently represent clues for the diagnosis. The only sign that enables a reliable clinical diagnoisis of Lyme borreliosis is a typical erythema migrans. Laboratory confirmation of a borrelial infection is needed for all manifestations of Lyme borreliosis, with the exception of typical skin lesions.

General Remarks

Lyme borreliosis, caused by *Borrelia burgdorferi* sensu lato (s.l.), presents with a variety of clinical signs and symptoms and with several variations in the course of the disease. This may frequently result in an uncritical interpretation of manifestations mistakenly attributed to Lyme borreliosis [1]. Most often the diagnosis of Lyme borreliosis is based on erroneous interpretations of serologic or PCR test results and an equation of infection with disease [2, 3]. On the other hand, some patients with typical clinical signs still remain undiagnosed and untreated. In spite of possible variations in the clinical course, certain rules could be useful for identification of patients and confirmation of borrelial infection. Lyme borreliosis should not become a domain in which everyone interprets findings according to their own feelings and intentions. This temptation exists not only with Lyme borreliosis, but also with several other illnesses presenting with numerous clinical features and limited laboratory confirmation. Such behavior regarding Lyme borreliosis is coupled not only with incomplete information about the disease, but most often with inadequate familarity with the existing knowledge. This may lead to more restricted recognition of the disease by some (predominantly academic) physicians, and others to the fantasy that substantial numbers of patients with chronic symptoms such as arthralgia, myalgia, headache, fatigue and so on – symptoms quite frequently present in the general population – are suffering from chronic Lyme borreliosis, and thus require long-term treatment with antibiotics. The latter approach appears to be much more frequent than the former, and has been expanding fairly rapidly, not only in the USA but also in several countries in Europe. It is mostly a consequence of the pronounced expectations of patients with nonspecific and/or devastating signs and symptoms and their desire to get a 'decent' diagnosis offering efficacious and relatively simple treatment. Therapy in these cases is often coupled with limited proficiency of the care providers and unfortunately in some cases also with malevolent activities of some individuals who are not able to avoid the temptations of financial opportunities in the management of 'chronic Lyme disease'.

Not knowing what to do is frustrating, not doing what is known is tragic, intentionally doing things that are not efficient and can even be harmful is ethically intolerable.

Diagnosing Lyme Borreliosis

The terms Lyme borreliosis and Lyme disease are generally used synonymously. However, the term Lyme disease was coined to name an enlarging spectrum of symptoms that were obviously linked to each other by an etiology that was unknown until the early 1980s; the first observations of Lyme arthritis and Lyme carditis were made in the USA [4, 5]. After the discovery of the borrelial origin of these disorders, the more specific term Lyme borreliosis was introduced, and now appears to be the more appropriate term to describe a disorder that exists in moderate climates all over the northern hemisphere.

When diagnosing Lyme borreliosis it is important to acknowledge some simple facts that are often neglected or not properly recognized [1–3]. One such fact is that Lyme borreliosis is a disease. Disease is defined as 'any deviation from or interruption of the normal structure or function of any body part, organ, or system that is manifested by a characteristic set of symptoms and signs and whose etiology, pathology, and prognosis may be known or unknown' [6]. Therefore, there is no disease without signs and/or symptoms, and consequently there is no diagnosis of Lyme borreliosis in the absence of clinical manifestations. The mere proof of an infection with borreliae is not sufficient, because the infection may not always result in illness. It appears that the proportion of symptomatic infections is much higher in the USA, at about 90% [7], than in Europe, where fewer than 50% of infections result in clinical illness [8–10]. In addition, demonstration of antibodies to *B. burgdorferi* s.l. does not discriminate between active infection and an immunologic imprint of previous (symptomatic or asymptomatic) infection. Because signs and symptoms form the basis for recognition of the disease, good knowledge of clinical features is important in diagnosing Lyme borreliosis [2]. Case definitions for Lyme borreliosis are beneficial in everyday clinical practice, and especially for comparing the findings of different researchers. Unfortunately, clinically useful definitions are rare. Those of the Centers for Disease Control and Prevention (CDC) in the USA [11] were made primarily for epidemiologic purposes and are, with the exception of the definition of erythema migrans (EM), not applicable in clinical practice, whereas European definitions [12, 13] are somewhat complicated for a busy clinician. Guidelines for diagnosis and treatment (management) are also useful. They are available as the Infectious Diseases Society of America (IDSA) guidelines for the USA [14], were termed clinical case definitions by the European Union Concerted Action on Lyme Borreliosis (EUCALB), and as laboratory guidelines by a working group of the European Society for Clinical Microbiology and Infectious Diseases (ESCMID) [12, 13].

Another often neglected fact is that the clinical presentations of Lyme borreliosis in America and Europe differ in some respects, making it inappropriate to uncritically apply the findings from one side of the Atlantic to the other side [15]. Another important aspect is that, because of the much higher publication frequency of USA researchers and physicians in the field of Lyme borreliosis, it is quite possible that the diagnosis of Lyme borreliosis in Europe is predominantly assessed through 'American eyes'. The opinions offered in the present report are based primarily on European data and experience, and most probably fit better to the situation in Europe.

The only sign that enables a reliable clinical diagnosis of Lyme borreliosis is a typical EM [1–3, 12–14, 16–19]. However, according to current knowledge, even this is valid only for Europe and is less straightforward in the USA where skin lesions of STARI (Southern tick-associated rash illness; Masters' disease) are very similar to EM [20, 21]. Ear lobe lymphocytoma, meningoradiculoneuritis (Garin-Bujadoux-Bannwarth syndrome) and acrodermatitis chronica atrophicans (ACA) are also highly supportive of the diagnosis [2, 3, 13]. The large majority of numerous other symptoms and signs, especially when expressed individually, have only minimal or even symbolic diagnostic value. Laboratory confirmation of a borrelial infection is needed for all manifestations of Lyme borreliosis, with the exception of typical skin lesions [1–3, 12–14, 16–19]. An apparently favorable effect of treatment with antibiotics is of small diagnostic value, because the natural course of Lyme borreliosis in an individual patient is difficult to predict (is variable) and, moreover, the majority of clinical manifestations will resolve spontaneously [2, 3]. Individual case reports of unusual clinical manifestations may serve as a trigger for scientific evaluation, but it is incorrect to conclude that these are 'new' signs of Lyme borreliosis or new (newly discovered) clinical manifestations of the disease. Moreover, coincidence should be ruled out by controlled prospective clinical studies, since the presence of borrelial antibodies in serum and/or the presence of specific nucleic acid sequences of *B. burgdorferi* s.l. in a patient's specimen, and in some circumstances even the isolation of borreliae from involved tissue or organ, do not alone prove the etiology [1–3].

Little information exists on the frequency of coinfections of tick-borne pathogens and their effects on the clinical manifestations, diagnosis, treatment and outcome of Lyme borreliosis. Dual infection with *Babesia microti* and *B. burgdorferi* sensu stricto (s.s.) can result in more serious disease than infection with either agent alone [22]. A combination of Lyme borreliosis with tick-borne encephalitis could cause diagnostic dilemmas, and consequently a delay in antibiotic treatment [23]. Coinfection with the agent of human granulocytic anaplasmosis, *Anaplasma phagocytophilum*, affects the choice of antibiotic for treatment of early Lyme borreliosis [24].

Only the main clinical manifestations of Lyme borreliosis will be dealt with in this chapter.

Clinical Manifestations

A complete presentation of the disease is an extremely unusual observation, in which a skin lesion follows a tick bite, the lesion is then followed by heart and nervous system involvement, and later on by arthritis; late involvement of eye, nervous system, joints and skin may also occur. Information on the relative frequency of individual clinical manifestations of Lyme borreliosis is limited. The disease has traditionally been divided into stages; however, although this may be valuable for didactic reasons, it is somewhat theoretical and often not in agreement with clinical findings.

Skin Involvement

Skin is the most frequently involved tissue in Lyme borreliosis, and skin manifestations frequently represent clues for the diagnosis. EM, borrelial lymphocytoma (formerly lymphadenosis benigna cutis) and ACA are today rated as classic manifestations of Lyme borreliosis. These manifestations were well known as distinct skin disorders long before the discovery of the causative agent [17, 25–27]. In addition, Lyme borreliosis may be associated with several other skin manifestations, such as scleroderma circumscripta, lichen sclerosus et atrophicus and cutaneous B cell lymphoma.

Erythema Migrans

Short Definition

Several definitions of EM have been proposed for different purposes. Best known among these are the definitions of the CDC [11], EUCALB [12] and the ESCMID study group [13]. In Slovenia, a modified CDC definition has been used since 1988. EM is defined as

Table 1. Frequency of the main clinical manifestations of Lyme borreliosis in patients registered at the Lyme borreliosis outpatient clinic in Ljubljana, Slovenia, in 2000

Manifestation	Adults	Children	Total
Erythema migrans	621 (83.4)	218 (79.3)	839 (82.3)
Borrelial lymphocytoma	4 (0.5)	4 (1.5)	8 (0.8)
Lyme neuroborreliosis	48 (6.4)	40 (14.5)	88 (8.6)
Lyme carditis	2 (0.3)	0	2 (0.2)
Lyme arthritis	21 (2.8)	13 (4.7)	34 (3.3)
ACA	49 (6.6)	0	49 (4.8)
Total	745	275	1,020

Figures in parentheses are percentages.

an erythematous skin lesion that develops days to weeks after infection at the site where borreliae were inoculated into the skin. It typically begins as a red macula or papule and expands over a period of days to weeks to usually an oval or round lesion, with or without central clearing. For a reliable diagnosis, a single primary lesion must reach ≥5 cm in size. A lesion <5 cm qualifies for the diagnosis of EM only if: (1) it develops at the site of a tick bite, (2) a time interval between the bite and the onset of the lesion is reported, and (3) the lesion is enlarging (fulfillment of all 3 requirements is needed). Secondary lesions may also occur. Multiple EM is defined as the presence of 2 or more skin lesions, at least 1 of which must fulfil the size criteria for solitary EM given above.

Frequency

EM is by far the most frequent manifestation of Lyme borreliosis. In the USA, more than 70% of patients registered with Lyme borreliosis had EM [28]. Among 1,471 patients shown to have Lyme borreliosis in an epidemiologic study in southern Sweden, EM was seen in 77% of all cases, and was accompanied by other signs of the disease such as nervous system involvement, arthritis, lymphocytoma and/or carditis in only 6.5% [29]. Mandatory notification in Europe has been instituted in only a limited number of countries. In Slovenia, where notification of Lyme borreliosis has been mandatory for more than 20 years and where during the past 10 years the incidence of the disease has been more than 100 per 100,000 inhabitants, rising to 224 per 100,000 in 2006, EM represents about 90% of registered cases [30, 31]. The relative frequency of individual clinical manifestations in patients registered at the Lyme borreliosis outpatient clinic at the Department of Infectious Diseases, University Medical Center Ljubljana, Slovenia, are shown in table 1.

Etiology

In North America, EM is caused by *B. burgdorferi* s.s., this species apparently being the sole cause of human Lyme borreliosis there. Reports from Europe, based on the characterization of borreliae isolated from skin, revealed that EM is most often caused by *B. afzelii* (up to 96%, most often 70–90%), less frequently by *B. garinii* (up to 33%, most often 10–20%), rarely by *B. burgdorferi* s.s. and only exceptionally by other species such as *B. bissettii*, *B. spielmanii* and as yet unidentifiable species [32–44]. Among 488 skin isolates from Slovenian patients with EM, 433 (89%) were typed as *B. afzelii*, 53 (11%) as *B. garinii* and only 2 as *B. burgdorferi* s.s. [38]. However, in a Finnish series of 82 patients with EM, 21.5% were skin culture positive (a rather low isolation rate), and all the isolates were typed as *B. garinii* [45]. It seems that the predominance of *B. afzelii* is valid for western and central Europe, but may not be for eastern Scandinavia, eastern Europe and Asia. It is of interest that the proportions of the main *Borrelia* species isolated from EM skin lesions do not completely match with the proportions found in ticks. Studies in Slovenia and Germany found that *B. garinii* and *B. burgdorferi* s.s. were relatively more frequently isolated from ticks than *B. afzelii*, and that this differed from the *Borrelia* species isolated from the skin of patients with EM in the same region [39, 46].

Information obtained predominantly from PCR [34, 47, 48] but also from culture results [49, 50] indicates that an individual patient with Lyme borreliosis may simultaneously harbor more than 1 *Borrelia* strain of the same species and even more than 1 *Borrelia* species.

Borreliae enter the skin during the blood meal of an infected *Ixodid* tick. Most probably, the bacteria initially accommodate to the new environment and then spread into the skin and other tissue. Results of experimental infection suggest that borreliae may disseminate in the skin over a long period of time without causing disease, unless the host's defenses are imbalanced [3].

Tick Bite

In the USA, only about 1 in 4 patients (14–32%) with EM recall a previous tick bite at the site of the skin lesion [15, 28, 51, 52]. In several European studies, the proportion of patients recalling a tick bite is substantially higher [15, 53–56]. Among 892 adult patients diagnosed with typical EM at the Ljubljana Lyme borreliosis clinic in 1993, 73% reported a tick bite at the site where the EM skin lesion expanded, and in 2000 the corresponding rate was 311 of 535 (58%) [56]. Patients with EM who do not recall a tick bite were most probably bitten, but were not aware of it. The history of an insect bite followed by skin lesion and interpreted as EM is often insecure, and cannot exclude an unnoticed tick bite.

Histologic Findings

Commonly mild superficial perivascular infiltration by lymphocytes and some histiocytes is usually present, and is sometimes accompanied by plasma cells, rarely by neutrophils, in the dermis at the site of the EM lesion and also in the clinically normal-looking skin bordering the lesion [57]. The epidermis is usually unaffected. The presence of T cells and increased numbers of Langerhans cells suggest that cell-mediated immune mechanisms are involved in the initial host response to *B. burgdorferi* s.l. [3]. High levels of mRNA expression of the T cell-active chemokines CXCL9 and CXCL10 and low levels of the B cell-active chemokine CXCL13 have been established in EM. CD3+ T cells and CXCL9 have been visualized using immunohistologic methods [58].

Clinical Characteristics

EM affects all ages and both sexes with a slight predomination of females in Europe, but not in the USA. The lesion usually appears on the skin at the site of a tick bite. Days to weeks thereafter, a small red macula or papule appears. In 1 study of adult European patients with *B. afzelii* isolated from skin, the median time from bite to rash onset was 17 days, whereas the median time in *B. burgdorferi* s.s. patients in the USA was 11 days [15]. Because of the close temporal proximity of tick bites and onset of EM, this manifestation of Lyme borreliosis has a pronounced seasonal occurrence. The erythema slowly enlarges and central clearing usually begins – in adult patients in Europe typically by the end of the first week – resulting in a ring-like lesion that spreads outward (EM). Untreated lesions persist and expand over days to several months. EM skin lesions are typically oval or round, but can have an irregular shape. Their diameter may range from a few centimeters to more than a meter. In adult patients EM is most often located on the lower extremities; in children the upper part of the body is relatively more often involved [3, 15–17, 19, 53–56].

About half of adult European patients report local symptoms at the site of EM, usually mild itching, burning or pain; a smaller proportion (20–51%) have systemic symptoms such as fatigue and malaise, headache, myalgia and arthralgia, which are usually intermittent and often vary in intensity and location. In European patients with EM, fever is an exception, being present or recalled in fewer than 5% [17, 19, 54–56, 59], whereas in the USA it is documented in about 16% and recalled by more than one third of patients [28]. Although the frequencies of local symptoms appear similar in the USA and Europe [15], the proportion of patients with systemic symptoms is higher in the USA, where as many as 80% of patients evaluated for EM have simultaneous systemic complaints [28, 60]. In a study on culture-proven EM, 82 of 119 (69%) adult patients in the USA, in whom *B. burgdorferi* s.s. was causing disease, reported systemic symptoms, in contrast to 43 of 85 (51%) Slovenian patients with *B. afzelii* isolated from their skin lesion. The comparison also revealed several other differences, including briefer duration of EM in the USA (median 4 days vs. 14 days in European patients), greater frequency of abnormal findings on physical examination (57 vs. 14%) including lymphadenopathy (39 vs. 9%) and fever (15 vs. 1%), and differences in seroreactivity; central clearing was more likely in European patients (68 vs. 35%). The frequency of multiple EM was greater in the USA than in the Slovenian patients (13 vs. 7%), but the difference was not significant [15]. Several distinctions have also been found in European patients when comparing culture-confirmed EM caused by *B. afzelii* with EM caused by *B. garinii* [33, 61, 62]. According to some authors, the presence of systemic symptoms associated with a solitary EM skin lesion might indicate dissemination of the etiologic agent; however, this most probably applies more to patients in North America than in Europe. According to the somewhat limited information in Europe, the yield from blood cultures of patients with EM is low and spirochetemia is often clinically silent. The isolation rate from blood was found to be only about 1% in adult patients and 9% in children with solitary EM [59, 63], which is in contrast to reports from the USA where as many as 50% of patients with EM had a positive blood culture [64]. Possible explanations for these distinctions are the much larger volume of blood cultured in the USA than in Europe, and differences in the species causing EM. All blood isolates in the USA belong to *B. burgdorferi* s.s., but only a subset of subtypes of this species is prone to disseminate and to cause spirochetemia. In Europe, *B. afzelii* predominates, not only among skin isolates but also among blood isolates (≥80%) of patients with EM [38, 59, 63]. In 1 study, only 7 of 35 (20%) adult patients with EM and *B. burgdorferi* s.l. isolated from blood reported constitutional symptoms [59]. Comparison of 12 blood culture-positive and 122 blood culture-negative children with solitary EM found no differences in pretreatment characteristics, including the frequency of the associated systemic symptoms [63]. The fact that in Europe only some of the patients with multiple EM report systemic symptoms indicates that the absence of systemic symptoms is not a reliable indication of the lack of dissemination. For example, nearly 50% of adult Slovenian patients and 70% of children with multiple EM do not report any systemic complaints [unpublished data, 65]. Multiple EM is defined as the presence of 2 or more skin lesions in an individual patient and is interpreted as a consequence of hematogeneous dissemination of borreliae from the primary EM skin lesion. The secondary lesions are similar in morphology to the initial solitary lesion, but lack the indurated center usually seen in primary lesions at the site of the tick bite; secondary lesions are also smaller and are only exceptionally associated with local itching or pain. It seems that they are more frequent in children than in adults, and are apparently a more common finding in EM in the USA (up to 50% [60]) than in Europe (3–8% of adult patients) [15, 19, 53–56]. It is of interest that in children with multiple EM, a mild predominantly lymphocytic pleocytosis was seen in 18–26% of patients, although none had clear clinical evidence of central nervous system (CNS) involvement [65, 66], and fewer than half of these patients reported systemic symptoms [66]. European patients with EM are mostly seronegative in convalescent-phase serum samples, whereas the majority of such patients in the USA are seropositive. However, in both groups routine medical laboratory tests do not reveal signs of inflammation or any other abnormalities [4, 15, 51–55, 60].

Diagnosis

Diagnosis of a typical EM is clinical [1–3, 14, 16]. For atypical lesions, proof is required by the demonstration of borreliae in skin [2, 3]. However, even 'typical' EM may not be considered pathognomonic for Lyme borreliosis, especially in the southern part of the USA, where skin lesions consistent with EM but with no microbiologic evidence for *Borrelia* infection have been established [20, 21].

Differential Diagnosis
EM is sometimes misdiagnosed as fungal infection and vice versa, especially when lesions are present in inguinal or axillary regions. Skin lesions that do not show central clearing may resemble erysipelas, although in patients with erysipelas the onset of the lesion is typically preceded by rigors and high fever and is accompanied by high fever, malaise and laboratory signs of inflammation, which are – at least in Europe – not present in patients with EM. When a skin lesion appears immediately or during the first 24 h after a tick bite, it is usually the result of a hypersensitivity reaction and not a borrelial infection. In Lyme borreliosis there is typically a symptom-free interval of at least some days from the bite to the onset of a skin lesion. Other differential diagnoses may include reaction to an insect bite, urticaria, contact eczema, folliculitis, cellulitis, granuloma annulare, tinea corporis (ring worm), fixed drug eruption or pseudolymphoma [2, 3, 12, 67].

Borrelial Lymphocytoma

Basic Description and Histologic Findings
Borrelial lymphocytoma is a solitary swelling with a diameter of up to a few centimeters, consisting of a dense lymphocytic infiltration of cutis and subcutis as a result of borrelial infection [17, 68–72]. The infiltration is polyclonal with a predominance of B lymphocytes and may show germinal centers [17, 57, 68, 69, 72, 73]. In contrast to the other 2 main skin manifestations of Lyme borreliosis, EM and ACA, where high levels of the T cell-active chemokines CXCL9 and CXCL10 have been established, in borrelial lymphocytoma high levels of the B cell-active chemokine CXCL13 are found [58]. In children, borrelial lymphocytoma is most frequently located on the ear lobe and in adults in the region of the areola mammae [17, 68–72]. When located on the ear lobe, the involved skin is bluish red; at other locations, the skin color is usually normal. Borrelial lymphocytoma usually appears later, has slower evolution and is of longer duration than EM, but also resolves spontaneously although sometimes only after more than a year [17, 68–70, 72]. Other signs of Lyme borreliosis may develop in the course of (untreated long-lasting) borrelial lymphocytoma [17, 68, 69, 71, 72].

Frequency
Borrelial lymphocytoma is a rare manifestation of European Lyme borreliosis. There are no reliable reports on autochthonous borrelial lymphocytoma from North America. Data on the exact frequency of this manifestation in Europe are limited. In a well-designed epidemiologic study in southern Sweden, borrelial lymphocytoma was

found in 16 of 232 (7%) children and in 25 of 1,239 (2%) adults registered with Lyme borreliosis [29]. In Slovenia, only 18 of 1,582 (1.1%) patients registered with Lyme borreliosis in the years 1986–1988 had borrelial lymphocytoma [74]. The proportion of patients with borrelial lymphocytoma diagnosed at the Ljubljana Lyme borreliosis clinic during 1999 is shown in table 1. Similar ratios were also found for the following years [unpublished data].

Etiology
Information on the genospecies of borreliae that cause borrelial lymphocytoma is limited. The large majority of isolates from borrelial lymphocytoma tissue have been found to be *B. afzelii*, but in some patients *B. garinii* and *B. burgdorferi* s.s. have been isolated, and in 1 patient the presence of *B. bissettii* was established [38, 70, 71, 75–77].

Clinical Characteristics
After the recognition that solitary lymphocytoma (lymphadenosis benigna cutis) is a manifestation of Lyme borreliosis, only 5 studies [68–71, 73] with large numbers of patients, including 1 with a predominantly pathologic orientation [73], and a few reports on a very limited number of patients have been published [78–80]. A review of 36 patients with a solitary borrelial lymphocytoma diagnosed at the Department of Infectious Diseases of the University Medical Center Ljubljana (the department cares for both children and adults) over a 5-year period revealed that in most of these patients the onset of borrelial lymphocytoma was in the second half of the year and that distribution according to sex was well balanced. The lesion was localized on the ear lobe in 47% of patients, on the breast in 42%, and on the nose, arm, shoulder or scrotum in 11%. Patients with ear lobe borrelial lymphocytoma were younger than those with the lesion on the breast (median 12 vs. 42 years); of 17 patients with ear-lobe borrelial lymphocytoma only 3 were adults and all the others were 10 years or younger; in breast borrelial lymphocytoma, all patients but 1 were 18 years or older [69]. This accords with observations of other researchers and with further reports from the same group [68, 70, 71, 73]. The reasons for such distinctive localizations and for differences in location of the lesion according to age are not completely understood. Asbrink and Hovmark [81] hypothesized that borreliae prosper at a temperature below 37°C, which would explain why the ear lobe and the nipple, the cooler parts of the body, are most frequently affected. However, there are some additional explanations. Lymphocytoma on the ear lobe is easy to notice and can be easily recognized from its characteristic appearance, provided the physician is familiar with the disorder. Changes in the nipples and nodules in the breast often scare the patient into seeking medical help, although the physician has to use various diagnostic measures to achieve a possibility of correct diagnosis. Nodules found in other areas of the skin, whether in the dermis or subcutis, are usually no cause for consulting a physician. Even if the patient seeks medical attention in such cases, it is difficult to establish a clinical diagnosis without other manifestations of a borrelial infection. It is also difficult to inter-

pret the differences in localization of borrelial lymphocytoma in children and adults. Possibly, one reason may be the different sites of tick bites. It is known that ticks are usually found on vegetation a few centimeters up to one meter above ground. This explains why children more often have tick bites on the head and neck than adults [29], and consequently why EM is localized much more frequently on the face of children than adults and also why ear lobe borrelial lymphocytoma is found predominantly in children. Yet, the localization of the tick bite does not explain why borrelial lymphocytoma on the breast is an exception in children. It seems that there are local tissue factors which support the development of borrelial lymphocytoma on the breast in adults [69]. In the same study, a tick bite was reported by 29 of 36 (81%) patients, a median of 30 days before borrelial lymphocytoma developed. In 24 (83%) of the patients the tick bite was in close vicinity to the location of the subsequent borrelial lymphocytoma, indicating that in the great majority of patients the spirochetes may spread from the site of the bite to the site where the disorder appears. This is well known in EM, which spreads out from the site of inoculation. In addition, borrelial lymphocytoma was located within the EM in 24 of 25 patients with concomitant EM. The onset of EM, the typical early manifestation of Lyme borreliosis, preceded borrelial lymphocytoma in 19 out of 25 cases. Only 3 of 17 (18%) patients with ear lobe borrelial lymphocytoma had mild systemic symptoms, such as moderate headache, general malaise and fatigue, and 8 (47%) patients reported mild local itching; also in 8 (47%) members of this group, enlarged regional lymph nodes were found on examination. In contrast, 12 out of 15 (80%) patients with breast borrelial lymphocytoma reported constitutional symptoms, and all but 1 reported localized discomfort in the region of the areola mammae – the patients were bothered by clothing and the area was slightly painful to touch. Mild itching, breast tension, burning and pain of the thoracic wall on the affected side were complained of by 9 (60%), 8 (53%), 6 (40%) and 4 (27%) patients, respectively. On inspection, the nipples were found to be asymmetric and, with 1 exception, showed no discoloration; they were edematous, painful to touch, and completely hardened in 8 (53%) patients and partly so in 4 patients. Infiltration was regularly found in the area of areola mammae, within a diameter of up to 3 cm. At presentation, 26 of 36 (72%) patients had borrelial antibodies in serum. Routine laboratory blood tests did not reveal any significant abnormality [69].

Among 85 adult patients with solitary borrelial lymphocytoma diagnosed at the Department of Infectious Diseases, University Medical Center Ljubljana, during a period of 15 years [71], there were 36 (42%) females and 49 (58%) males with a median age of 49 (15–74) years. Borrelial lymphocytoma was located on the breast (nipple/areola mammae region) in 68 (80%) patients, on the ear lobe in 8 (9%) and at other locations in 9 (11%). A concomitant EM enabling clinical diagnosis of Lyme borreliosis was registered or reported in 67 (79%) patients. Fifteen (18%) patients had no accompanying symptoms, 34 (40%) reported local and constitutional symptoms, 23 (27%) recounted local symptoms only and 13 (15%) had solely constitutional symptoms. Clinical findings indicating early disseminated borrelial infection were observed at the first visit in 12 (14%) patients: 6 (7%) had multiple EM , 1 had meningitis, 1 meningoradiculitis and arthritis, 1 radiculoneuritis and arthritis, 1 peripheral facial palsy and concomitant meningitis, and 2 arthritis. In addition, 1 of the patients with borrelial lymphocytoma on the breast had ACA. A seropositive response to borrelial antigens was found in only 30 (35%) patients at the initial examination. In 11 of 46 (24%) patients, infection with *B. burgdorferi* s.l. was confirmed by isolation of the agent from lymphocytoma tissue. Eight of 9 (89%) typed borrelial strains were *B. afzelii*, and 1 (11%) was *B. bissettii* [71].

Diagnosis

A reasonably consistent diagnosis of ear lobe lymphocytoma is usually possible on clinical grounds that can often be further supported by the presence or a reliable history of EM (usually in the region of the lymphocytoma), the occurrence of other manifestations of Lyme borreliosis, and/or by the demonstration of borrelial infection – usually by positive serology [17, 69, 70]. The isolation rate of *Borrelia* from lesional skin is difficult to assess because of the limited information; nevertheless, it appears to be considerably lower than from the skin of EM, but similar to that from the skin of patients with ACA. According to 2 reports, borreliae were isolated from skin biopsies of lymphocytoma in 4 of 11 (36%) patients and 11 of 46 (24%) patients [70, 71].

Differential Diagnosis

Differential diagnosis in ear lobe borrelial lymphocytoma is much more limited than in patients with breast lymphocytoma or lymphocytoma at other (atypical) locations; thus, the need for histologic examination is much greater in patients with lymphocytoma at locations other than the ear lobe [69]. Diagnostic difficulties in ear lobe borrelial lymphocytoma are usually the result of unawareness, whereas the main differential diagnostic possibility in breast lymphocytoma is a malignancy [17, 69]. It is sometimes difficult to distinguish the difference between borrelial lymphocytoma, B cell lymphoma and other pseudolymphomas [17, 69–71, 82, 83].

Acrodermatitis Chronica Atrophicans

Frequency

ACA is a chronic skin manifestation of Lyme borreliosis seen almost exclusively in Europe [3, 14, 16]. Reports on this skin condition from the USA are rare, and are predominantly limited to descriptions of the manifestation in immigrants from Europe [84, 85].

ACA is much less frequently observed than EM, but is more common than borrelial lymphocytoma [17]. In an epidemiologic study on Lyme borreliosis in southern Sweden, it was found in only 47 of 1,471 (3%) patients who fulfilled the criteria for Lyme borreliosis [29]. The proportion of patients with ACA diagnosed at the Ljubljana

Lyme borreliosis clinic in 1999 is shown in table 1. Similar ratios were also found for the following years [unpublished data].

Etiology

According to the results of PCR and isolation of borreliae from skin, the large majority of ACA cases are caused by *B. afzelii* [76, 86–90]; however, in some patients *B. garinii* and *B. burgdorferi* s.s. have been isolated from the skin lesion [77, 91]. Analysis of the genetic profiles of 22 strains of *B. burgdorferi* s.l. cultivated from skin biopsies of Slovenian patients with ACA lesions revealed 17 (77%) *B. afzelii* strains, 4 (18%) *B. garinii* and 1 (5%) *B. burgdorferi* s.s., indicating that *B. afzelii* is the predominant, but not the exclusive, etiologic agent of ACA [91]. This was confirmed later in a larger study. According to Ružić-Sabljić et al., among 74 isolates from the skin of patients with ACA, 89% were *B. afzelii*, 7% *B. garinii* and 4% *B. burgdorferi* s.s. [38].

Tick Bite

Because of the long incubation time and the long duration of the skin lesions prior to diagnosis, it is understandable that no reliable data exist on the frequency and location of tick bites. Most patients report being repeatedly bitten every year or being, or having been, outdoor workers in endemic areas, but almost no patient specifically recalls a tick bite at the affected body site [67]. The only exceptions are patients in whom ACA was preceded by an EM lesion in the same location several months to many years before. However, such a history is reported by no more than 10–20% of these patients [67, 92], and only some of them recall a tick bite prior to the onset of their EM skin lesion.

Histologic Findings

Findings depend upon the phase of the illness, which is rather academically divided into an early edematous (infiltrative) and a late atrophic phase. The disease starts with a nonspecific perivascular lymphocytic infiltrate. In early lesions, the epidermis is frequently thinned. The upper and middle portions of the dermis show a band-like and perivascular infiltrate consisting of lymphocytes and plasma cells, often in combination with more or less pronounced edema [57]. Dilated blood vessels can be found in the superficial dermis. Periarticular fibroid nodules seen in some patients with ACA are located in the deeper portions of the reticular cutis extending into the subcutaneous fat. Clinically, they resemble rheumatoid nodules, but have a different histologic structure with a homogeneous eosinophilic center surrounded by irregular fascicles of collagen typically arranged in an onion-like concentric fashion. Perivascular infiltrates of lymphocytes and plasma cells are present predominantly in the peripheral parts of the lesion, and fibrosis is present. In the late stage of ACA, cutaneous atrophy with more or less pronounced inflammation is present. The epidermis often has only a few layers of cells. Dilated blood vessels surrounded by lymphocytes and plasma cells can be found in the superficial cutis [57, 92, 93]. In very long-standing atrophic lesions, the inflammatory infiltrates are sparse or may even be absent.

The collagen fibers are strongly reduced in numbers and degeneration of elastic fibers is present [57]. In general, histologically constant findings in active ACA lesions are telangiectases and a lymphocytic infiltrate with a moderate-to-rich admixture of plasma cells [93]. The histopathologic pattern is not diagnostic in itself, but characteristic enough to alert the experienced pathologist [94].

Clinical Characteristics

ACA is a chronic borrelial skin manifestation that in contrast to EM and borrelial lymphocytoma does not disappear spontaneously [16, 17]. It is most often located on acral parts of the body, usually on the extensor part of hands or feet. Initially, the lesion is usually unilateral, later on it may become more or less symmetrical. The initial changes usually manifest themselves several months or years after the introduction of borreliae into the body. Some patients remember having had other signs of Lyme borreliosis – such as EM, neurologic involvement, heart involvement or arthritis before the onset or diagnosis of ACA – but most patients do not. Asbrink et al. [95] reported that in 9 out of 50 patients (18%) spontaneous healing of EM was followed at the same location by ACA lesions after a latency period of 6 months to 8 years. Thus, ACA can be the first and the only clinical sign of Lyme borreliosis [17, 95, 96].

ACA is more often diagnosed in women than in men, and occurs only very exceptionally in children. Patients are usually over 40 years old; in several reports the median value was over 60 years [17, 95, 96]. The onset is insidious, hardly appreciable: mildly bluish-red discoloration of the skin appears (usually on the foot, knee or dorsal part of one of the hands, mostly pronounced over metacarpophalangeal joints) and enlarges very slowly over periods of months to years. The involved region is usually edematous; swelling may occasionally dominate the clinical picture. Initially, the erythema and swelling may vary in intensity. In some patients, the cutaneous manifestations are confined to a heel that is swollen, sometimes discolored and painful. A common typical sign is that one of the feet (sometimes both) gradually increases in size, and the need for larger shoes arises [96]. After the initial months to years, the edema slowly vanishes and gradually atrophy becomes more and more prominent. The skin becomes increasingly violaceous, thin and wrinkled, with prominently visible underlying vessels. When exposed to a cold environment, the skin becomes pronouncedly bluish. The violaceous color also becomes more visible when involved arms or legs are in a dependent position. Healing of damage to the skin is impaired. In some patients, a concomitant migrating erythema, similar to EM, can be seen at the periphery of ACA lesions [96].

Up to one fifth of patients may have fibrous indurations in the involved regions [67, 95]; they may be band-like (usually in ulnar or tibial regions) or nodular (most often prepatellary or in the vicinity of the olecranon). The indurations are more frequent in the initial years of the evolution of ACA than in the late phase with pronouncedly atrophic skin.

In some patients with ACA, sclerotic lesions develop that are clinically and histologically indistinguishable from localized scleroderma (morphea) or lichen sclerosus et atrophicus. According to Asbrink and Hovmark [81], about 10% of patients with typical inflammatory ACA have sclerotic lesions. In one of the studies from that group, in addition to ACA lesions, lichen sclerosus et atrophicus-like lesions were found clinically in 5 of 32 (16%) examined patients. Four of these patients displayed a histopathologic picture compatible with lichen sclerosus et atrophicus, suggesting a relationship between these 2 skin conditions [93].

Peripheral nerves and joints are quite often involved in the regions of affected skin [16, 17, 95]. An association between ACA and peripheral neuropathy was established in systematic studies in the 1960s and 1970s. In these reports, nearly half the patients with ACA showed signs of predominately sensory polyneuropathy, often most pronounced in the limbs, with cutaneous involvement [96, 97]. After the recognition that ACA is a manifestation of borrelial infection, it became obvious that the majority of untreated patients with ACA have some kind of mild (mostly) or moderate neuropathy, as indicated by clinical and/or neurophysiologic examination [98, 99]. Peripheral nervous involvement is more frequent in the late phase of ACA. Sensory and motor mononeuropathy or polyneuropathy or patchy dysesthesia may develop at the site of the cutaneous lesions. Patients with ACA quite often complain of hyperesthesia/dysesthesia, muscle cramps, weakness in the muscles and/or sensations of heaviness, mainly in the affected limb(s).

In contrast to peripheral neuropathy, there are far fewer data on CNS involvement in patients with ACA. According to published information, CNS involvement and cerebrospinal fluid (CSF) abnormalities are rare [96].

In an investigation of 50 patients with ACA, radiographic examination revealed subluxation and/or luxations of small joints of the hands or feet in 11 (22%) patients; 4 (8%) patients showed periosteal thickening of bones (similar to dactylitis syphilitica in the late phase of syphilis) [95, 96]. The affected joints and bones were usually located underneath the skin lesions. The patients with skeletal involvement had had their disease for a longer period than the patients with skin lesions alone [81, 95, 96]. In 17 of 86 (20%) patients, episodic attacks of joint effusions of a knee were found to have preceded or have occured simultaneously with the ACA lesions [81]. Periarticular manifestations – such as knee or olecranon bursitis, epicondylitis, retro- or subcalcaneal bursitis, and Achilles tendinitis on the same extremity as the cutaneous involvement – have been reported; they usually precede, but sometimes also accompany ACA [81, 100].

According to some reports, enlarged regional lymph nodes are a common finding in patients with ACA [101]. Some patients report headaches, myalgia and/or arthralgia [92].

Diagnosis

For proper diagnosis, appropriate clinical findings should be corroborated with the establishment of borrelial infection. Patients with ACA usually have high serum concentrations of borrelial IgG antibody; the absence of borrelial antibody in a patient with clinically suspicious ACA should be the reason for rechecking the diagnosis and searching for an alternative explanation, because 'seronegative' ACA patients are almost nonexistent [16, 17, 95, 96]. Histologic examination of the involved skin is also needed in suspected ACA, for exclusion of other possibilities and for consolidating the diagnosis of ACA. The histologic findings depend on the duration and severity of the skin involvement; more or less pronounced lymphocytic and plasma cell infiltration of dermis (and sometimes subcutis) is frequently seen, with or without atrophy [17, 95, 96]. Thus, the diagnosis of ACA is based on clinical, serologic and histologic criteria. Routine laboratory tests may find mild-to-moderately elevated erythrocyte sedimentation rates, and raised γ-globulin and C-reactive protein concentrations, but these are usually in normal range and are not of substantial diagnostic help [17, 96]. Diagnosis of ACA can be further supported by the isolation of borreliae from the involved skin; isolation is successful in about one third of patients who have not previously received antibiotics [91].

Differential Diagnosis

ACA is a relatively frequent borrelial skin manifestation that usually causes many diagnostic problems [17, 95, 96]. It can be the first and only sign of Lyme borreliosis, although a detailed history may reveal antecedent signs of the disease. Previous EM on the extremity on which months to years later a skin lesion compatible with ACA develops has been reported by about 10–20% of patients. In some patients, the history reveals preceding nervous system or joint involvement [17, 95, 96].

ACA is often overlooked or misinterpreted, not only by patients, but also by their physicians. Frequent visits to the doctor without establishing a proper diagnosis are more often the rule than the exception. Difficulties in recognition are usually the result of limited acquaintance with the disease, but can also be a consequence of atypical clinical features. ACA has many differential diagnoses, which partly depend on the stage of the disease. ACA skin lesions on lower extremities are often falsely interpreted to be a result of vascular insufficiency (chronic venous insufficiency, superficial thrombophlebitis, hypostatic eczema, arterial obliterative disease, acrocyanosis, livedo reticularis, lymphedema, etc.), a consequence of old age ('old skin') or chilblains. Fibrous nodules are often misinterpreted as rheumatoid nodules and sometimes as skin involvement in the course of gout (tophi) or even as erythema nodosum. It is not unusual for patients with ACA to visit their doctor because of difficulties with shoes associated with deformations of joints, or because of dysesthesias, hyperesthesias or paresthesias. General physicians and the specialists to whom these patients are quite frequently referred often fail to appreciate ACA skin lesions, do not take them seriously or are not able to associate the skin lesions with the involvement of joints and/or peripheral nervous system [17, 95, 96].

ACA should be considered as a possible diagnosis in a patient with bluish-red discoloration of a limb with or without swelling and/or atrophy [67].

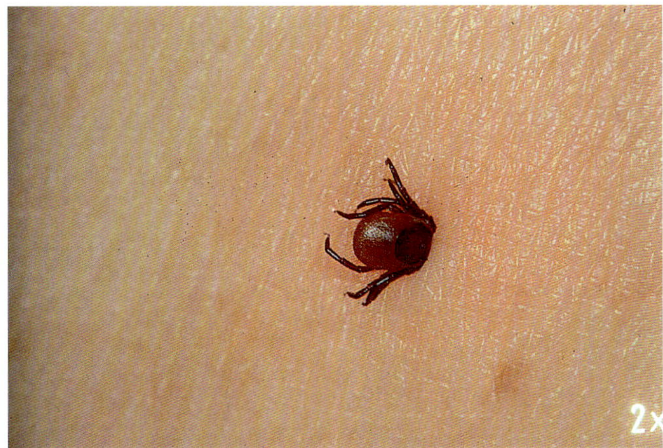

Fig. 1. Adult tick on a human host (kindly supplied by Prof. D. Lipsker).

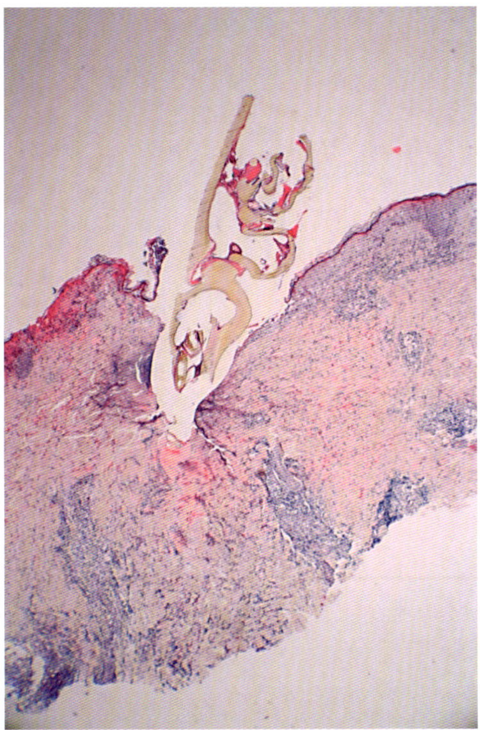

Fig. 2. Cutaneous biopsy of a tick bite. Mouth piece of the tick (yellow) is within the human dermis (kindly supplied by Prof. D. Lipsker).

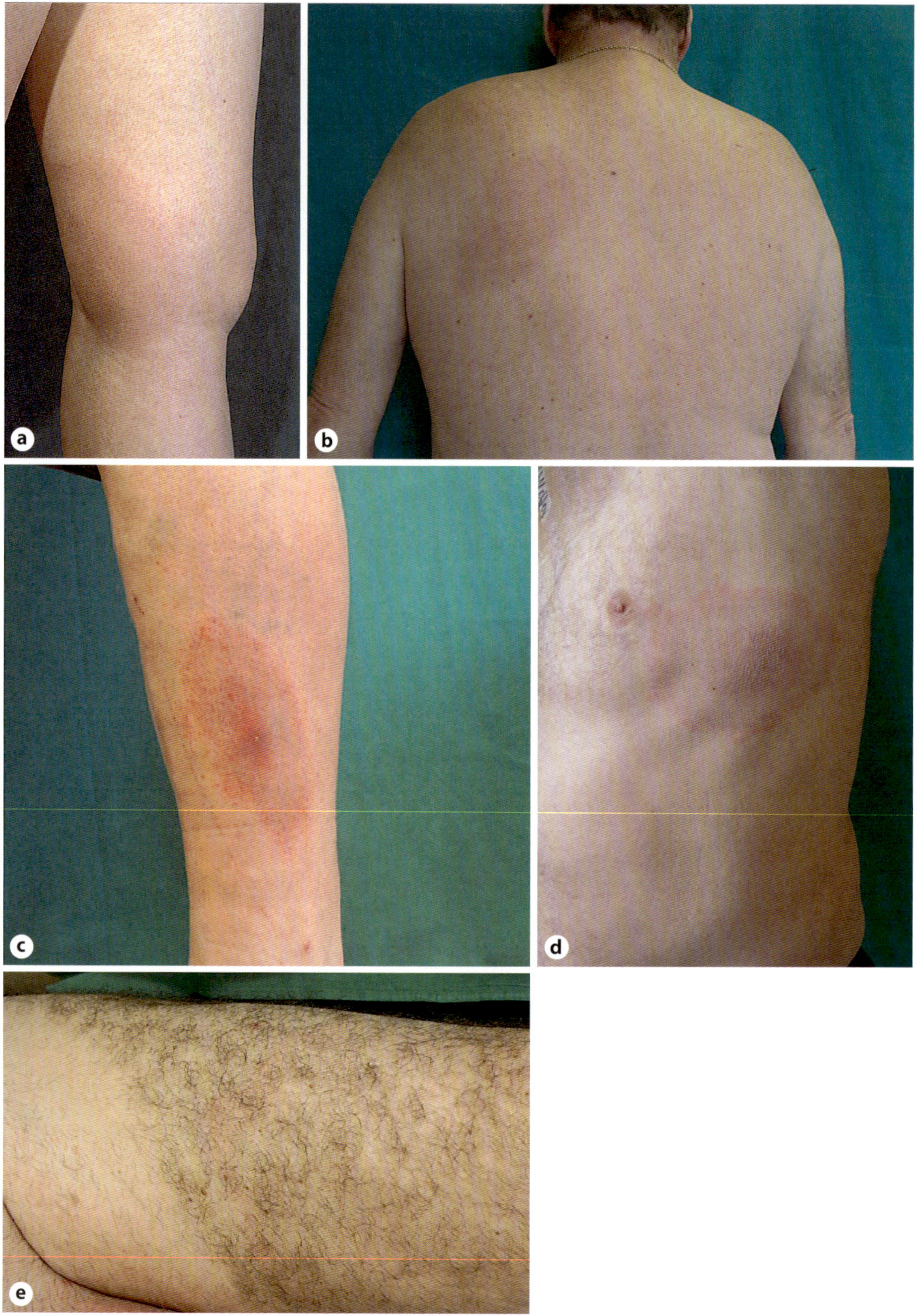

Fig. 3. Examples of erythema migrans with or without central clearing. Erythema migrans is a slowly expanding red macule or plaque. Usually, but not always, the periphery of the lesion is more visible and can be slightly raised. Many variants exist, including lesions with more inflammation as well as small lesions. In other patients, the erythema is hardly visible (**e**) (kindly supplied by Prof. D. Lipsker).

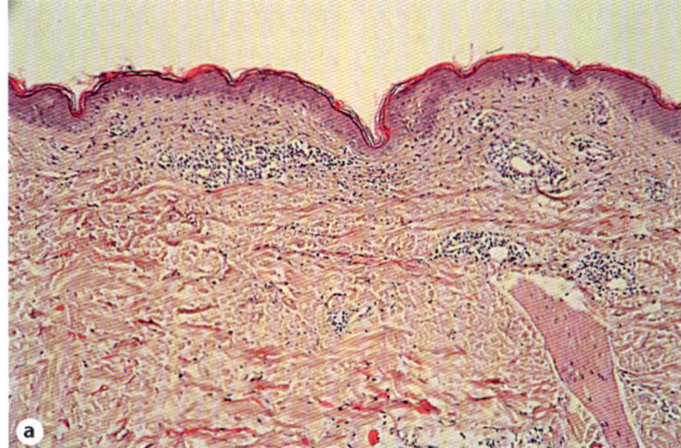

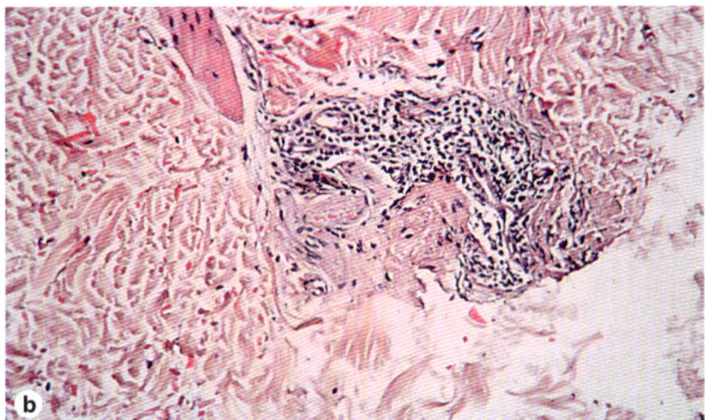

Fig. 4. Biopsy specimen of erythema migrans. A perivascular and perisudoral lymphocytic infiltrate is common, and some findings will help lead experienced dermatopathologists to the diagnosis. Clues are interstitial spreading, the presence of plasma cells and perineural involvement (kindly supplied by Prof. D. Lipsker).

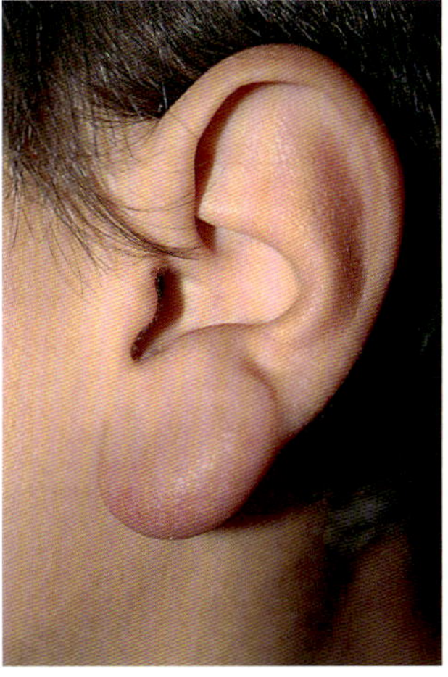

Fig. 5. A redish-blue nodule on the ear lobe is a typical finding in borrelial lymphocytoma (kindly supplied by Prof. D. Lipsker).

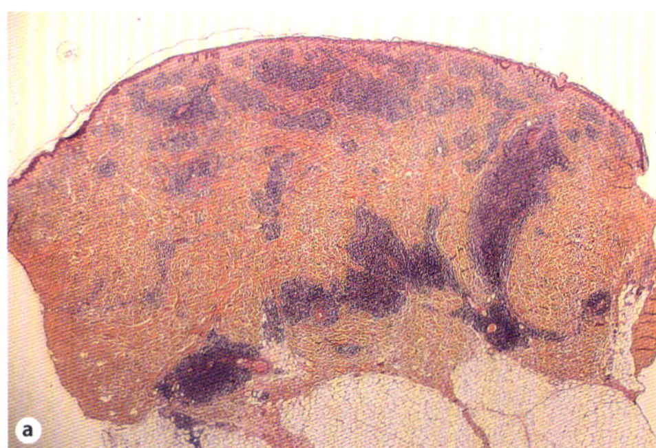

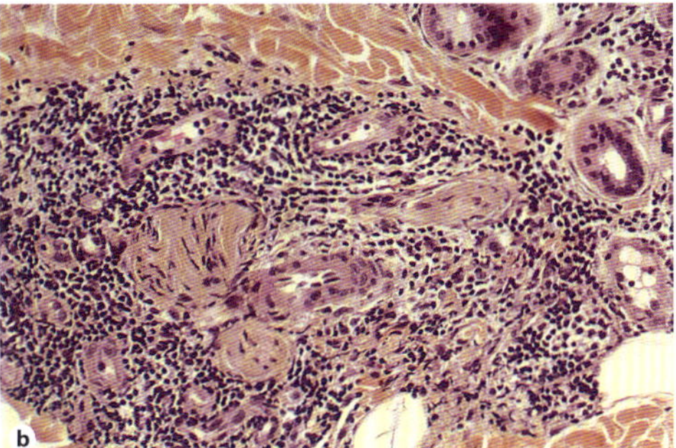

Fig. 6. Biopsy specimen of borrelial lymphocytoma. A dense perivascular and perisudoral lymphocytic infiltrate is present and perinervous involvement, as well as the presence of some plasma cells, should raise suspicion of borrelial lymphocytoma (kindly supplied by Prof. D. Lipsker).

Fig. 7. Acrodermatitis chronica atrophicans manifests first as a red violaceous inflammatory patch (**a**), mainly localized on an extremity. Within months to years it atrophies, and thus the skin becomes wrinkly, and superficial vessels become visible through a transparent epidermis and dermis (**b**, **c**) (kindly supplied by Prof. D. Lipsker).

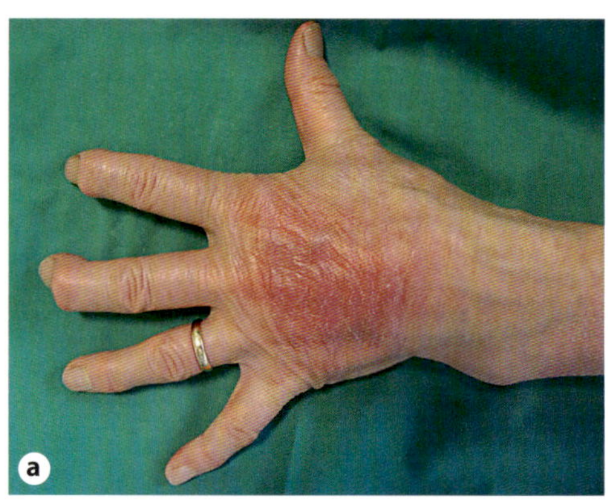

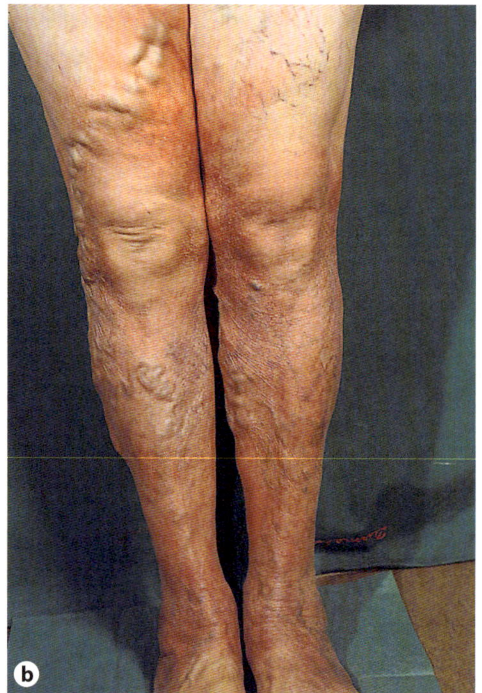

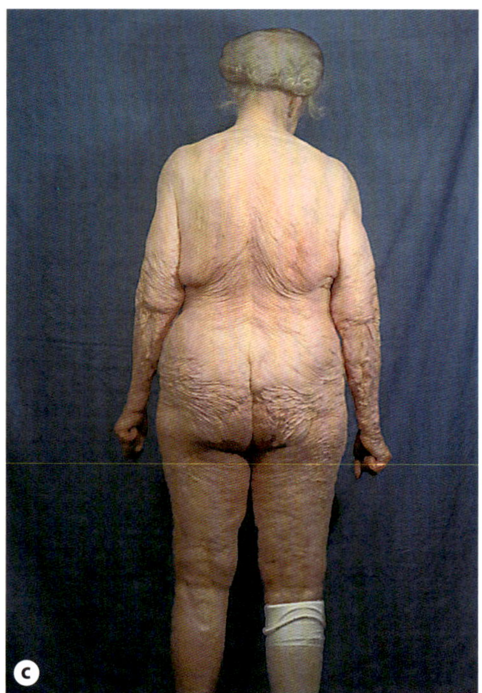

8

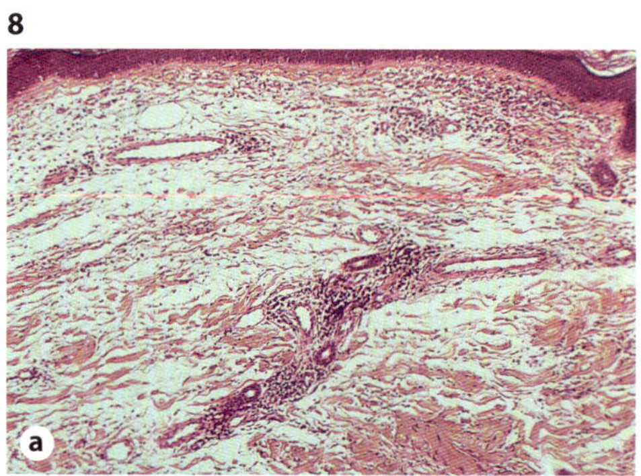

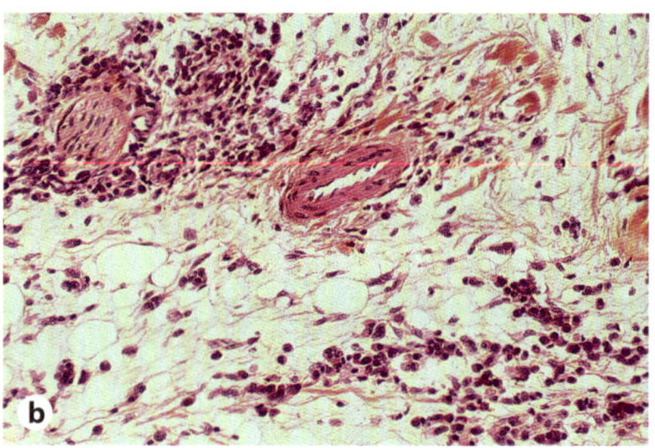

Other Skin Manifestations of Potential Borrelial Etiology

Scleroderma circumscripta and Lichen sclerosus et atrophicus

Soon after the recognition that Lyme disease is a multisystem disorder, several dermatologic entities were proposed as candidate manifestations of the disease. EM was accepted very early as being the essential part of the disease, and has been recognized as a clinical hallmark of Lyme borreliosis; somewhat later, ACA and solitary lymphocytoma (lymphadenosis benigna cutis) were clearly demonstrated to be representations of skin manifestations of Lyme borreliosis. Discussions on the potential borrelial etiology of scleroderma circumscripta and lichen sclerosus et atrophicus (sclerotic skin lesions of unknown etiology) have been continuing.

Borrelial etiology of these 2 entities has been implicated on the basis of humoral and cellular immune responses to *B. burgdorferi* s.l., immunohistologic findings or silver staining, as well as demonstration of borrelial DNA in and isolation of borreliae from lesional tissue. However, findings reported in the literature are markedly discordant. The highest prevalence of antibodies to *B. burgdorferi* s.l. was found among scleroderma circumscripta patients in Austria (33–54%) and Switzerland (up to 38%), whereas no differences were found in the frequency or level of borrelial antibodies compared with controls in most other European countries [67], the USA [102] and Japan [103]. Lymphoproliferative responses to *B. burgdorferi* s.l., reflecting the cellular immune response of patients, were elevated in about one third of 39 Austrian patients with scleroderma circumscripta [104], whereas analyses of 52 Swiss patients gave inconclusive results [105]. Because of pronounced limitations in specificity and sensitivity of lymphocyte proliferation assays, these findings cannot be reliably interpreted; therefore, the use of this diagnostic approach for the diagnosis of borrelial infection has been discouraged [14]. There have been several attempts to demonstrate borreliae in the skin lesions. As reviewed by Mullegger [67] in 2004, spirochetes were found by immunohistology or silver staining of lesional tissue from about 20 patients with scleroderma circumscripta and a similar number with lichen sclerosus et atrophicans. Those methods, however, are susceptible to artifacts and interpretation faults, and the findings could not be reproduced by other investigators. In the same review, Mullegger [67] reported that PCR studies of lesional skin gave positive results in 21 of 140 scleroderma circumscripta patients and 15 of 40 lichen sclerosus et atrophicans patients in Europe (particularly Germany and Italy) and Ja-

Fig. 8. Even at late and atrophic stages (**a**), diagnosis of acrodermatitis chronica atrophicans should be suspected histologically as plasma cells remain abundant (**b**). There are numerous clinical and pathological variants, mimicking granuloma annulare or interstitial granulomatous dermatitis, but the presence of plasma cells and a perineural involvement are rarely missing (kindly supplied by Prof. D. Lipsker).

pan [106], whereas *B. burgdorferi* s.l.-specific DNA could not be amplified in any of 98 scleroderma circumscripta and 48 lichen sclerosus et atrophicans patients in the USA [106, 107]. With the exception of positive PCR findings in some additional patients, nothing substantially new has happened during the past 4 years (2004–2008). Various types of primer have been used in the PCR studies, for example, primers specific for flagellin, ospA, or rRNA genes of *B. burgdorferi* s.l. The negative studies appear to be more comprehensive in that usually more than 1 primer set was applied to a larger collection of cases [67]. Some of the PCR-positive cases were seronegative; however, a positive PCR in a seronegative patient with a manifestation lasting for several months or even years should be regarded with skepticism [14, 108]. The attempt to isolate *B. burgdorferi* s.l. from lesional skin [67] was successful in 5 scleroderma circumscripta patients from Austria and southern Germany [109–111], but failed in most other studies [112, 113]. For lichen sclerosus et atrophicans, the demonstration of *B. burgdorferi* s.l. by cultivation has succeeded in probably only 1 patient so far [114]. The isolation of the causative agent (borreliae) from the lesion is the most reliable demonstration of the etiology of the process, and indicates that culture-positive scleroderma circumscripta and lichen sclerosus et atrophicans lesions were really caused by *B. burgdorferi* s.l. Although such findings might indicate that a subset of scleroderma circumscripta and lichen sclerosus et atrophicus is of borrelial origin, it may well be that this subset of patients in fact have ACA with sclerotic lesions. Sclerotic lesions, which are clinically and histologically indistinguishable from localized scleroderma (morphea) or lichen sclerosus et atrophicus, develop in about 10% of patients with typical inflammatory ACA [93, 96].

Cutaneous Lymphoma

A possible association between primary cutaneous B cell lymphomas and *B. burgdorferi* s.l. infection was first suspected because of raised serum borrelial antibody titers in several small series of patients with primary cutaneous B cell lymphoma. This was later supported by more definite evidence, including demonstration of borrelial DNA by PCR in 18–35% of European patients with various types of primary cutaneous B cell lymphoma [67, 115], and by isolation of *B. burgdorferi* s.l. from skin lesions in 2 further patients [116]. In addition, the results of a recent case-control study in Denmark and Sweden suggest an association between *B. burgdorferi* s.l. infection and risk of mantle cell lymphoma [117]. These European results are in contrast to findings in the USA and Asia, where neither molecular [118] nor epidemiologic [119] studies could demonstrate an etiopathogenetic role for *B. burgdorferi* s.l. in cutaneous B cell lymphoma. This discrepancy was interpreted as possibly due to differences between *B. burgdorferi* s.l. strains on the different continents. As shown in ACA, *B. burgdorferi* s.l. can persist in the skin for many years, despite the presence of an active host immune system, possibly by modulation of surface antigens by the spirochete [17]. In analogy to *Helicobacter pylori*-associated MALT (mucosa-associated lymphoid tissue) lymphomas, it is conceivable that the chronic stimulation of skin-associated lymphoid tissues in response to *B. burgdorferi* s.l. infection may be operative in the pathogenesis of a subset of primary cutaneous B cell lymphoma [67, 120].

The association of borrelial infection and cutaneous B cell lymphomas might have substantial practical consequences concerning management of these lymphomas. Although from a scientific point of view the magnitude and even the existence of this association are still uncertain, everyday clinical practice has been influenced. The European Organization for Research and Treatment of Cancer and the International Society for Cutaneous Lymphoma recently published consensus recommendations on management of cutaneous B cell lymphomas in which the authors stated that 'because an association between *B. burgdorferi* infection has been reported in a significant minority of European cases of primary cutaneous marginal zone lymphoma, but not in Asian cases or cases from the United States [115, 118, 120, 121], in European areas with endemic *B. burgdorferi* infection, the presence of *B. burgdorferi* should be investigated by serology and polymerase chain reaction techniques on skin biopsy specimens' [122]. In the article, treatment with antibiotics is proposed for patients with primary cutaneous marginal zone lymphoma and evidence of *B. burgdorferi* s.l. infection [122]. The proposal is based on analogy with antibiotic treatment of gastric mucosa-associated lymphoid tissue lymphomas to eradicate *Helicobacter pylori* [123–125] and on several recent reviews suggesting that primary cutaneous marginal-zone lymphoma associated with *B. burgdorferi* s.l. infection should first be treated with antibiotics before more aggressive therapies are used [67, 126]. However, the efficacy of antibiotic treatment in borrelia-associated primary cutaneous marginal-zone lymphoma is poorly documented [116, 122, 127–131]. Six of 14 (43%) reported patients achieved clinical response after various antibiotic regimens; data on 8 patients suggest that systemic treatment with cephalosporins is superior to oral treatment with high-dose tetracyclines [122].

We may hope that in the next few years more information will be available on the association of *Borrelia* infection and cutaneous B cell lymphoma, which at the moment seems to be operative in a subset of European patients with this type of lymphoma.

Nervous System Involvement

Lyme Neuroborreliosis

Lyme neuroborreliosis is the involvement of the central and/or peripheral nervous systems in an infection with *B. burgdorferi* s.l.

Etiology

In America, all manifestations of Lyme borreliosis, including Lyme neuroborreliosis, are caused by *B. burgdorferi* s.s.

Table 2. Genospecies of *B. burgdorferi* s.l. as agents of Lyme neuroborreliosis in European patients [modified from 136]

Mode of detection	Reference No.	Genospecies				All
		B. garinii	*B. afzelii*	*B. burgdorferi* s.s.	others	
Isolation from CSF	134	21	10	4	1[1]	36
	133	3				3
	135	25	14	1		40
	32	5	1			6
	38	26	8	1		35
	136	23	10	3		36
	39	38	15	18	1[2]	72
Total		141	58	27	2	228 (75)
PCR (CSF)	137	11	1		1[1]	13
	138	4	1	2		7
Total		15	2	2	1	20 (7)
Serology	133	18	2	3	5[3]	28
	132	16	7	2	3[4]	28
Total		34	9	5	8	56 (18)
Total		190 (63)	69 (23)	34 (11)	11 (4)	304 (100)

Figures in parentheses are percentages.
[1] *B. garinii* and *B. afzelii*. [2] *B. bissettii*. [3] Inconclusive. [4] *B. valaisiana*.

In Europe, Lyme neuroborreliosis is most often caused by *B. garinii*, less frequently by *B. afzelii*, rarely by *B. burgdorferi* s.s. and only exceptionally by other *Borrelia* species such as *B. valaisiana* [132], *B. bissettii* [39–41] or as yet unidentifiable species [133]. The information is based on results of typing borreliae isolated from CSF of patients with Lyme neuroborreliosis [32, 38, 39, 133–136], demonstration of distinct nucleic acid sequences of *Borrelia* species in the CSF [137, 138] and on species-specific serologic responses [132, 133]. In all the approaches, the principal species found in patients with Lyme neuroborreliosis was *B. garinii*, followed by *B. afzelii* (table 2). However, the design of some of the cited studies does not allow one to draw very precise conclusions on the proportion of the etiologic agents, because of several potential biases in the collection of isolates and in their selection for typing.

A comparison of patients with *B. garinii* or *B. afzelii* isolated from CSF found that patients with *B. garinii* infection have a clinical presentation distinct from that of patients with *B. afzelii* [136]. In contrast to the *B. garinii* group, the large majority of the *B. afzelii* group did not fulfil the European criteria for Lyme neuroborreliosis [12, 13]. The findings of the study might indicate that although *B. afzelii* is able to pass through the blood-brain barrier, it has restricted ability to initiate substantial inflammation of the CNS [136]. The significance of this genospecies and of *B. valaisiana* and *B. bissettii* in Lyme neuroborreliosis remains to be elucidated.

Frequency

Although in the 1980s early neurologic Lyme disease was reported to occur in approximately 10–15% of untreated patients with Lyme disease in the USA [139, 140], the frequency of this manifestation has become less in more recent reports [14, 16, 141], possibly because of bias of ascertainment in the early studies and/or improved recognition and treatment of patients with EM [14]. In the USA, cranial neuropathy is the most common manifestation of early neurologic Lyme disease [142]. Peripheral facial palsy is the most common of the cranial neuropathies, and bilateral involvement of nerve VII may occur [143, 144]. In areas where Lyme disease is endemic, about 1 in 4 patients who present with nerve VII palsy in nonwinter months can be shown to have Lyme disease [145]. By far the most common borrelial CNS disorder in the USA is lymphocytic meningitis [146]; Lyme encephalitis seems to be extremely rare. Although there are no firm incidence numbers, estimates are that no more than 1 patient per 1 million population at risk will develop this disorder in any year [146].

Whereas there are several (minor) differences between American and European Lyme borreliosis, the general trends in the frequency of clinical manifestations in Europe are most probably similar. Among 1,471 patients with Lyme borreliosis in an epidemiologic study in southern Sweden, the most frequent clinical manifestation was EM (77%), followed by Lyme neuroborreliosis (16%) and arthritis (7%) [29]. According to data from the National Institute of Public Health in Slovenia, Lyme neuroborreliosis represented 24% of all cases of Lyme borreliosis in 1988 [30], whereas during the past 10 years about 90% of patients were registered with EM and only 4–7% with Lyme neuroborreliosis [31]. Data from the Ljubljana Lyme borreliosis clinic are shown in table 1. In Slovenia, about 20% of adult patients and 25% of children with peripheral facial palsy are associated with Lyme borreliosis [147, unpublished data].

Tick Bites

In meningopolyneuritis (Garin-Bujadoux-Bannwarth syndrome), the most prominent clinical manifestation of Lyme neuroborreliosis in adult European patients, between one and two thirds of patients remember arthropod bites preceding the onset of the neurologic involvement [148]. According to the study of Kristoferitsch [149], a median of 3 weeks (range 1–18 weeks) elapses from the bite to the onset of neurologic symptoms. However, the causal relationship between an individual tick bite and Lyme neuroborreliosis is rather uncertain; it is most reliable when a bite is followed by an EM. This skin lesion has been reported to precede or sometimes accompany meningopolyneuritis in 34–64% of patients [148–151], and has been found in 18 of 33 (55%) patients with *B. garinii* or *B. afzelii* isolated from CSF [136]. Close topical association between the cutaneous region involved by the EM (and thus by the tick bite) and the initial radicular lesion has been established in European patients [148, 151–

156], in contrast to American patients in whom no such association was found [146, 157].

Histology

Knowledge of histopathologic findings in the CNS is limited. In patients with meningoradiculoneuritis, lymphocytic involvement of leptomeninges, ganglia, and afferent and efferent rootlets is present. The CNS may show focal microgliosis [57, 158, 159].

In peripheral neuropathy accompanied by ACA, lymphocytes and plasma cells are present around blood vessels in the perineurium, with occasional sparse lymphocytes in the vessel wall. Vessel walls show no signs of necrosis, but may become thickened and obliterated; thrombosis may develop [57]. Fibers within the nerve eventually lose myelin. The most striking finding is axonal degeneration [57, 98].

Neuropathologic and neurophysiologic evidence in patients with peripheral nervous system involvement resulting from borrelial infection [146], and in experimentally infected rhesus macaque monkeys [160], indicates that this infection causes changes in multiple peripheral nerves that are affected individually (mononeuropathia multiplex type of involvement) as a consequence of local damage to vessels (but without evidence of vessel wall necrosis, the usual requirement to be termed vasculitis) [146].

Clinical Characteristics

Early Lyme Neuroborreliosis

Lyme neuroborreliosis may appear early, during the first few weeks or months, or late in the course of Lyme borreliosis. The initial clinical report of early Lyme neuroborreliosis was in 1922 [161], although it was not classified as such until more than 65 years later. Early Lyme neuroborreliosis typically comprises lymphocytic meningitis and involvement of cranial and peripheral nerves [3, 156, 157, 162]. Usually the most pronounced clinical symptom is pain as a result of radiculoneuritis. The pain is usually severe and most pronounced during the night; patients may be deprived of sleep for several weeks. When located in the thoracic or abdominal region, the pain is often belt-like. Radicular pain is seen more often in European than in American patients, and is usually more frequent and more pronounced in adults than children [16, 157, 162]. Although painful radiculoneuritis is clinically the most typical and pronounced manifestation of peripheral nervous system involvement in adults with early European Lyme neuroborreliosis, other types of peripheral nerve involvement may be present. Involvement of motoric nerves may lead to paresis, usually asymmetric [162, 163] and, in contrast to general opinion, not always clinically prominent [164].

Patients with borrelial meningitis usually suffer from mild intermittent headache, but in some patients the headache may be excruciating. In adult European patients, there is often no fever, nausea is usually mild or absent, and vomiting is frequently absent. Meningeal signs are usually only mildly expressed or may be absent [162, 163]. Physicians not used to patients with borrelial meningitis are often surprised by abnormal CSF findings. These comprise lymphocytic pleocytosis up to several hundred $\times 10^6$ cells/l, normal or slight-to-moderately elevated protein concentration, and normal or mildly depleted glucose concentration. Overall, the course of borrelial meningitis resembles relatively mild but unusually protracted viral meningitis with intermittent improvements and deterioration [3].

Any cranial nerve may be affected in early Lyme neuroborreliosis, but facial nerves are by far the most frequently involved (about 80%), resulting in unilateral or bilateral peripheral facial palsy [3, 143, 145–147, 157]. Patients with borrelial peripheral facial palsy often show lymphocytic pleocytosis, even those without any sign or symptom of meningitis [3, 16, 146, 147]. According to general opinion, prognosis of borrelial peripheral facial palsy is good not only in antibiotic-treated patients, but also in those who are not treated [16, 157, 163]. According to data from the USA, more than 90% of patients show improvement leading to, or close to, normal [143, 145, 146]. However, in clinical and neurophysiologic examinations, mild sequelae were found in as many as half of Swedish children who had peripheral facial palsy associated with Lyme neuroborreliosis 3–5 years earlier [165]. Results from another Swedish study revealed that one fifth of children with acute facial palsy have permanent mild-to-moderate dysfunction of the facial nerve, but that other neurologic symptoms or health problems do not accompany the sequelae of the facial palsy, and that treatment of Lyme neuroborreliosis seems to have no correlation with clinical outcome of peripheral facial palsy [166]. Shortly after onset of symptoms, intrathecal antibodies may not be detectable and CSF pleocytosis may be absent in patients (predominantly children) with isolated facial palsy [3]. Patients who present with peripheral facial palsy as the sole neurologic manifestation of Lyme borreliosis only very rarely have (a history of recent) EM. Involvement of most other cranial nerves has been described, but particularly III (oculomotor), VI (abducens) and VIII (vestibulo-auditory). Critical appraisal of the literature suggests that the involvement of some cranial nerves (for example, optic nerve) occurs extremely rarely, if ever [146, 167].

In adult European patients, early Lyme neuroborreliosis usually begins gradually with increasing pain, later on accompanied by palsies and other neurologic signs and symptoms that will, if untreated, not diminish for many weeks [3]. In children, painful radiculoneuritis is rare, but isolated meningitis and peripheral facial palsy are more common than in adults. In Slovenia, about 20% of adult patients and 25% of children with peripheral facial palsy have associated Lyme borreliosis [147, unpublished data]. Pseudotumor cerebri is an unusual manifestation of Lyme neuroborreliosis seen primarily in children [168, 169].

Late Lyme Neuroborreliosis

With the exception of peripheral neuritis in association with ACA, late Lyme neuroborreliosis is most probably very rare. Peripheral neuritis occurs in more than half of patients with long-lasting (advanced) ACA skin lesions [162, 170]. Critical appraisal of the literature suggests that peripheral neuritis without ACA is an extremely rare condition; that is, among patients with peripheral neuropathy, the proportion of those with Lyme neuroborreliosis is negligible.

Up to 10% of European patients with untreated meningopolyneuritis (Garin-Bujadoux-Bannwarth syndrome) develop features of disseminated encephalomyelitis that may in some respects resemble those seen in multiple sclerosis [162].

Subtle encephalopathy has been reported predominantly by American authors [16, 157, 171].

Diagnosis

Lyme neuroborreliosis may appear during the first few weeks or months after infection or not until late in the course of Lyme borreliosis. Early Lyme neuroborreliosis, which is better defined and much more frequent than late Lyme neuroborreliosis [1, 3, 12, 13, 18], typically comprises lymphocytic meningitis and involvement of cranial and peripheral nerves [157]. Clinical diagnosis is straightforward when the triad is complete or when 1 or more manifestations of the triad are associated with the presence of or a reliable history of EM [1, 3, 12, 13, 18, 157].

The diagnosis of early Lyme neuroborreliosis is normally based on clinical characteristics, the presence of lymphocytic pleocytosis and demonstration of CNS borrelial infection, as evidenced by seroconversion, intrathecal borrelial antibody production, isolation of borreliae from CSF samples or demonstration of borrelial DNA in CSF samples [12, 13, 108, 136]. In practice, seroconversion is rarely found to be a useful criterion because by the time that neurologic signs appear, the majority of patients are seropositive. In addition, seroconversion confirms recent borrelial infection, but it does not confirm CNS involvement. The main limitations of PCR for demonstration of borrelial DNA in CSF samples are low sensitivity, the possibility of false-positive findings and the lack of procedure standardization [13, 108]. Isolation of the etiologic agent from patient samples is the most reliable method for diagnosis of borrelial infection, and isolation of the etiologic agent from CSF is the most reliable method for diagnosis of Lyme neuroborreliosis. Isolation also provides live microorganisms that can be further characterized; however, isolation from CSF samples is a markedly low-yield procedure, and results are obtainable only after several weeks [1, 3, 108, 136, 172]. Demonstration of intrathecally synthesized borrelial antibodies has generally been used for establishment of a diagnosis of Lyme neuroborreliosis in everyday European clinical practice. The problem with this diagnostic approach is insensitivity during the first few weeks of CNS involvement and long persistence of the antibodies; intrathecal borrelial antibody production can be detected for several months or years, even after appropriate antibiotic treatment [12, 13, 108, 136].

A diagnosis of Lyme neuroborreliosis involving the peripheral nervous system is even more difficult because of the limited possibilities of demonstrating borrelial infection of peripheral nerves. For a reliable diagnosis, (an objective) proof of the involvement of the nervous system is necessary (clinical, neurophysiologic and neuropathologic approaches are generally available for demonstration of peripheral nervous system involvement), together with demonstration of (active) borrelial infection (usually the only available approach in this group of patients is demonstration of borrelial antibodies in serum; however, serology has many limitations) and proof that the borrelial infection really is the cause of the peripheral nervous system involvement. Because of the many obstacles with all 3 requirements (the second and especially the third are even harder to fulfil than the first), it is obvious that reliable diagnosis of peripheral nervous system involvement as a consequence of borrelial infection profoundly depends upon the concomitant presence of CNS Lyme neuroborreliosis (in which borrelial CNS involvement can be demonstrated by corresponding findings in CSF examination) and/or the presence of some other manifestations of Lyme borreliosis such as EM (for example, in patients with cranial nerve involvement) or ACA.

Differential Diagnosis
Differential diagnosis comprises a list of differential diagnoses for each main manifestation of Lyme neuroborreliosis [meningitis, radiculo(neuritis), cranial nerve involvement and so on]. However, an exact history and meticulous clinical examination often substantially narrow the differential possibilities.

Cardiac Involvement

Lyme Carditis

Lyme carditis is heart involvement related to a *Borrelia* infection that usually presents with the acute onset of varying degrees of intermittent atrioventricular (A-V) heart block, sometimes in association with clinical evidence of myopericarditis.

Frequency
Information on the relative frequency of Lyme carditis is incomplete. Lyme carditis had earlier been reported to occur in 0.3–4% of untreated European patients with Lyme borreliosis and in 4–10% of corresponding patients in the USA [14, 173–175]. However, the frequency of this manifestation is reported to be much lower in more recent series [176, 177]. No evidence of carditis was found among 233 cases with definite Lyme disease in 2 prospective studies on the evaluation of a recombinant OspA vaccine in the USA [178, 179]; in a Swedish epidemiologic study, only 7 of 1,471 (0.5%) patients diagnosed with Lyme borreliosis had Lyme carditis [29], and at the Ljubljana Lyme borreliosis clinic, where between 600 and 900 patients with different manifestations of Lyme borreliosis are diagnosed each year, Lyme carditis represents up to 0.5% of cases [unpublished data]. This diminution in the frequency of Lyme carditis, like the one observed for acute neurologic manifestations, could be the result of a bias of ascertainment in early studies and/or improved recognition and treatment of patients with EM [14].

Etiology

There are no direct data on the *Borrelia* species causing Lyme carditis. In the USA, Lyme carditis should be caused by *B. burgdorferi* s.s., the only species causing Lyme borreliosis in humans there; in Europe, the main candidates are *B. afzelii*, *B. garinii* and *B. burgdorferi* s.s. A heart isolate of 1990 [180] was later identified as *B. burgdorferi* s.s., but this has not been published.

Tick Bites

In a series of 20 patients with Lyme carditis presented by Steere et al. [174], 2 reported a tick bite, and in a series of 66 European patients with Lyme carditis collected by van der Linde [175], tick bite prior to the onset of Lyme carditis was recalled by 31 (47%) patients.

Histology

Information on histologic findings is limited, and is based on rare cases of heart tissue examination obtained at autopsy and on material acquired by endomyocardial biopsy. Histopathologic findings include an interstitial infiltrate of lymphocytes and plasma cells involving the myocardium, pericardium and endocardium. Aggregates of lymphocytes may be seen in the myocardium. Muscle fibers are usually intact, but individual myocardial fibers show sporadic infiltration with lymphocytes. The endocardium shows band-like infiltrates of lymphocytes and plasma cells [174, 175, 181, 182]. Examination of the heart conducting system in 1 patient revealed localized edema and slight lymphocytic infiltration of sinoatrial and A-V nodes, fibers with contraction band necrosis in an edematous area of the sinoatrial node, focal edema in the bundle of Hiss, and a fibrotic lesion in the left bundle branch [57]. Vasculitis involving the small and large intramyocardial vessels can be present [173]. The small vessels frequently show endothelial cell edema, whereas large vessels show adventitial infiltrates with loose reticulin and increased collagen deposition [158, 183]. Spirochetal forms located inside and near cellular infiltrates, between muscle fibers, and in the myocardium [158, 184, 185] have been found in endomyocardial biopsy [184] and autopsy specimens [181]. They have also been cultured from biopsy specimens [180]. Whether the presence of live borreliae is required for continued disease or whether the disease results (predominantly) from immune-mediated mechanisms remains to be determined [173].

Clinical Characteristics

Lyme carditis typically occurs between June and December, usually within 2 months (range 4 days–7 months) after the onset of infection, and more often affects men than women [14, 174, 176, 186]. The cardiac manifestations are often coincident or in close temporal proximity with other features of Lyme borreliosis such as EM [174, 186, 187], Lyme neuroborreliosis [174, 187] or arthritis [174, 185]. In a large European series of patients who had Lyme carditis, EM was found in 67%, joint complaints in 51% and Lyme neuroborreliosis in 27% [185]. However, there are patients who present with

Lyme carditis (usually with complete heart block) as the sole manifestation of Lyme borreliosis.

Cardiac involvement may be asymptomatic. When symptomatic, the most common complaints include light-headedness, syncope, dyspnea, palpitations and/or chest pain [173]. Patients with symptomatic cardiac involvement associated with Lyme borreliosis usually present with the acute onset of varying degrees of intermittent A-V heart block, sometimes in association with clinical evidence of myopericarditis [174, 176, 183, 185–187]. Electrophysiologic studies have usually demonstrated block occurring above the bundle of Hiss, often involving the A-V node, but heart block may occur at multiple levels [174, 176, 185]. Cases of pericarditis, endocarditis, myocardial infarction, coronary artery aneurism, QT-interval prolongation and congestive heart failure have also been associated with Lyme borreliosis [173], but for some of these the causal association remains uncertain.

Lyme carditis is characterized by changing A-V blocks as a result of conduction disturbances [18, 174, 176, 185]. The course is usually favorable. In both antibiotically treated and untreated patients, complete heart block usually disappears within a week, whereas symptoms of heart involvement and ECG abnormalities usually vanish within 3–6 weeks [14, 174, 176, 185]. Hospitalization and permanent ECG surveillance are needed in patients who have first-degree A-V block with P-Q interval longer than 0.30 s, second- or third-degree A-V blocks, quickly changing A-V blocks or hemodynamically important arrhythmias [3, 176, 185]. In a case of complete heart block, insertion of temporary heart pacemaker may be life-saving. Complications are rare and include partial improvement of conduction disturbances with a consequent persistent (first-degree A-V) block, and possible induction of chronic cardiomyopathy [180]. Complete heart block would be the only reason for a lethal outcome in patients with Lyme borreliosis, and fortunately it is an extremely rare event [3, 16, 188].

Diffuse ST segment and T wave changes on surface electrocardiograms were noted in 65% of patients in the series of patients with Lyme carditis of Steere [174]; although nonspecific, these findings may indicate diffuse myocardial involvement [173]. Myocardial involvement may lead to cardiomegaly, left-ventricular dysfunction or clinical congestive heart failure and is thought to be present in 10–15% of patients with Lyme carditis [185, 186]. In most cases, myocardial dysfunction is mild and self-limited [174, 189].

It has been suggested that borreliae may play a causative role in chronic heart failure. This hypothesis originated from a 1990 Austrian case report on a 54-year-old man with a 4-year history of dilated cardiomyopathy, high levels of *B. burgdorferi* s.l. IgG antibodies in serum, and isolation of *B. burgdorferi* s.l. from an endomyocardial biopsy specimen [180]. The hypothesis was supported in some later reports on a limited number of patients [190, 191], whereas in other reports, apparently more convincing ones, it was not backed up [192]. Further studies are warranted to clarify the potential role of *B. burgdorferi* s.l. in acute and chronic congestive heart failure [173]. According to the recent IDSA guidelines [14], severe or fulminant congestive heart failure or development of valvular heart disease are not associated with Lyme disease [176] and, at least in the USA, there is no convincing evidence that Lyme disease is a cause of chronic cardiomyopathy [192, 193].

Diagnosis

Lyme carditis usually presents with the acute onset of varying degrees of intermittent A-V heart block, sometimes in association with clinical evidence of myopericarditis [174, 176, 183, 185–187].

Diagnosis of Lyme carditis should be based on demonstration of heart involvement manifested by either conduction disturbances (established by electrocardiographic and/or electrophysiologic findings) and/or myo(peri)carditis (demonstrated pathohistologically in endomyocardial biopsy specimens, or suggested by electrocardiographic, echocardiographic and/or MRI findings), and corroborated with the demonstration of borrelial infection by 1 or more of the following: (1) isolation of borreliae from an endomyocardial biopsy specimen and/or demonstration of borrelial DNA in the specimen; (2) by seroconversion to borrelial antigens; (3) by the presence of *Borrelia* antibodies in serum; (4) by the presence of EM and/or Lyme neuroborreliosis together with or in close temporal proximity to Lyme carditis. In practice, there are several obstacles to the proposed diagnostic approaches. Endomyocardial biopsy is not a routine diagnostic procedure in patients with suspected Lyme carditis because the potential yield is suboptimal, due to the focality of myocarditis, and the procedure carries an inherent risk [173]. In addition, seroconversion is rarely found to be a useful criterion, because at the time of the appearance of Lyme carditis the majority of patients are seropositive [175, 176]. Moreover, seroconversion confirms recent borrelial infection, but does not confirm heart involvement and, in addition, seropositivity cannot distinguish between recent and delayed infection or between active and past infection. In practice, therefore, the most reliable method of demonstrating borrelial infection to enable the interpretation of heart involvement to be Lyme carditis is the presence of another typical manifestation(s) of Lyme borreliosis. Because Lyme carditis usually occurs within 2 months after onset of infection, EM [174, 186, 187] or Lyme neuroborreliosis [174, 187] quite often occur concomitantly or in close proximity to the carditis. In fact, concurrent EM, which enables a reliable diagnosis of early Lyme borreliosis, is present in up to 85% of cases [186].

The diagnosis of Lyme carditis should be further substantiated by the absence or exclusion of other (obvious) explanations for cardiac abnormalities.

Differential Diagnosis

The differential diagnosis of Lyme carditis is extremely broad and includes diseases that can cause conduction disturbances, endomyocarditis and pericarditis that may be due to infectious agents (viral, bacterial, mycotic and parasitic), as well as noninfectious causes. Because of a large number of potential other causes, the attribution of rhythm disturbances to the infection is highly problematic [175], and is usually supported with only indirect demonstration of infection (often limited to demonstration of specific antibodies in serum). The clinical manifestations of other diseases, specific laboratory tests, epidemiologic data and general information, such as age and state of health at the onset of the illness, can help in differentiating from Lyme carditis [175].

Joint Involvement

Lyme Arthritis

Lyme arthritis, the main joint manifestation in the course of Lyme borreliosis, is an inflammatory arthritis associated with *B. burgdorferi* s.l. infection. It is predominantly a monoarticular or oligoarticular form of arthritis, and typically involves the knee.

Frequency

Although Lyme arthritis was reported to occur in 60% of untreated patients with Lyme disease in the USA about 20 years ago [194], the frequency of this manifestation has been ≤10% in recent series [141, 178, 179, 195], probably because of improved recognition and earlier treatment of patients with early Lyme disease [14]. However, this is in contrast to the much higher frequency of arthritis among Lyme disease cases reported to the CDC [142]. For example, during 2003–2005, the CDC received reports of 64,382 Lyme disease cases. Records for 32,095 (50%) of these patients met the criteria for evaluation of symptoms. A history of EM was reported for 70%, arthritis for 30%, facial palsy for 8%, radiculopathy for 3%, meningitis or encephalitis for 2%, and heart block for <1% [142]. Possible explanations for the higher proportion of arthritis cases in national reporting include reporting bias favoring the tabulation of seropositive Lyme disease cases, confusion between arthritis and arthralgia by the treating health care provider, and inaccuracy of Lyme disease diagnosis. In addition, surveillance report forms differ by state, and reported seropositivity in support of a diagnosis of Lyme arthritis is not necessarily based on recommended two-tier testing [14, 142].

The existence of Lyme arthritis in Europe was recognized only after the reports from the USA. Although joint abnormalities in patients with ACA had been repeatedly described in the European dermatologic literature since 1922 [100], and even the term 'akrodermatitis atrophicans arthropathica' had been proposed [196], a causal relation of joint and bone abnormalities with ACA had been questioned [101]. Joint symptoms had been mentioned in case reports of patients in Europe with erythema chronicum migrans [100, 197] and lymphocytic meningitis [100, 198, 199], yet the association of arthritis with EM and neurologic disease was not recognized until Lyme arthritis was described in the USA [5].

From the very beginning of understanding that arthritis is a manifestation of Lyme borreliosis, there has been a firm conviction that this is less common in Europe than in the USA [100]. However, information on the (relative) frequency of Lyme arthritis in Europe is limited. In an epidemiologic study in southern Sweden, 98 of 1,491 (7%) patients diagnosed with Lyme borreliosis had Lyme arthritis [29], and among Lyme borreliosis cases at the Ljubljana Lyme borreliosis clinic arthritis is present in 2–5% of adult patients [unpublished data]. However, in a nationwide survey in Germany where 3,935 patients were reported to be diagnosed with Lyme borreliosis in a 1-year period (March 1998 to February 1999), the most frequent clinical manifestation was EM in 50.9% of the patients, 24.5% had Lyme arthritis (14.7% mono- or oligoarthritis, 9.8% polyarthritis) and 18.4% had neuroborreliosis [200]. Possible explanations for the relatively high proportion of Lyme arthritis in that survey, especially in comparison with the frequency of neuroborreliosis, could be at least partly similar to those for the national reporting system in the USA.

Etiology

Since the isolation rate of borreliae from joint fluid and synovia is notoriously low [108], data on the etiology of Lyme arthritis are based predominantly on detection and typing of borrelial DNA in synovial fluid or synovial tissue by PCR. Information on the etiology in Europe is limited. Because of the apparently (much) higher prevalence of Lyme arthritis in the USA than in Europe, there was a conviction that in Europe the arthritis was due to infection with *B. burgdorferi* s.s., the strain causing Lyme borreliosis in North America. However, the association of European Lyme arthritis and *B. burgdorferi* s.s. does not appear to be firm. PCR-based analyses of samples from European patients with Lyme arthritis gave inconsistent results, indicating that *B. burgdorferi* s.s. appears to be either the sole, the major or just one of the pathogens involved. In the Netherlands, borrelial DNA was detected in synovial tissue and synovial fluid in 3 of 4 patients with Lyme arthritis; in all 3, *B. burgdorferi* s.s. was identified by reverse line blot [201]. However, among 10 consecutive PCR-positive patients with Lyme arthritis from northeastern France, 2 species were identified in synovial samples: *B. burgdorferi* s.s. in 9 cases and *B. garinii* in 1 case [202]. The conclusion that *B. burgdorferi* s.s. is the principal but not the only *Borrelia* species involved in Lyme arthritis was further substantiated by another report of 2 cases of treatment-resistant Lyme arthritis, in which DNA amplification of the flagellin gene followed by dot-blot hybridization in the synovial fluid identified *B. garinii* as the causative agent [203]. A study from Munich, using ospA type-specific PCRs, found *B. burgdorferi* s.l. DNA in synovial fluid in 13 of 20 patients with the diagnosis of Lyme arthritis (positive serologic findings and fulfilled clinical criteria): *B. burgdorferi* s.s. was established in 27%, *B. afzelii* in 33% and *B. garinii* in 40%. The conclusion of the authors was that in Europe *B. burgdorferi* s.l. strains causing Lyme arthritis are considerably heterogeneous, and that there is no prevalence of particular genospecies or OspA types among these strains [204]. Similar results have been reported by Eiffert et al. [205], where PCR was used to identify a part of the ospA gene in 7 of 11 synovial fluid samples of patients with Lyme arthritis: sequencing the amplified DNA found *B. burgdorferi* s.s. in 3 patients, *B. garinii* in 3 patients and *B. afzelii* in 1 patient.

Pathogenesis

In spite of abundant research, several issues in the pathogenesis of Lyme arthritis remain obscure. As in other manifestations of Lyme borreliosis, the presence of the causative agent (most information on Lyme arthritis is for *B. burgdorferi* s.s.) and immune mechanisms are involved; in Lyme arthritis, the immune mechanisms are probably even more important than in most other manifestations of Lyme borreliosis. After transmission in the bite of an infected tick, the borreliae change expression of several immunostimulatory outer-surface lipoproteins thought to play a role in dissemination to synovial tissue and in the pathogenesis of inflammation in the joint itself [206]. *B. burgdorferi* s.l. does not produce proteases, and therefore does not cause the rapid joint destruction seen in classic septic arthritis [207]. The acute arthritis results from borrelia-induced infiltration of mononuclear cells into the synovial tissue and the accumulation of neutrophils, immune complexes, complement and cytokines in the synovial fluid. In untreated Lyme arthritis, host factors involved may include TLR2 and MyD88 [208]. Other arthritogenic factors may comprise adhesion molecules such as P66 that bind the extracellular matrix, decorin-binding proteins A and B, Bgp and BKK [209]. Matrix metalloproteinases may be involved in the pathogenesis of erosive features in the joint in long-standing infection, and possibly also in antibiotic-refractory arthritis [210, 211].

A small subset of patients who have already received standard antibiotic treatment may have persistent Lyme arthritis. In general, 3 main models for the immunopathogenesis of antibiotic-refractory Lyme arthritis have been proposed [207]: persistent infection, T cell epitope mimicry and bystander activation. None of them has enabled a reliable and complete explanation for all patients: the etiology is most probably multifactorial and may vary from patient to patient [207].

Histologic Findings

The pathologic alternatives in Lyme arthritis correspond to a nonspecific synovitis.

The inflammatory infiltrate shows predominately lymphocytes, often in follicular structures with incomplete germinal centers, and plasma cells. Mast cells can easily be found in the areas of increased vascularization [57, 158, 212].

Chronically inflamed hypertrophic synovial villi with deposition of fibrinaceous eosinophilic material in the synovia are seen in specimens of synovectomized patients. Unlike other nonspecific inflammation of joints, in Lyme arthritis the synovium is rarely scarred. Obstruction of small blood vessels with synovial fibrin deposition is quite often seen [57, 100, 212, 213].

Clinical Characteristics

The spectrum of articular manifestations in Lyme arthritis can be, rather academically, classified into 3 categories: (1) arthralgias (musculoskeletal pain) without objective findings; (2) arthritis (intermittent or chronic) with objective clinical findings; (3) chronic joint and bone involvement under the affected skin in ACA [100]. The main and the most important rheumatic manifestation of Lyme borreliosis is arthritis, and the most elusive presentation is arthralgia that may precede, accompany or follow arthritis, but may sometimes be the only rheumatic manifestation of Lyme borreliosis.

The most complete description of the clinical evolution of Lyme arthritis is in the report by Steere et al. [194] on 55 untreated patients who had EM during the years 1976–1979, that is, before antibiotic treatment of Lyme disease was established in the USA. Of these 55 patients, 11 (20%) had no musculoskeletal symptoms after the resolution of EM, arthritis developed in 34 (62%; in about half, the arthritis was preceded by arthralgias), and arthralgias alone were seen in 10 (18%) patients. Those with arthralgias had brief episodes of pain in joints, tendons, enthesis, bones or muscles without objective signs of inflammation. The symptoms tended to be migratory, with onset from 1 day to 8 weeks (mean, 2 weeks) after the onset of EM. Symptoms lasting from 1 month to as long as 6 years (mean, 3.1 years) had a relapsing/remitting pattern, and were often accompanied by fatigue [194]; however, patients with arthralgias associated with Lyme borreliosis (who may or may not have Lyme arthritis) generally did not experience widespread chronic pain [207]. No corresponding European report on the natural history of a large number of untreated EM patients exists, most probably as a consequence of antibiotic treatment of EM which has been widely practiced in Europe since 1951 [214], long before the complete clinical picture of Lyme borreliosis (including arthritis) and the etiology of the disease were established. It has been reported that only 1 of 16 Swedish patients developed arthritis after spontaneous healing of EM [215].

The succession or coexistence of intermittent attacks of musculoskeletal pain and arthritis have also been reported in Europe, and have been interpreted as particularly indicative of Lyme arthritis [100]. In 25 of 65 patients with Lyme arthritis in Germany [216], episodes of severe pain in joint and periarticular sites had either preceded arthritis for several weeks or months (8 patients), had preceded and continued after arthritis (5 patients), or had developed as late as arthritis (12 patients). Particular episodes lasted from some hours to several days, and were separated by days to months of remission. Episodes of arthralgias sometimes alternated with attacks of arthritis. Predominantly large but also small joints were affected in an often migratory pattern, but commonly only 1 or 2 sites were affected at any one time [100].

Arthralgias are a relatively frequent complaint early in the course of Lyme borreliosis, in patients with EM before therapy and in some patients even after antibiotic treatment, and more commonly accompany EM in the USA than in Europe. In the early studies, arthralgias were reported in as many as 48% of patients with EM in North America [60], but in only 22% at the most in European patients [53]. In a group of culture-positive adult patients in New York state with EM caused by *B. burgdorferi* s.s., arthralgias were reported in 48 of 119 (40%) prior to treatment, whereas in Slovenian patients with *B. afzelii* isolated from the skin lesion, the frequency was only 23 of 85 (27%) [15]. In a study in 1994 on 231 European patients with culture-confirmed EM at the Ljubljana Lyme borreliosis clinic, 27 (12%) patients reported arthralgias that as a rule were mild-to-moderately severe [55]. Arthralgias may be present in some patients after standard antibiotic treatment of EM, usually during the first few weeks after treatment, but normally vanish within 6 months after treatment. Whether they had arthralgias or not, patients treated for solitary EM with standard courses of antibiotics only very exceptionally develop later objective manifestations of Lyme borreliosis, including arthritis [14].

Lyme arthritis affects both children and adults. Several patients remember tick bite(s); however, temporal association between an individual tick bite and the onset of Lyme arthritis is often difficult to assess and is most reliable in patients who develop EM at the site of the bite. In patients from North America who had EM but did not receive antibiotic treatment and were followed up for a mean duration of 6 years (range 3–8 years), arthritis occurred from 4 days to 2 years after disease onset (mean 6 months) [194]. In a European series of patients [216], the period from tick bites or EM to the onset of arthritis ranged from 10 days to 16 months (median, 3 months). However, there are case reports of patients in whom tick bite and EM had preceded arthritis for much longer periods of time [100]. Since the latent period between infection and onset of Lyme arthritis is highly variable and mostly runs for several months, there is no seasonal peak in the occurrence of Lyme arthritis [100].

Lyme arthritis can be preceded or accompanied by other manifestations of Lyme borreliosis. In the initial description of Lyme disease in the USA, 13 of 51 (25%) patients reported having had EM before they developed arthritis [5]. Of 65 German patients with Lyme arthritis, 40 were without history of well-defined Lyme borreliosis or concurrent extra-articular disease manifestations, whereas 25 (38%) had at least 1 additional manifestation including EM (21 patients, 32%), Lyme neuroborreliosis (14 patients, 22%), ACA (5 patients, 8%) and carditis (1 patient) [100]. In a 1-year nationwide survey in Germany, 32% of patients with Lyme arthritis remembered having had an EM [200]. An epidemiologic study of Lyme borreliosis in southern Sweden found that among 98 patients diagnosed with Lyme arthritis, the arthritis was the sole main manifestation in 65 (66%) patients, whereas in the others it was associated with additional manifestation(s) such as EM (10 patients), Lyme neuroborreliosis (8 patients), ACA (8 patients) and borrelial lymphocytoma (1 patient); 6 patients with arthritis had at least 2 additional main manifestations of the disease [29].

Several European authors have emphasized that Lyme arthritis often begins in the extremity that was affected by a tick bite or EM [216–218]; for example, this correlation was observed in 15 of 18 patients in whom EM had preceded arthritis [216]. Such an observation has not been reported from the USA.

Lyme arthritis usually consists of intermittent attacks of inflammation of one or a few joints and is often preceded by intermittent migratory joint pain. Joint involvement is usually asymmetric, onset of arthritis is acute and with effusion, and skin over the affected joint is warm but of normal color [16]. The arthritis is frequently mono- or oligoarticular, only rarely polyarticular. In a European series of 65 patients with Lyme arthritis [100], the course was intermittent in 55 (85%), initially intermittent and later chronic in 4 (6%) and unremitting (chronic) in 6 (9%); the pattern of joint involvement was monoarticular in 39 (60%; onset of arthritis was monoarticular in as many as 55 patients), oligoarticular in 21 (32%) and polyarticular in 4 (6%) patients. One patient had isolated heel swelling [100].

Large joints are predominantly involved, most often the knee. In 28 patients with a relapsing/remitting course of Lyme arthritis presented in a classic series by Steere et al. [194], the knee was involved in all but 1 patient; shoulder, ankle, elbow, temporomandibular joint, wrist and hip were affected in the range of 28–43%, and metacarpophalangeal, proximal interphalangeal, distal interphalangeal and metatarsophalangeal joints were involved in 3 (11%) patients. One patient had sternoclavicular involvement. Similarly, in the European series of 65 patients with Lyme arthritis reported by Herzer [100, 216], involvement of the knee was by far the most common (outnumbering the frequency of any other joint involvement by ≥2.5 times), followed by ankle, wrist, finger, toe and elbow (seen in 10–30% of patients); involvement of midtarsal joints, sternoclavicular joint and hip occurred only exceptionally. Heel swelling was found in 6 (9%) patients (1 had heel swelling only) and sausage digits (dactylitis) in as many as 15 (23%). In a subgroup of 24 patients with knee involvement investigated by ultrasound, Baker cysts were found in as many as 12 (50%).

Joints are painful; however, some patients with pronounced joint (knee) effusions may have disproportionately mild pains [194]. Joint inflammation usually lasts a few days to weeks, sometimes several months [194]. The course of Lyme arthritis is very variable, usually recurring and may continue for several years. In the beginning, the attacks of arthritis are more frequent and short, later they may be more prolonged. Every year about 10–20% of patients have complete resolution of the attacks. About 10% of patients develop chronic arthritis with duration of a year or longer; in some of them erosions may develop [194, 219].

Although constitutional symptoms mostly occur early in Lyme borreliosis [60], they occasionally outlast the initial period and may accompany arthritis [194]. In the study by Herzer [100, 216], 9 of 65 patients with Lyme arthritis also had fatigue, malaise, low fever or night sweats.

Clinical characteristics of joint involvement in association with ACA are outlined in the section 'Skin Involvement'.

Lyme arthritis is one of the rare inflammatory joint diseases in which routine laboratory parameters are often completely normal. Only about half the patients with Lyme arthritis have moderately elevated erythrocyte sedimentation rate (>20 mm/h) with median values of approximately 20–30 mm/h [194, 216]. Concentration of C-reactive protein is usually in the normal range or slightly elevated. Findings of an erythrocyte sedimentation rate >80 mm/h or demonstration of pronounced elevation of other laboratory indicators of inflammation in a patient with arthritis points strongly against Lyme arthritis. Some patients have white cell blood counts slightly above 10×10^9 cells/l, some have elevated serum IgM. Cryoglobulins and circulating immune complexes may be present. Rheumatoid factors and antinuclear antibodies are usually negative, but in some patients may be positive in low titer [4, 16, 194, 216, 220].

Elevated white cell counts in synovial fluid, usually 10–35 $\times$ 10^9 cells/l (range 0.5–110 $\times$ 10^9 cells/l) with predominance of polymorphonuclear leukocytes (average 70–80%), are found [5, 100, 194, 216, 219]. Total protein concentration commonly ranges from 3.5 to 5.6 g/l [5, 100, 194, 216]. Cryoglobulins and abnormal C1q binding consistent with antigen-antibody complexes are commonly present in synovial fluid [220, 221].

There are no specific radiographic findings for Lyme arthritis. Soft tissue changes, particularly effusions, are commonly present. Erosions are rare and generally seen only in some long-lasting (persistent) cases. Osseous changes, including subarticular cysts and osteophytes are uncommon [100, 222].

In patients with Lyme arthritis, borrelial IgG antibodies in serum are almost always strongly positive; negative IgG serology essentially rules out Lyme arthritis [108, 207]. Investigation of paired sera with the aim of identifying seroconversion to *Borrelia* antigens is usually unsuccessful because almost all patients with Lyme arthritis are seropositive at presentation. Serologic investigation of paired samples of serum and synovial fluid for determination of intra-articular antibody production (parallel to determination of intrathecal antibody synthesis in Lyme neuroborreliosis) is of no value because of the lack of a blood/synovial barrier that would efficiently prevent diffusion of immunoglobulins from blood into synovial fluid and vice versa. In patients with arthritis and borrelial IgG antibodies in serum, the diagnosis of Lyme arthritis is substantially supported by demonstration of borrelial DNA in synovial fluid or in synovial tissue.

Diagnosis

Diagnosis of Lyme arthritis is based on the medical history and clinical features, laboratory findings, exclusion of other causes of arthritis and demonstration of serum IgG antibodies to *Borrelia* [1–3, 16, 18]. Unfortunately, serology has many methodologic limitations and several pitfalls in interpretation of the results. Demonstration of borrelial (IgG) antibodies in serum does not enable distinction between symptomatic and asymptomatic infection, between active and past infection, or between acute and chronic (short- and long-lasting) infection; it also does not enable location of the disease process. Thus, demonstration of borrelial antibodies in the serum of a patient with arthritis does not guarantee that the infection is active or that it is located in the joints – it does not indicate Lyme arthritis. Isolation of *Borrelia* from synovial fluid is rarely successful. Detection of borrelial DNA in synovial tissue or synovial fluid by PCR is much more sensitive (up to 85%) [14, 108, 201, 202, 204, 205, 223, 224]. However, a positive PCR finding in a seronegative patient is most probably of low diagnostic value, and should be regarded with skepticism [14, 108]. Cultures of synovial fluid and synovial tissue for the presence of *Borrelia* have been generally unsuccessful [108, 207].

The presence or a reliable history of other manifestations of Lyme borreliosis such as EM, Lyme neuroborreliosis or ACA is of substantial help for relatively straightforward diagnosis.

Differential Diagnosis

The differential diagnosis of Lyme arthritis is broad and generally includes inflammatory rheumatic diseases, bacterial (septic) arthritis, viral arthritis and crystal-induced arthritis [3, 18, 100, 219].

The acute presentation of (monoarticular) Lyme arthritis can be mistaken for bacterial (septic) or crystal-induced arthritis (gout, pseudogout) and sometimes also for sarcoid arthritis in *Borrelia*-seropositive persons. In Europe, adult patients with Lyme arthritis only very exceptionally have fever (>38 °C), do not have signs of sepsis, and usually have normal or slightly elevated laboratory indicators of inflammation, which – in addition to synovial fluid smears for the presence of bacteria and synovial fluid culture – permits a fairly reliable distinction of Lyme arthritis from septic arthritis. The presence of hyperuricemia and *Borrelia* IgG antibodies in serum may be conflicting diagnostic criteria in a patient with acute monoarticular arthritis unless crystals are demonstrated in synovial fluid. Acute sarcoid arthritis, which commonly affects the ankles, may be wrongly diagnosed as Lyme arthritis, especially in cases of sarcoidosis without erythema nodosum.

Migratory arthritis in Lyme borreliosis is similar to that of rheumatic fever, disseminated gonococcal infection and viral infections. Diffuse hand swelling, which may occur in some patients with early Lyme arthritis, may also occur in viral infections such as those with parvovirus B19 [100].

With regard to the intermittent course, Lyme arthritis may be mistakenly diagnosed as intermittent hydarthrosis or palindromic rheumatism in persons with borrelial antibodies in serum. Recurrent episodes of arthritis may precede (more) indicative signs of Whipple's disease [100].

In general, Lyme arthritis is most like pauciarticular juvenile arthritis in children and reactive arthritis in adults [3]. Thus, there may be difficulties in differentiation between Lyme arthritis and reactive arthritis, as well as between Lyme arthritis (in children) and HLA B27-positive juvenile oligoarthritis or antinuclear antibody-positive pauciarticular juvenile arthritis. The pattern of joint involvement in Lyme arthritis resembles that in seronegative spondyloarthropathies; in addition, heel involvement and sausage digits are not limited to seronegative spondyloarthropathies, but are also seen in some patients with Lyme arthritis [100]. Other differential diagnoses include psoriatic arthritis, early rheumatoid arthritis and systemic lupus erythematosus in patients who have borrelial antibodies in serum.

Musculoskeletal pain in Lyme borreliosis may be mistaken for psychogenic rheumatism or fibromyalgia. However, more often fibromyalgia in *Borrelia*-seropositive persons is wrongly diagnosed as Lyme borreliosis. In contrast to the rather distinctive intermittent and migratory pattern of musculoskeletal pain in Lyme borreliosis, fibromyalgia is characterized by more generalized chronic pain and by symmetric tender points [100].

Eye Involvement

Information on eye involvement in the course of Lyme borreliosis is limited. It appears to occur very rarely, and is often associated with other signs of Lyme borreliosis [16, 225, 226] such as EM, Lyme neuroborreliosis or Lyme arthritis, but can also be the sole manifestation of the disease. Ocular Lyme borreliosis may be underdiagnosed because of difficulties in the (serologic) diagnosis and because the clinical ocular features are often not recognized [227–229]. Some ophthalmologists are not acquainted with the possibility of ocular manifestations of this disease, nor are most other specialists and general practitioners. Intraocular material is usually not available from humans, therefore serology is the main aid in diagnosis. False seropositivity and asymptomatic seropositivity can lead to substantial overdiagnosis, particularly in highly endemic regions. Frequent association of eye involvement with other manifestations of Lyme borreliosis may be the consequence of diagnostic bias.

The interval from EM to the onset of eye involvement is variable and may be from a few days to years, conjunctivitis being representative of an early ocular lesion, whereas keratitis appears late in the course of Lyme borreliosis [16, 230].

Eyes can be affected primarily as the result of inflammation, such as conjunctivitis, keratitis, iridocyclitis, retinal vasculitis, chorioiditis, optic neuropathy, episcleritis, panuveitis, panophthalmitis (some of these manifestations appear to be extremely rare and not all are reliably proven to be the consequence of borrelial infection), or secondarily as a result of extra-ocular manifestations of Lyme borreliosis, including pareses of cranial nerves (VII, III, IV or VI cranial nerve), pseudotumor cerebri and orbital myositis [227, 229, 231, 232]. Inflammation, particularly when long-lasting, may lead to severe impairment or even complete loss of vision [16, 226, 228–230].

According to the reports on EM that were published soon after Lyme borreliosis was recognized, conjunctivitis was found in as many as 35 of 314 (11%) patients in the USA [230], whereas in Europe the proportion of patients with EM and conjunctivitis was lower: of 104 patients with EM in southern Germany only 1 had conjunctivitis [53], and it was found in 23 of 425 (5%) Slovenian patients diagnosed with EM before 1990 [230] and in 10 of 231 (4%) skin culture-confirmed patients diagnosed in 1994 [136]. In the majority of later series on EM, conjunctivitis was reported only rarely or not mentioned at all. Among 19 European patients with intraocular involvement interpreted as due to borrelial infection, 12 had chorioiditis (bilateral 8, unilateral 4; diffuse or disseminated 8, focal 4), 3 had neuroretinitis, 2 bilateral retinal vasculitis, 1 bilateral iridocyclitis and 1 keratitis [230]. Borrelial infection was demonstrated in all the patients by the presence of borrelial antibodies in serum, and in 9 it was also indicated by the presence of other objective manifestation(s) of Lyme borreliosis (3 patients had lymphocytic meningitis, 1 had meningoradiculitis with second-degree A-V block, 2 had peripheral facial palsy – 1 also had lymphocytic pleocytosis, and 3 had oligoarthritis). None of these 9 patients had EM, but 3 of the 10 remaining patients had a reliable history of EM. Patients were treated with antibiotics, and were followed for a median of 12 months (range 3–49 months). Visual acuity, which was initially found impaired in 18 patients (1 patient was not assessed), improved or normalized in the large majority of patients [230]. Huppertz et al. [233] reported that 3 of 84 (4%) children and adolescents with Lyme arthritis had ocular inflammation, including keratitis, anterior uveitis and uveitis intermedia. All 3 had symptoms of decreased visual acuity. Whereas anterior uveitis disappeared without sequelae, corneal scarring and permanent loss of visual acuity remained in the patients with keratitis and intermediate uveitis. The authors stressed that loss of vision appears to be symptomatic, making regular ocular screening of such patients unnecessary.

Several case reports and some series of patients with (presumed) ocular Lyme borreliosis have been published [226–229], indicating that uveitis (which may be associated with photophobia, macular edema, retinal vasculitis and decreased vision), neuroretinitis and choroiditis with retinal detachment may develop, and that interstitial keratitis, episcleritis and follicular conjunctivitis are possible anterior-segment manifestations. Transient worsening of symptoms as a result of a Jarisch-Herxheimer reaction after the intravenous administration of ceftriaxone has also been described [226].

Diagnosis of borrelial ocular involvement is difficult. It should be based on medical history (epidemiologic data and information on other antecedent or concurrent manifestations of Lyme borreliosis are of particular importance, but often fail to be noticed), complete physical not only ophthalmologic examination and demonstration of borrelial infection. In clinical practice, demonstration of serum antibodies is the most often used test. In addition to several problems of borrelial serology that are discussed elsewhere, concerns have been expressed that in some patients with isolated borrelial eye involvement the antibody response to this localized *Borrelia* infection might be inadequate [226–228]. Antibodies in ocular fluid could also be determined, and demonstration of intraocular production of borrelial antibodies could be of substantial diagnostic help [234]. However, eye puncture is not a procedure included in routine clinical practice, and the volume of obtainable ocular fluid is small. In the literature, there are many reports of eye involvement attributed to Lyme borreliosis, in which borrelial infection was indicated only by the presence of serum antibodies. It is very difficult if not impossible to prove that an individual ocular clinical sign (particularly without the presence of or a reliable history of other manifestations of Lyme borreliosis) is really a result of infection with *B. burgdorferi* s.l. without direct demonstration of the causative agent in the involved eye [225, 226, 228, 230]. Isolation of *Borrelia* from eye tissue has been reported only once [235], but there are several publications on the demonstration of borrelial DNA in eye structures and ocular fluid [226, 228, 236]. However, several patients with positive PCR findings were reported to be seronegative to borrelial antigens, a finding that needs critical interpretation [14, 108].

The ocular manifestations described resemble those seen in ocular syphilis in some ways, and are not pathognomonic for Lyme borreliosis. Differential diagnosis is rather broad [226, 230]. Granulomatous iridocyclitis or chorioiditis are seen in several diseases caused by bacteria (such as syphilis, tuberculosis and leprosy) and protozoa *(Toxoplasma gondii)*, and can be associated with fungal infections and immunologic processes of unclear etiology such as sarcoidosis and Vogt-Koyanagi-Harada syndrome, as well as with rheumatic disorders [230], particularly in children and adolescents with pauciarticular juvenile rheumatoid arthritis (typical ocular manifestation is chronic anterior uveitis) and juvenile spondyloarthropathy (acute anterior uveitis) [233]. Generally, the association of arthritis and uveitis is suggestive of HLA B27-positive spondyloarthropathies, and uveitis is a typical feature of antinuclear antibody-positive pauciarticular juvenile arthritis [100].

Other Rare (Potential) Manifestations of Lyme Borreliosis

Some case reports have implicated *B. burgdorferi* s.l. infection as a possible cause of 2 subtypes of scleroderma circumscripta, progressive facial hemiatrophia (suggested by silver staining) and eosinophilic fasciitis (Shulman syndrome, indicated by silver staining, immunohistology, PCR) [67, 237–239].

There are case reports on patients with myositis [240–242], the existence of which has also been demonstrated in an animal model in nonhuman primates [243], dermatomyositis [244, 245], nodular fasciitis [246], panniculitis [247–249] and osteomyelitis [250]. Most authors are of the opinion that borrelial infection is not causally associated with the syndrome of fibromyalgia [3, 16]. There are also reports on the effect on individual organs or organ systems, such as the liver, lymphatic system, respiratory tract, urinary tract and genitalia [16], but proof of the existence of such involvement in humans is weak.

Short Comment on Chronic Lyme Borreliosis and 'Chronic Lyme Borreliosis'

The designation chronic Lyme borreliosis should be reserved for patients with objective manifestations of late Lyme borreliosis (in Europe typically represented by ACA, chronic arthritis and rare cases of chronic Lyme neuroborreliosis without ACA) and not misused for: (1) symptoms of unknown cause with no (objective or valid) evidence of *B. burgdorferi* s.l. infection, (2) well-defined illness unrelated to borrelial infection (even with the presence of borrelial antibodies in serum), (3) symptoms of unknown cause, with antibodies against *B. burgdorferi* s.l. but no history of objective clinical findings that are consistent with Lyme borreliosis, or (4) post-Lyme borreliosis (post-Lyme disease) syndrome [251, 252]. A definition of post-Lyme disease syndrome was proposed in the recent IDSA clinical practice guidelines [14]. The problems associated with diagnosis and management of patients with 'chronic Lyme disease' (patients in categories 1, 2, 3 and especially 4) have been discussed in several articles, including a critical appraisal in the *New England Journal of Medicine* [251] and a recent review in *Infectious Disease Clinics of North America* [252]. The information in these reports is valid not only for North America, but also for Europe.

Lyme Borreliosis in Special Groups of Patients

Although Lyme borreliosis has been recognized for more than 30 years, knowledge of the course and outcome of the illness is limited in certain groups, including pregnant women and immunocompromised patients. Lyme borreliosis during pregnancy is discussed elsewhere in this book; here, we present some basic data on Lyme borreliosis in immunocompromised patients.

Lyme Borreliosis in an Immunocompromised Host

In general, it is well known that bacteria can induce infections of varying severity, and that the preinfection immune status is often crucial for the clinical course of a disease. Information on the course and outcome of *B. burgdorferi* s.l. infection in immunocompromised patients is very limited; as a consequence, neither the natural course nor the efficacy of treatment of Lyme borreliosis has been accurately assessed in this diverse group comprising several distinct types and severities of immunosuppression. Data in the literature are scant and predominantly restricted to individual case reports, such as a report on a *B. burgdorferi* infection in a patient with dermatomyositis [253], a description of a morphea-like skin condition apparently caused by *B. burgdorferi* in an immunocompromised patient [254], a case of Lyme borreliosis in a transplant recipient [255] and several cases of Lyme borreliosis in conjunction with human immune deficiency virus infection [256–258]. We were able to find only 3 reports on a series of cases of Lyme borreliosis in immunocompromised patients.

In the first report, several distinctions were revealed in a comparison of the course and outcome of borrelial infection in 67 adult patients with typical EM and an underlying immunocompromised condition with 67 previously healthy age- and sex-matched individuals with EM, who were examined and diagnosed in the period 1990–1996 at a single center. The duration of EM after starting antibiotic treatment was similar in the 2 groups, but the occurrence of early disseminated borrelial infection before treatment and the frequency of treatment failure were found more often in immunocompromised patients than in the control group (16/67 vs. 6/67, respectively). Treatment failure was defined as the occurrence of severe minor or major manifestations of Lyme borreliosis, persistence of *B. burgdorferi* s.l. in the skin and/or persistence of EM after treatment; the mode and duration of antibiotic treatment was the same in both groups of patients. Re-treatment was required in 13 (19%) immunocompromised patients, but in only 5 (7%) patients in the control group. However, in spite of the more severe course and the more frequent need for retreatment among patients whose immune system was impaired, both groups had a favorable outcome of borrelial infection after 1 year [259]. Persistence of *B. burgdorferi* s.l. in normal-looking skin at the site of previous EM 2 months after treatment was found in 1 of 20 immunocompromised patients and in none of 21 immunocompetent patients who had positive *Borrelia* culture from an EM lesion before treatment and were rebiopsed 2–3 months later at the same site. As stressed by the authors of the study, these results should be interpreted with caution because the causes of immune deficiency were somewhat heterogeneous. The findings in the small numbers of patients with individual underlying diseases could give only a hint of potential differences between distinct immunocompromised settings, but could not permit reliable statistical analysis; 1 of 7 patients (14%) with cirrhosis of the liver, 4 of 22 (18%) patients treated for diabetes, 2 of 8 (25%) with autoimmune disease, and 4 of 14 patients with underlying malignant disease presented with signs of disseminated Lyme borreliosis or developed treatment failure during the observational period of 1 year. The various types and levels of altered immunity in patients within individual immunocompromised subgroups might also have considerably influenced the results. Nevertheless, according to the results of the study, it appears that in patients with underlying malignant disease the likelihood of developing disseminated infection or treatment failure may be higher among those with hematologic malignancies: signs of disseminated borrelial infection or development of treatment failure were present in 3 of 7 patients (2/3 with chronic lymphatic leukemia, 1/2 with lymphoma and 0/2 with myeloproliferative disorders), in contrast to 1 of 7 patients with nonhematologic malignancies. The authors concluded that although in the majority of immunocompromised patients with EM the management can be the same as in immunocompetent patients with early Lyme borreliosis, more aggressive initial antibiotic treatment might be appropriate for some subgroups of patients with altered immunity; for example, in patients with hematologic malignancy [259].

A second study [260] investigated the impact of immunosuppression on EM in 33 patients with malignant or autoimmune disease, chronic infection or immunosuppressive therapy for organ transplantation by comparing findings in the immunosuppressed patients with those in 75 otherwise healthy patients with EM. The 2 groups were matched for sex, age and antibiotic therapy. Comparison did not reveal any significant difference between the 2 groups in pretreatment clinical parameters, such as presentation of the skin lesion and presence of extracutaneous signs and symptoms, in the disease course during a median follow-up of 9 months after treatment, or in serum borrelial antibodies before treatment and at the end of follow-up. Further, it appeared that immunosuppression did not influence clinical presentation, response to therapy or production of *B. burgdorferi* antibodies in patients with EM. The authors concluded that it is not necessary to treat immunosuppressed patients with EM differently from immunocompetent patients [260]. Again, one of the several drawbacks of this retrospective study was the pronounced heterogeneity in types and levels of altered immunity.

The third report comprised 6 adult recipients of solid-organ transplants who had chronic drug-induced immunosuppression and presented with solitary EM. These patients appeared to have only localized infection of the skin, even though they were immunosuppressed; all had a mild and smooth course of illness, as well as a favorable outcome of the illness after treatment with antibiotics administered at the same dosage and for the same duration as used in treatment of early localized Lyme borreliosis in immunocompetent patients. However, the number of patients in the study was too small to enable valid generalization of the findings. Potential application of the observations might be appropriate for European patients with solitary EM caused by *B. afzelii* (in this study 3 of 4 *Borrelia* isolates from lesional skin were typed as *B. afzelii* and 1 as *B. garinii*; a skin sample from 1 patient was culture negative), but the observations may not apply to patients with *B. burgdorferi* infection in the USA (localized infection of the skin is more commonly associated with *B. afzelii* infection in Europe than with *B. burgdorferi* infection in the USA [15]) or to patients with disseminated *Borrelia* infection [261].

Laboratory Diagnosis of Lyme Borreliosis

An important observation in Lyme borreliosis is that there is usually no clinical laboratory parameter in the peripheral blood that is indicative of this infectious disease. Almost all patients have normal CRP values and usually normal white blood cell counts [1–3, 16, 18].

The marked impression of EM on the skin could be expected to represent a typical histologic reaction, but the histologic picture in EM is generally nonspecific with some perivascular infiltration, mainly of lymphocytes and sometimes plasma cells. In borrelial lymphocytoma, the respective skin area, in contrast to EM, frequently shows lymphocytic infiltration in the dermis with plasma cells, macrophages and eosinophils. The histopathologic picture of ACA is also characterized by a lymphocytic infiltration, and also by telangiectases. The cellular infiltration is again mixed with plasma cells and is present not only in the dermis, but also not infrequently in the subcutis. Histology in ACA may be supportive of the diagnosis, but it is not typical enough to be exclusive, and in borrelial lymphocytoma the histologic picture is not unique and may be difficult to differentiate from malignant lymphomas.

In Lyme neuroborreliosis, the CSF usually shows moderate-to-intense lymphocytic pleocytosis, but some patients have only elevated CSF protein. Lymphocytic pleocytosis is absent in several patients with peripheral facial palsy and in patients with isolated peripheral neuropathy, and may be absent very early in CNS involvement particularly in children [262]. Intrathecal IgM and IgG production and oligoclonal IgG bands are common findings in patients with CNS involvement of a few weeks or longer and are supportive of the diagnosis. Concentration of CSF glucose is usually normal. Patients with 'chronic' peripheral polyneuropathy, usually a feature of ACA, have normal CSF findings.

Thus, without a specific marker, full proof of the borrelial etiology of any of the given disorders in Lyme borreliosis is missing. The specific etiology of any infectious disease is usually best documented by direct detection of the agent, but this is not straightforward in suspected Lyme borreliosis.

Direct Detection of the Agent

Culture

Culture of *B. burgdorferi* s.l. strains is possible in complex media [263, 264], with success depending on the type of specimen. For example, cultivation of *B. burgdorferi* s.l. from skin biopsies of EM is usually very successful, at 60–80% [38, 77, 108]. However, the clinical conditions EM and ACA will mostly be identified by inspection, to some extent with the help of histology in the latter case, and cultivation is only rarely requested. In CSF the success of culture is usually around 10% or less, possibly increasing to 30% in children in the very early phase of neurologic disorders [262]. Borreliae have also been isolated from the blood of patients with EM, most successfully in the USA by using high-volume blood cultures [64], from cardiac tissue of patients with dilated cardiomyopathy [180], and from synovial fluid of patients with Lyme arthritis [265]. Although some results suggest that even early Lyme borreliosis such as EM is very frequently a disseminated infectious disease, most medical laboratories would not be able to manage the relatively sophisticated demands of *Borrelia* culture. Thus, blood, cardiac tissue and synovial fluid are less suitable sources for culture of *B. burgdorferi* s.l.

Nucleic Acid Amplification Techniques

Genus- and species-specific PCR methods can be used to detect low copy numbers of *B. burgdorferi* s.l. Unlike culture, PCR detects borrelial DNA of both viable and nonviable organisms, which means that a positive PCR cannot explicitly establish whether an infection is active or not. PCR appears to be a valuable tool, particularly in the diagnosis of patients with arthritis, since it can detect borrelial DNA in 85% of synovial fluid samples and even more if the synovial membrane is examined [224].

Urine has been investigated by several groups [266]; however, results are contradictory and studies indicate that more attention to methods of DNA extraction may help improve this situation [267]. A further problem is illustrated by a study in which a proportion of urine samples of healthy individuals whose serum contained *Borrelia*-specific antibodies also reacted positive in a *Borrelia*-specific PCR. Thus, as with serologic findings, PCR results should always be interpreted with caution and the clinical significance of a PCR-positive finding in urine remains to be established.

Lastly, reference should be made to the fact that a negative result for culture and/or PCR does not exclude active infection.

Indirect Detection of Borrelial Infection: Serology

Currently, there are almost uncountable numbers of commercial test kits on the market for detection of IgG and IgM antibodies against *B. burgdorferi* s.l. The test systems comprise immunofluorescence assay (IFA), enzyme-linked immunosorbent assay (ELISA) and immunoblot.

IFA were the first serodiagnostic tests used for detection of antibodies against *B. burgdorferi* s.l., and are still used in many countries. Nevertheless, although IFA can be automated today, ELISA are the most frequently used tests. Since the two-tier testing principle was introduced, ELISA has become the most commonly used serodiagnostic screening method for Lyme borreliosis. Sonicate and recombinant ELISA are in use. Most assays are either enriched with VlsE (variable-like sequence expressed) antigen or use VlsE or C6 as a single antigen for detection of specific IgG antibodies. OspC antigen as a single ELISA antigen is used for detection of specific IgM antibodies in serum. VlsE and C6 were originally considered markers for active infection; however, the strong immune reaction to these antigens is also present in convalescent and healthy persons and thus does not differentiate between active and past infection.

Immunoblot, or Western blot, is important in characterization of immune responses to specific *B. burgdorferi* s.l. proteins, and is generally used in the two-tier testing procedure. The interpretation criteria for immunoblot results are based on diagnostic antigens. Standardization of criteria for interpretation of immunoblot results in Europe was the subject of a study by EUCALB [268]. This multicenter study, involving 6 European laboratories using different immunoblot protocols, identified 8 bands that were discriminatory in all the laboratories, though with variations in significance. From these bands, 5 closely related European rules were formulated giving acceptable sensitivity and specificity, though there was no single rule that could be applied in all laboratories. This panel of European rules provides a framework for immunoblot interpretation that may be adapted in relation to the characteristics of Lyme borreliosis in local areas. Another source for the selection of diagnostic antigens is the work of Wilske and colleagues [269, 270]. Since complete standardization of immunoblotting protocols in Europe cannot be achieved, there was hope that new recombinant immunoblots would help to solve this problem [271]. However, even this hope was not fulfilled, particularly with recombinant IgM blots, which proved to be more sensitive than recombinant IgM ELISA.

Table 3. Laboratory support in the diagnosis of Lyme borreliosis; modified according to the EUCALB clinical case definitions in Lyme borreliosis [12]

Initial clinical diagnosis	Essential laboratory evidence	Supporting laboratory evidence
EM	none if typical	culture from skin biopsy; significant change in levels of specific antibodies or presence of specific IgM[1]
Borrelial lymphocytoma	specific IgG antibodies	histology; culture from skin biopsy
ACA	high level of specific serum IgG antibodies	histology; culture from skin biopsy
Early Lyme neuroborreliosis	lymphocytic pleocytosis in CSF; intrathecally produced specific antibodies[2]	intrathecal total IgM and IgG; specific oligoclonal bands in CSF; significant change in levels of specific antibodies[1]; culture from CSF
Chronic Lyme neuroborreliosis	lymphocytic pleocytosis in CSF; intrathecally produced specific antibodies[2]; specific serum IgG	specific oligoclonal bands in CSF
Lyme arthritis	high level of specific serum antibodies	detection of borrelial DNA in synovial fluid and/or tissue (culture from synovial fluid and/or tissue)
Lyme carditis	significant change in levels of specific IgG antibodies[1]	culture from endomyocardial biopsy

[1] Specific antibody levels in serum may increase in response to progression of infection or treatment, or may decrease due to abrogation of the infection process. Samples collected a minimum of 3 months apart may be required in order to detect a decrease in IgG levels.
[2] Intrathecally produced specific antibodies are determined by investigating simultaneously drawn samples of CSF and serum.

With the introduction of VlsE and C6 peptides in the serology of Lyme borreliosis and the similar success in detecting *Borrelia*-specific IgG and IgM antibodies by using VlsE and OspC as single antigens in ELISA systems, it appears logical to replace the two-tier test principle, as indicated by results of recent studies [272]. However, even if the two-tier principle is abandoned, there is still no method or technique for identification of active infection. In addition, the high seroprevalence of specific antibodies in the general population in highly endemic areas will cause the problem of relevance to clinical disease. Moreover, persons such as hunters continuously exposed to ticks show an age-related seroprevalence as high as 83% in those over 70 years old [273]. Thus, physicians must take local seroprevalence into account when interpreting the clinical relevance of positive serology in patients. After more than 20 years of

‘Lyme serology’ it appears that for diagnostic purposes serology has created more problems than it has solved. It is possible that the immune response to *Borrelia* infection still requires further elucidation. The results of a recent study appear to offer reasons for optimism with respect to diagnostic support [274].

Nevertheless, serologic tests for detection of intrathecal production of specific antibodies are very beneficial in the diagnosis of Lyme neuroborreliosis. Differing concentrations of immune globulins and specific antibodies in serum and CSF must be taken into account in detection of intrathecally produced specific antibodies; this is expressed as the CSF/serum index as follows:

$$\text{CSF/serum index} = \frac{\text{ELISA units in CSF} \times \text{total IgG in serum}}{\text{ELISA units in serum} \times \text{total IgG in CSF}}$$

Thus, the index expresses the proportion of pathogen-specific IgG antibodies in the total IgG content in the CSF compared with the serum. An index >1.0 would, strictly mathematically, prove the intrathecal production of specific antibodies. With respect to small volume variations when diluting samples, an index ≥1.5 is considered significantly elevated.

Table 3 refers to EUCALB recommendations listing the suspected clinical conditions and the weight of laboratory results required to confirm the clinical suspicion [12].

References

1 Nadelman RB, Wormser GP: Lyme borreliosis. Lancet 1998;352:557–565.

2 Strle F: Principles of the diagnosis and antibiotic treatment of Lyme borreliosis. Wien Klin Wochenschr 1999;111:911–915.

3 Stanek G, Strle F: Lyme borreliosis. Lancet 2003;362:1639–1647.

4 Steere AC, Malawista SE, Hardin JA, Ruddy S, Askenase W, Andiman WA: Erythema chronicum migrans and Lyme arthritis: the enlarging clinical spectrum. Ann Intern Med 1977;86:685–698.

5 Steere AC, Malawista SE, Snydman DR, Shope RE, Andiman WA, Ross MR, Steele FM: Lyme arthritis: an epidemic of oligoarticular arthritis in children and adults in three Connecticut communities. Arthritis Rheum 1977;20:7–17.

6 The Free Dictionary: Medical dictionary. www.thefreedictionary.com.

7 Steere AC, Sikand VK, Schoen RT, Nowakowski J: Asymptomatic infection with *Borrelia burgdorferi*. Clin Infect Dis 2003;37:528–532.

8 Gustafson R, Svenungsson B, Gardulf A, Stiernstedt G, Forsgren M: Prevalence of tick-borne encephalitis and Lyme borreliosis in a defined Swedish population. Scand J Infect Dis 1990;22:297–306.

9 Fahrer H, van der Linden SM, Sauvain MJ, Gern L, Zhioua E, Aeschlimann A: The prevalence and incidence of clinical and asymptomatic Lyme borreliosis in a population at risk. J Infect Dis 1991;163:305–310.

10 Zhioua E, Gern L, Aeschlimann A, Sauvain MJ, van der Linden S, Fahrer H: Longitudinal study of Lyme borreliosis in a high risk population in Switzerland. Parasite 1998;5:383–386.

11 Anonymous: Case definitions for infectious conditions under public health surveillance: Lyme disease (revisited 9/96). MMWR Morb Mortal Wkly Rep 1997;46(suppl RR-10):20–21.

12 Stanek G, O'Connell S, Cimmino M, Aberer E, Kristoferitsch W, Granstrom M, Guy E, Gray J: European Union Concerted Action on Risk Assessment in Lyme borreliosis: clinical case definitions for Lyme borreliosis. Wien Klin Wochenschr 1996;108:741–747.

13 Brouqui P, Bacellar F, Baranton G, Birtles RJ, Bjoersdorff A, Blanco JR, Caruso G, Cinco M, Fournier PE, Francavilla E, Jensenius M, Kazar J, Laferl H, Lakos A, Lotric Furlan S, Maurin M, Oteo JA, Parola P, Perez-Eid C, Peter O, Postic D, Raoult D, Tellez A, Tselentis Y, Wilske B: Guidelines for the

diagnosis of tick-borne bacterial diseases in Europe. Clin Microbiol Infect 2004;10:1108–1132.
14 Wormser GP, Dattwyler RJ, Shapiro ED, Halperin JJ, Steere AC, Klempner MS, Krause PJ, Bakken JS, Strle F, Stanek G, Bockenstedt L, Fish D, Dumler S, Nadelman R: The clinical assessment, treatment, and prevention of Lyme disease, human granulocytic anaplasmosis, and babesiosis: clinical practice guidelines by the Infectious Diseases Society of America. Clin Infect Dis 2006;43:1089–1134.
15 Strle F, Nadelman RB, Cimperman J, Nowakowski J, Picken RN, Schwartz I, Maraspin V, Aguero-Rosenfeld ME, Varde S, Lotric-Furlan S, Wormser GP: Comparison of culture-confirmed erythema migrans caused by *Borrelia burgdorferi* sensu stricto in New York state and *Borrelia afzelii* in Slovenia. Ann Intern Med 1999;130:32–36.
16 Steere AC: Lyme disease. N Engl J Med 1989;321: 586–596.
17 Asbrink E, Hovmark A: Early and late cutaneous manifestations in *Ixodes*-borne borreliosis (erythema migrans borreliosis, Lyme borreliosis). Ann NY Acad Sci 1988;539:4–15.
18 Steere AC: Lyme disease. N Engl J Med 2001;345: 115–125.
19 Weber K, Neubert U, Buchner SA: Erythema migrans and early signs and symptoms; in Weber K, Burgdorfer W (eds): Aspects of Lyme Borreliosis. Heidelberg, Springer, 1993, pp 105–121.
20 Masters E, Granter S, Duray P, Cordes P: Physician-diagnosed erythema migrans and erythema migrans-like rashes following Lone Star tick bites. Arch Dermatol 1998;134:955–960.
21 Masters EJ, Grigery CN, Masters BE: STARI, or Masters Disease: Lone star tick-vectored Lyme-like illness. Infect Dis Clin North Am 2008;22:361–376.
22 Krause PJ, Telford SR 3rd, Spielman A, Sikand V, Ryan R, Christianson D, Burke G, Brassard P, Pollack R, Peck J, Persing DH: Concurrent Lyme disease and babesiosis: evidence for increased severity and duration of illness. JAMA 1996;275:1657–1660.
23 Cimperman J, Maraspin V, Lotric-Furlan S, Avsic-Zupanc T, Picken RN, Strle F: Concomitant infection with tick-borne encephalitis virus and *Borrelia burgdorferi* sensu lato in patients with acute meningitis or meningoencephalitis. Infection 1998;26: 160–164.
24 Nadelman RB, Horowitz HW, Hsieh TC, Wu JM, Aguero-Rosenfeld ME, Schwartz I, Nowakowski J, Varde S, Wormser GP: Simultaneous human granulocytic ehrlichiosis and Lyme borreliosis. N Engl J Med 1997;337:27–30.
25 Herxheimer K, Hartmann K: Über Acrodermatitis chronica atrophicans. Arch Dermatol Syph 1902; 61:57–76.
26 Afzelius A: Verhandlungen der Dermatologischen Gesellschaft zu Stockholm, 28 Oct 1909. Arch Dermatol Syph 1910;101:404.
27 Lipschütz B: Über eine seltene Erythemform (Erythema chronicum migrans). Arch Dermatol Syph 1913;118:349–356.
28 Dandache P, Nadelman RB: Erythema migrans. Infect Dis Clin North Am 2008;22:235–260.
29 Berglund J, Eitrem R, Ornstein K, Lindberg A, Ringer A, Elmrud H, Carlsson M, Runehagen A, Svanborg C, Norrby R: An epidemiologic study of Lyme disease in southern Sweden. N Engl J Med 1995;333:1319–1327.
30 Anonymous: Epidemiologic Surveillance of Infectious Diseases in Slovenia (in Slovene). Ljubljana, Institute of Public Health of the Republic of Slovenia, Slovenia, 2000.
31 Anonymous: Epidemiologic Surveillance of Infectious Diseases in Slovenia (in Slovene). Ljubljana, Institute of Public Health of the Republic of Slovenia, 2008.
32 Ornstein K, Berglund J, Nilsson I, Norrby R, Bergstrom S: Characterization of Lyme borreliosis isolates from patients with erythema migrans and neuroborreliosis in southern Sweden. J Clin Microbiol 2001;39:1294–1298.
33 Carlsson SA, Granlund H, Jansson C, Nyman D, Wahlberg P: Characteristics of erythema migrans in *Borrelia afzelii* and *Borrelia garinii* infections. Scand J Infect Dis 2003;35:31–33.
34 Cerar T, Ružić-Sabljić E, Glinsek U, Zore A, Strle F: Comparison of PCR methods and culture for the detection of *Borrelia* spp. in patients with erythema migrans. Clin Microbiol Infect 2008;14:653–658.
35 Zore A, Ružić-Sabljić E, Maraspin V, Cimperman J, Lotrič-Furlan S, Pikelj A, Jurca T, Logar M, Strle F: Sensitivity of culture and polymerase chain reaction for the etiologic diagnosis of erythema migrans. Wien Klin Wochenschr 2002;114:606–609.
36 Kuiper H, Cairo I, van Dam A, de Jongh B, Ramselaar T, Spanjaard L, Dankert J: Solitary erythema migrans: a clinical, laboratory and epidemiological study of 77 Dutch patients. Br J Dermatol 1994;130: 466–472.
37 Ciceroni L, Ciarrochi S, Ciervo A, Mondarini V, Guzzo F, Caruso G, Murgia R, Cinco M: Isolation and characterization of *Borrelia burgdorferi* sensu lato strains in an area of Italy where Lyme borreliosis is endemic. J Clin Microbiol 2001;39:2254–2260.
38 Ružić-Sabljić E, Maraspin V, Lotrič-Furlan S, Jurca T, Logar M, Pikelj-Pečnik A, Strle F: Characterization of *Borrelia burgdorferi* sensu lato strains isolated from human material in Slovenia. Wien Klin Wochenschr 2002;114:544–550.

39 Fingerle V, Schulte-Spechtel UC, Ružić-Sabljić E, Leonhard S, Hofmannd H, Weber K, Pfister K, Strle F, Wilske B: Epidemiological aspects and molecular characterization of *Borrelia burgdorferi* s.l. from southern Germany with special respect to the new species *Borrelia spielmanii* sp. nov. Int J Med Microbiol 2008;298:279–290.
40 Picken RN, Cheng Y, Strle F, Picken MM: Patient isolates of *Borrelia burgdorferi* sensu lato with genotypic and phenotypic similarities of strain 25015. J Infect Dis 1996;174:1112–1115.
41 Strle F, Picken RN, Cheng Y, Cimperman J, Maraspin V, Lotrič-Furlan S, Ružić-Sabljić E, Picken MM: Clinical findings for patients with Lyme borreliosis caused by *Borrelia burgdorferi* sensu lato with genotypic and phenotypic similarities to strain 25015. Clin Infect Dis 1997;25:273–280.
42 Foldvari G, Farkas R, Lakos A: *Borrelia spielmanii* erythema migrans, Hungary. Emerg Infect Dis 2005;11:1794–1795.
43 Maraspin V, Ružić-Sabljić E, Strle F: Lyme borreliosis and *Borrelia spielmanii*. Emerg Infect Dis 2006; 12:1177.
44 Ružić-Sabljić E, Zore A, Strle F: Characterization of *Borrelia burgdorferi* sensu lato isolates by pulsed-field gel electrophoresis after MluI restriction of genomic DNA. Research Microbiol 2008;159:441–448.
45 Oksi J, Marttila H, Soini H, Aho H, Uksila J, Viljanen MK: Early dissemination of *Borrelia burgdorferi* without generalized symptoms in patients with erythema migrans. APMIS 2001;109:581–588.
46 Picken RN, Cheng Y, Strle F, Cimperman J, Maraspin V, Lotrič-Furlan S, Ružić-Sabljić E, Han D, Nelson JA, Picken MM, Trenholme GT: Molecular characterization of *Borrelia burgdorferi* sensu lato from Slovenia revealing significant differences between tick and human isolates. Eur J Clin Microbiol Infect Dis 1996;15:313–323.
47 Picken MM, Picken RN, Han D, Cheng Y, Strle F: Single-tube nested polymerase chain reaction assay based on flagellin gene sequences for detection of *Borrelia burgdorferi* sensu lato. Eur J Clin Microbiol Infect Dis 1996;6:489–498.
48 Seinost G, Golde WT, Berger BW, Dunn JJ, Qiu D, Dunkin DS, Dykhuizen DE, Luft BJ, Dattwyler RJ: Infection with multiple strains of *Borrelia burgdorferi* sensu stricto in patients with Lyme disease. Arch Dermatol 1999;135:1329–1333.
49 Ružić-Sabljić E, Arnez M, Lotrič-Furlan S, Maraspin V, Cimperman J, Strle F: Genotypic and phenotypic characterisation of *Borrelia burgdorferi* sensu lato strains isolated from human blood. J Med Microbiol 2001;50:896–901.
50 Ružić-Sabljić E, Arnez M, Logar M, Maraspin V, Lotrič-Furlan S, Cimperman J, Strle F: Comparison of *Borrelia burgdorferi* sensu lato strains isolated from specimens obtained simultaneously from two different sites of infection in individual patients. J Clin Microbiol 2005;43:2194–2200.
51 Nadelman RB, Nowakowski J, Forseter G, Goldberg NS, Bittker S, Cooper D, Aguero-Rosenfeld M, Wormser GP: The clinical spectrum of early Lyme borreliosis in patients with culture-confirmed erythema migrans. Am J Med 1996;100:502–508.
52 Smith RP, Schoen RT, Rahn DW, Sikand VK, Nowakowski J, Parenti DL, Holman MS, Persing DH, Steere AC: Clinical characteristics and treatment outcome of early Lyme disease in patients with microbiologically confirmed erythema migrans. Ann Intern Med 2002;136:421–428.
53 Weber K, Neubert U: Clinical features of early erythema migrans disease and related disorders. Zentralbl Bakteriol Mikrobiol Hyg [A] 1986;263: 209–228.
54 Asbrink E, Olsson I, Hovmark A: Erythema chronicum migrans Afzelius in Sweden: a study on 231 patients. Zentralbl Bakteriol Mikrobiol Hyg [A] 1986;263:229–236.
55 Strle F, Nelson JA, Ružić-Sabljić E, Nowakowski J, Picken RN, Schwartz I, Maraspin V, Aguero-Rosenfeld ME, Varde S, Lotrič-Furlan S, Wormser GP: European Lyme borreliosis: 231 culture-confirmed cases involving patients with erythema migrans. Clin Infect Dis 1996;23:61–65.
56 Strle F, Videcnik J, Zorman P, Cimperman J, Lotrič-Furlan S, Maraspin V: Clinical and epidemiological findings for patients with erythema migrans: comparison of cohorts from the years 1993 and 2000. Wien Klin Wochenschr 2002;114:493–497.
57 De Koning J, Duray PH: Histopathology of human Lyme borreliosis; in Weber K, Burgdorfer W (eds): Aspects of Lyme Borreliosis. Heidelberg, Springer, 1993, pp 70–92.
58 Mullegger RR, Means TK, Shin JJ, Lee M, Jones KL, Glickstein LJ, Luster AD, Steere AC: Chemokine signatures in the skin disorders of Lyme borreliosis in Europe: predominance of CXCL9 and CXCL10 in erythema migrans and acrodermatitis and CXCL13 in lymphocytoma. Infect Immun 2007;75: 4621–4628.
59 Maraspin V, Ružić-Sabljić E, Cimperman J, Lotrič-Furlan S, Jurca T, Picken RN, Strle F: Isolation of *Borrelia burgdorferi* sensu lato from blood of patients with erythema migrans. Infection 2001;29: 65–70.
60 Steere AC, Bartenhagen NH, Craft JE, Hutchinson GJ, Newman JH, Rahn DW, Sigal LH, Spieler PN, Stenn KS, Malawista SE: The early clinical manifestations of Lyme disease. Ann Intern Med 1983;99: 76–82.

61 Logar M, Ružić-Sabljić E, Maraspin V, Lotrič-Furlan S, Cimperman J, Jurca T, Strle F: Comparison of erythema migrans caused by *Borrelia afzelii* and *Borrelia garinii*. Infection 2003;31:404–409.

62 Bennet L, Fraenkel CJ, Garpmo U, Halling A, Ingman M, Ornstein K, Stjernberg L, Berglund J: Clinical appearance of erythema migrans caused by *Borrelia afzelii* and *Borrelia garinii* – effect of the patient's sex. Wien Klin Wochenschr 206;118:531–537.

63 Arnez M, Ružić-Sabljić E, Ahcan J, Radsel-Medvescek A, Pleterski-Rigler D, Strle F: Isolation of *Borrelia burgdorferi* sensu lato from blood of children with solitary erythema migrans. Pediatr Infect Dis J 2001;20:251–255.

64 Wormser GP, McKenna D, Carlin J, Nadelman RB, Cavaliere LF, Holmgren D, Byrne DW, Nowakowski J: Hematogenous dissemination in early Lyme disease. Ann Intern Med 2005;142:751–755.

65 Arnez M, Pleterski-Rigler D, Ahcan J, Ružić-Sabljić E, Strle F: Demographic features, clinical characteristics and laboratory findings in children with multiple erythema migrans in Slovenia. Wien Klin Wochenschr 2001;113:98–101.

66 Arnez M, Pleterski-Rigler D, Luznik-Bufon T, Ružić-Sabljić E, Strle F: Children with multiple erythema migrans: are there any pre-treatment symptoms and/or signs suggestive for central nervous system involvement? Wien Klin Wochenschr 2002;114:524–529.

67 Mullegger RR: Dermatological manifestations of Lyme borreliosis. Eur J Dermatol 2004;14:296–309.

68 Asbrink E, Hovmark A, Olsson I: Lymphadenosis benigna cutis solitaria – borrelia lymphocytoma in Sweden. Zentralbl Bakteriol 1989;(suppl 18):156–163.

69 Strle F, Pleterski-Rigler D, Stanek G, Pejovnik-Pustinek A, Ruzic E, Cimperman J: Solitary borrelial lymphocytoma: report of 36 cases. Infection 1992;20:201–206.

70 Strle F, Maraspin V, Pleterski-Rigler D, Lotrič-Furlan S, Ružić-Sabljić E, Jurca T, Cimperman J: Treatment of borrelial lymphocytoma. Infection 1996; 24:80–84.

71 Maraspin V, Cimperman J, Lotrič-Furlan S, Ružić-Sabljić E, Jurca T, Picken RN, Strle F: Solitary borrelial lymphocytoma in adult patients. Wien Klin Wochenschr 2002;114:515–523.

72 Hovmark A, Asbrink E, Weber K, Kaudewitz P: Borrelial lymphocytoma; in Weber K, Burgdorfer W (eds): Aspects of Lyme Borreliosis. Heidelberg, Springer, 1993, pp 122–130.

73 Colli C, Leinweber B, Mullegger R, Chott A, Kerl H, Cerroni L: *Borrelia burgdorferi*-associated lymphocytoma cutis: clinicopathologic, immunophenotypic, and molecular study of 106 cases. J Cutan Pathol 2004;31:232–240.

74 Strle F: Lyme borreliosis in Slovenia. Zentralbl Bakteriol 1999;289:643–652.

75 Picken RN, Strle F, Ružić-Sabljić E, Maraspin V, Lotrič-Furlan S, Cimperman J, Cheng Y, Picken MM: Molecular subtyping of *Borrelia burgdorferi* sensu lato isolates from five patients with solitary lymphcytoma. J Invest Dermatol 1997;108:92–97.

76 Busch U, Hizo-Teufel C, Bohmer R, Fingerle V, Rossler D, Wilske B, Preac-Mursic V: *Borrelia burgdorferi* sensu lato strains isolated from cutaneous Lyme borreliosis biopsies differentiated by pulsed-field gel electrophoresis. Scand J Infect Dis 1996;28: 583–589.

77 Ružić-Sabljić E, Strle F, Cimperman J, Maraspin V, Lotrič-Furlan S, Pleterski-Rigler D: Characterisation of *Borrelia burgdorferi* sensu lato strains isolated from patients with skin manifestations of Lyme borreliosis residing in Slovenia. J Med Microbiol 2000;49:47–53.

78 Weber K, Schierz G, Wilske B, Preac-Mursic V: Das Lymphozytom – eine Borrelize? Z Hautkr 1985;60: 1585–1598.

79 Weber K, Neubert U, Thurmayr R: Antibiotic therapy in early erythema migrans disease and related disorders. Zentralbl Bakteriol Mikrobiol Hyg [A] 1986;263:377–388.

80 Hovmark A, Asbrink E, Olsson I: The spirochetal etiology of lymphadenosis benigna cutis solitaria. Acta Derm Venereol 1986;66:479–484.

81 Asbrink E, Hovmark A: Cutaneous manifestations in *Ixodes*-borne borrelia spirechetosis. Int J Dermatol 1987;26:215–225.

82 Boye T: What kind of clinical, epidemiological, and biological data is essential for the diagnosis of Lyme borreliosis? Dermatological and ophtalmological courses of Lyme borreliosis. Med Mal Infect 2007; 37(suppl 3):S175–S188.

83 Lipsker D: Dermatological aspects of Lyme borreliosis. Med Mal Infect 2007;37:540–547.

84 DiCaudo DJ, Su WP, Marshall WF, Malawista SE, Barthold S, Persing DH: Acrodermatitis chronica atrophicans in the United States: clinical and histopathologic features of six cases. Cutis 1994;54:81–84.

85 Lavoie PE, Wilson AJ, Tuffanelli DL: Acrodermatitis chronica atrophicans with antecedent Lyme disease in a California. Case report. Mol Pathol 1997; 50:186–193.

86 Wienecke R, Zochling N, Neubert U, Schlupen EM, Meurer M, Volkenandt M: Molecular subtyping of in erythema migrans and acrodermatitis chronica atrophicans. J Invest Dermatol 1994;103:19–22.

87 Ohlenbusch A, Matuschka FR, Richter D, Christen HJ, Thomssen R, Spielman A, Eiffert H: Etiology of the acrodermatitis chronica atrophicans lesion in Lyme disease. J Infect Dis 1996;174:421–423.

88 Rijpkema SG, Tazelaar DJ, Molkenboer MJ, Noordhoek GT, Plantinga G, Schouls L, Schellekens JF: Detection of *Borrelia afzelii*, *Borrelia burgdorferi* sensu stricto, *Borrelia garinii* and group VS116 by PCR in skin biopsies of patients with erythema migrans and acrodermatitis chronica atrophicans. Clin Microbiol Infect 1997;3:109–116.
89 Lunemann JD, Zarmas S, Priem S, Franz J, Zschenderlein R, Aberer E, Klein R, Schouls L, Burmester GR, Krause A: Rapid typing of *Borrelia burgdorferi* sensu lato species in specimens from patients with different manifestations of Lyme borreliosis. J Clin Microbiol 2001;39:1130–1133.
90 Maraspin V, Ružić-Sabljić E, Strle F: Isolation of *Borrelia burgdorferi* sensu lato from a fibrous nodule in a patient with acrodermatitis chronica atrophicans. Wien Klin Wochenschr 2002;114:533–534.
91 Picken RN, Strle F, Picken MM, Ružić-Sabljić E, Maraspin V, Lotric-Furlan S, Cimperman J: Identification of three species of *Borrelia burgdorferi* sensu lato (*B. burgdorferi* sensu stricto, *B. garinii*, and *B. afzelii*) among isolates from acrodermatitis chronica atrophicans lesions. J Invest Dermatol 1998;110:211–214.
92 Asbrink E: Erythema chronicum migrans Afzelius and acrodermatitis chronica atrophicans: early and late manifestations of *Ixodes ricinus*-borne *Borrelia* spirochetes. Acta Derm Venereol Suppl (Stockh) 1985;118:1–63.
93 Asbrink E, Brehmer Andersson E, Hovmark A: Acrodermatitis chronica atrophicans – a spirochetosis: clinical and histopathological picture based on 32 patients. Am J Dermatopathol 1986;8:209–219.
94 Brehmer-Andersson E, Hovmark A, Asbrink E: Acrodermatitis chronica atrophicans: histopathologic findings and clinical correlations in 111 cases. Acta Derm Venereol 1998;78:207–213.
95 Asbrink E, Hovmark A, Olsson I: Clinical manifestations of acrodermatitis chronica atrophicans in 50 Swedish patients. Zentralbl Bakteriol Mikrobiol Hyg [A] 1986;263:253–261.
96 Asbrink E, Hovmark A, Weber K: Acrodermatitis chronica atrophicans; in Weber K, Burgdorfer W (eds): Aspects of Lyme Borreliosis. Heidelberg, Springer, 1993, pp 193–204.
97 Hopf HC: Peripheral neuropathy in acrodermatitis chronica atrophicans (Herxheimer). J Neurol Neurosurg Psychiat 1975;38:452–458.
98 Kristoferitsch W, Sluga E, Graf M, Partsch H, Neumann R, Stanek G, Budka H: Neuropathy associated with acrodermatitis chronica atrophicans: clinical and morphological features. Ann NY Acad Sci 1988;539:35–45.
99 Kindstrand E, Nilsson BY, Hovmark A, Pirskanen R, Asbrink E: Peripheral neuropathy in acrodermatitis chronica atrophicans – effect of treatment. Acta Neurol Scand 2002;106:253–257.
100 Herzer P: Joint manifestations; in Weber K, Burgdorfer W (eds): Aspects of Lyme Borreliosis. Heidelberg, Springer, 1993, pp 168–184.
101 Hauser W: Zur Kenntnis der Acrodermatitis chronica atrophicans. Arch Dermatol Syph 1955; 199;350–393.
102 Hoesly JM, Mertz LE, Winkelmann RK: Localized scleroderma (morphea) and antibody to *Borrelia burgdorferi*. J Am Acad Dermatol 1987;17:455–458.
103 Akimoto S, Ishikawa O, Miyachi Y: The absence of antibodies against *Borrelia burgdorferi* in the sera of Japanese patients with localized scleroderma. J Rheumatol 1996;3:573–574.
104 Breier F, Klade H, Stanek G, Poitschek C, Kirnbauer R, Dorda W, Aberer E: Lymphoproliferative responses to *Borrelia burgdorferi* in circumscribed scleroderma. Br J Dermatol 1996;134:285–291.
105 Buechner SA, Lautenschlager S, Itin P, Bircher A, Erb P: Lymphoproliferative responses to *Borrelia burgdorferi* in patients with erythema migrans, acrodermatitis chronica atrophicans, lymphadenosis benigna cutis, and morphea. Arch Dermatol 1995;131:673–677.
106 Fujiwara H, Fujiwara K, Hashimoto K, Mehregan AH, Schaumburg-Lever G, Lange R, Schempp C, Gollnick H: Detection of *Borrelia burgdorferi* DNA (*B. garinii* or *B. afzelii*) in morphea and lichen sclerosus et atrophicus tissues of German and Japanese but not of US patients. Arch Dermatol 1997;133:41–44.
107 Dillon WI, Saed GM, Fivenson DP: *Borrelia burgdorferi* DNA is undetectable by polymerase chain reaction in skin lesions of morphea, scleroderma, or lichen sclerosus et atrophicus of patients from North America. J Am Acad Dermatol 1995;33:617–620.
108 Aguero-Rosenfeld ME, Wang G, Schwartz I, Wormser GP: Diagnosis of Lyme borreliosis. Clin Microbiol Rev 2005;18:484–509.
109 Aberer E, Stanek G, Ertl M, Neumann R: Evidence for spirochetal origin of circumscribed scleroderma (morphea). Acta Derm Venereol 1987;67:225–231.
110 Weber K, Preac-Mursic V, Reimers CD: Spirochetes isolated from two patients with morphea. Infection 1988;16:25–26.
111 Breier FH, Aberer E, Stanek G, Khanakaha G, Schlick A, Tappeiner G: Isolation of *Borrelia afzelii* from circumscribed scleroderma. Br J Dermatol 1999;140:925–930.
112 Ranguin G, Boisnic S, Souteyrand P, Baranton G, Piette JC, Godeau P, Francès C: No evidence for a spirochetal origin of localized scleroderma. Br J Dermatol 1992;127:218–220.

113 Alonso-Llamazares J, Persing DH, Anda P, Gibson LE, Rutledge BJ, Iglesias L: No evidence for *Borrelia burgdorferi* infection in lesions of morphea and lichen sclerosus et atrophicus in Spain: a prospective study and literature review. Acta Derm Venereol 1997;77:299–304.
114 Breier F, Khanakah G, Stanek G, Kunz G, Aberer E, Schmidt B, Tappeiner G: Isolation and polymerase chain reaction typing of *Borrelia afzelii* from a skin lesion in a seronegative patient with generalized ulcerating bullous lichen sclerosus et atrophicus. Br J Dermatol 2001;144:387–392.
115 Cerroni L, Zöchling N, Pütz B, Kerl H: Infection by *Borrelia burgdorferi* and cutaneous B-cell lymphoma. J Cutan Pathol 1997;24:457–461.
116 Kutting B, Bonsmann G, Metze D, Luger TA, Cerroni L: *Borrelia burgdorferi*-associated primary cutaneous B cell lymphoma: complete clearing of skin lesions after antibiotic pulse therapy or intralesional injection of interferon alfa-2a. J Am Acad Dermatol 1997;36:311–314.
117 Schöllkopf C, Melbye M, Munksgaard L, Ekström Smedby K, Rostgaard K, Glimelius B, Chang ET, Roos G, Hansen M, Adami HO, Hjalgrim H: *Borrelia* infection and risk of non-Hodgkin lymphoma. Blood 2008;111:5524–5529.
118 Wood GS, Kamath NV, Guitart J, Heald P, Kohler S, Smoller BR, Cerroni L: Absence of *Borrelia burgdorferi* DNA in cutaneous B-cell lymphomas from the United States. J Cutan Pathol 2001;28:502–507.
119 Munksgaard L, Frisch M, Melbye M, Hjalgrim H: Incidence patterns of Lyme disease and cutaneous B-cell non-Hodgkin's lymphoma in the United States. Dermatology 2000;201:351–352.
120 Goodlad JR, Davidson MM, Hollowood K, Ling C, MacKenzie C, Christie I, Batstone PJ, Ho-Yen DO: Primary cutaneous B-cell lymphoma and *Borrelia burgdorferi* infection in patients from the highlands of Scotland. Am J Surg Pathol 2000;24:1279–1285.
121 Li C, Inagaki H, Kuo TT, Hu S, Okabe M, Eimoto T: Primary cutaneous marginal zone B-cell lymphoma: a molecular and clinicopathologic study of 24 Asian cases. Am J Surg Pathol 2003;27:1061–1069.
122 Senff NJ, Noordijk EM, Youn H, Kim YH, Bagot M, Berti E, Cerroni L, Dummer R, Duvic M, Hoppe RT, Pimpinelli N, Rosen ST, Vermeer MH, Whittaker S, Willemze R: European Organization for Research and Treatment of Cancer and International Society for Cutaneous Lymphoma consensus recommendations for the management of cutaneous B-cell lymphomas. Blood 2008;112:1600–1609.
123 Bayerdorffer E, Neubauer A, Rudolph B, Thiede C, Lehn N, Eidt S, Stolte M: Regression of primary gastric lymphoma of mucosa-associated lymphoid tissue type after cure of *Helicobacter pylori* infection: MALT Lymphoma Study Group. Lancet 1995;345:1591–1594.
124 Neubauer A, Thiede C, Morgner A, Alpen B, Ritter M, Neubauer A, Wundisch T, Ehninger G, Stolte M, Bayerdorffer E: Cure of *Helicobacter pylori* infection and duration of remission of low-grade gastric mucosa-associated lymphoid tissue lymphoma. J Natl Cancer Inst 1997;89:1350–1355.
125 Roggero E, Zucca E, Pinotti G, Pascarella A, Capella C, Savio A, Pedrinis E, Paterlini A, Venco A, Cavalli F: Eradication of *Helicobacter pylori* infection in primary lowgrade gastric lymphoma of mucosa-associated lymphoid tissue. Ann Intern Med 1995;122:767–769.
126 Dreno B: Standard and new treatments in cutaneous B-cell lymphomas. J Cutan Pathol 2006;33(suppl 1):S47–S51.
127 Zenahlik P, Fink-Puches R, Kapp KS, Kerl H, Cerroni L: Therapy of primary cutaneous B-cell lymphomas. Hautarzt 2000;51:19–24.
128 Hoefnagel JJ, Vermeer MH, Jansen PM, Heule F, van Voorst Vader PC, Sanders CJ, Gerritsen MJ, Geerts ML, Meijer CJ, Noordijk EM, Willemze R: Primary cutaneous marginal zone B-cell lymphoma: clinical and therapeutic features in 50 cases. Arch Dermatol 2005;141:1139–1145.
129 Bogle MA, Riddle CC, Triana EM, Jones D, Duvic M: Primary cutaneous B-cell lymphoma. J Am Acad Dermatol 2005;53:479–484.
130 Monari P, Farisoglio C, Calzavara Pinton PG: *Borrelia burgdorferi*-associated primary cutaneous marginal-zone B-cell lymphoma: a case report. Dermatology 2007;215:229–232.
131 Roggero E, Zucca E, Mainetti C, Bertoni F, Valsangiacomo C, Pedrinis E, Borisch B, Piffaretti JC, Cavalli F, Isaacson PG: Eradication of *Borrelia burgdorferi* infection in primary marginal zone B-cell lymphoma of the skin. Hum Pathol 2000;31:263–268.
132 Ryffel K, Peter O, Rutti B, Suard A, Dayer E: Scored antibody reactivity determined by immunoblotting shows an association between clinical manifestations and presence of *Borrelia burgdorferi* sensu stricto, *B. garinii*, *B. afzelii*, and *B. valaisiana* in humans. J Clin Microbiol 1999;37:4086–4092.
133 Peter O, Bretz AG, Postic D, Dayer E: Association of distinct species of *Borrelia burgdorferi* sensu lato with neuroborreliosis in Switzerland. Clin Microbiol Infect 1997;3:423–431.
134 Hizo-Teufel C, Fingerle V, Nitschko H, Wilske B, Preac-Mursic V: Three species of *Borrelia burgdorferi* sensu lato *(B. burgdorferi* sensu stricto, *B. afzelii* and *B. garinii)* identified from cerebrospinal fluid isolates by pulsed-field gel electrophoresis and PCR. J Clin Microbiol 1996;34:1072–1078.
135 Ružić-Sabljić E, Lotrič-Furlan S, Maraspin V, Cimperman J, Pleterski-Rigler D, Strle F: Analysis of *Borrelia burgdorferi* sensu lato isolated from cerebrospinal fluid. APMIS 2001;109:707–713.

136 Strle F, Ružić-Sabljić E, Cimperman J, Lotricč-Furlan S, Maraspin V: Comparison of findings for patients with *Borrelia garinii* and *Borrelia afzelii* isolated from cerebrospinal fluid. Clin Infect Dis 2006;43:704–710.

137 Lebech AM, Hansen K, Rutledge BJ, Kolbert CP, Rys PN, Pershing DH: Diagnostic detection and direct genotyping of *Borrelia burgdorferi* by polymerase chain reaction in cerebrospinal fluid in Lyme neuroborreliosis. Mol Diagn 1998;3:131–141.

138 Ornstein K, Berglund J, Bergstrom S, Norrby R, Barbour AG: Three major Lyme *Borrelia* genospecies *(Borrelia burgdorferi* sensu stricto, *B. afzelii* and *B. garinii)* identified by PCR in cerebrospinal fluid from patients with neuroborreliosis in Sweden. Scand J Infect Dis 2002;34:341–346.

139 Steere AC, Schoen RT, Taylor E: The clinical evolution of Lyme arthritis. Ann Intern Med 1987;107: 725–731.

140 Reik L, Steere AC, Bartenhagen NH, Shope RE, Malawista SE: Neurologic abnormalities of Lyme disease. Medicine 1979;58:281–294.

141 Gerber MA, Shapiro ED, Burke GS, Parcells VJ, Bell GL: Lyme disease in children in southeastern Connecticut. Pediatric Lyme Disease Study Group. N Engl J Med 1996;335:1270–1274.

142 Centers for Disease Control and Prevention: Lyme disease – United States, 2003–2005. MMWR 2007; 6:573–576.

143 Clark JR, Carlson RD, Sasaki CT, Pachies AR, Steere AC: Facial paralysis in Lyme disease. Laryngoscope 1985;95:1341–1345.

144 Shapiro ED, Gerber MA: Lyme disease and facial nerve palsy. Arch Pediatr Adolesc Med 1997;151: 1183–1184.

145 Halperin JJ, Golightly M: Lyme borreliosis in Bell's palsy. Long Island Neuroborreliosis Collaborative Study Group. Neurology 1992;42:1268–1270.

146 Halperin JJ: Nervous system Lyme disease. Infect Dis Clin North Am 2008;22:261–274.

147 Lotrič-Furlan S, Cimperman J, Maraspin V, Ružić-Sabljić E, Logar M, Jurca T, Strle F: Lyme borreliosis and peripheral facial palsy. Wien Klin Wochenschr 1999;111:970–975.

148 Pfister HW, Kristoferitsch W, Meier C: Early neurological involvement (Bannwarth's syndrome); in Weber K, Burgdorfer W (eds): Aspects of Lyme Borreliosis. Heidelberg, Springer, 1993, pp 152–167.

149 Kristoferitsch W: Neuropathien bei Lyme-Borreliose. Wien, Springer, 1989.

150 Stiernstedt GT, Granstrom M, Hederstedt B, Skoldenberg B: Diagnosis of spirochetal meningitis by enzyme-linked immunosorbent assay and indirect immunofluorescence assay in serum and cerebrospinal fluid. J Clin Microbiol 1985;21:819–825.

151 Pfister HW, Einhaupl KM, Wilske B, Preac-Mursic V: Bannwarth's syndrome and the enlarged neurological spectrum of arthropod-borne borreliosis. Zentralbl Bakteriol Mikrobiol Hyg [A] 1987;263: 343–347.

152 Bammer H, Schenk K: Meningomyeloradikulitis nach Zeckenbiss mit Erythem. Dtsch Z Nervenheilkunde 1965;187:25–34.

153 Schaltenbrand G: Durch Arthropoden übertragene Infektionen der Haut und des Nervensystems. Verh Dtsch Ges Inn Med 1967;72:975–1005.

154 Erbsloh F, Kohlmeyer K: Über polytope Erkrankungen des peripheren Nervensystems bei Lymphozytarer Meningitis. Fortschr Neurol Psychiatr 1968;36:321–342.

155 Horstup P, Ackermann R: Durch Zecken übertragene Meningopolyneuritis (Garin-Bujadoux-Bannwarth). Fortschr Neurol Psychiatr 1973;41: 583–606.

156 Kristoferitsch W, Spiel G, Wessely P: Meningopolyneuritis (Garin-Bujadoux-Bannwarth): clinical aspects and laboratory findings. Nervenarzt 1983;54:640–646.

157 Pachner AR, Steere AC: The triad of neurologic manifestations of Lyme disease: meningitis, cranial neuritis, and radiculoneuritis. Neurology 1985;111:47–53.

158 Duray PH: Clinical pathologic correlations of Lyme disease. Rev Infect Dis 1989;11(suppl 6): S1487–S1493.

159 Meurers B, Kohlhepp W, Gold R, Rohrbach E, Mertens HG: Histopathological findings in the central and peripheral nervous systems in neuroborreliosis: a report of three cases. J Neurol 1990;237:113–116.

160 Roberts ED, Bohm RP Jr, Lowrie RC Jr, Habicht G, Katona L, Piesman J, Philipp MT: Pathogenesis of Lyme neuroborreliosis in the rhesus monkey: the early disseminated and chronic phases of disease in the peripheral nervous system. J Infect Dis 1998; 178:722–732.

161 Garin C, Bujadoux R: Paralisie par les tiques. J Med Lyon 1922;71:765–767.

162 Kristoferitsch W: Neurological manifestations of Lyme borreliosis: clinical definition and differential diagnosis. Scand J Infect Dis 1991;77 (suppl):64–73.

163 Hansen K: Lyme neuroborreliosis: improvements of the laboratory diagnosis and a survey of epidemiological and clinical features in Denmark 1985–1990. Acta Neurol Scand 1994;89(suppl 151):7–44.

164 Pfadenhauer K, Schonsteiner T, Stohr M: Thoracoabdominal manifestation of stage II Lyme neuroborreliosis. Nervenarzt 1998;69:296–299.

165 Bagger-Sjoback D, Remahl S, Ericsson M: Longterm outcome of facial palsy in neuroborreliosis. Otol Neurotol 2005;26:790–795.

166 Skogman BH, Croner S, Odkvist L: Acute facial palsy in children – a 2-year follow-up study with focus on Lyme neuroborreliosis. Int J Pediatr Otorhinolaryngol 2003;67:597–602.
167 Sibony P, Halperin J, Coyle PK, Patel K: Reactive Lyme serology in optic neuritis. J Neuroophthalmol 2005;25:71–82.
168 Steenhoff AP, Smith MJ, Shah SS, Coffin SE: Neuroborreliosis with progression from pseudotumor cerebri to aseptic meningitis. Pediatr Infect Dis J 2006;25:91–92.
169 Feder HM Jr: Lyme disease in children. Infect Dis Clin North Am 2008;22:315–326.
170 Kristoferitsch W. Chronic peripheral neuropathy; in Weber K, Burgdorfer W (eds): Aspects of Lyme Borreliosis. Heidelberg, Springer, 1993, pp 219–227.
171 Logigian EL, Kaplan RF, Steere AC: Chronic neurologic manifestations of Lyme disease. N Engl J Med 1990;323:1438–1444.
172 Cerar T, Ogrinc K, Cimperman J, Lotrič-Furlan S, Strle F, Ružić-Sabljić E: Validation of cultivation and PCR methods for diagnosis of Lyme neuroborreliosis. J Clin Microbiol 2008;46:3375–3379.
173 Fish AE, Pride YB, Pinto DS: Lyme carditis. Infect Dis Clin North Am 2008;22:275–288.
174 Steere AC, Batsford WP, Weinberg M, Alexander J, Berger , Wolfson S, Malawista SE: Lyme carditis: cardiac abnormalities of Lyme disease. Ann Intern Med 1980;93:8–16.
175 Van der Linde MR: Lyme carditis; in Weber K, Burgdorfer W (eds): Aspects of Lyme Borreliosis. Heidelberg, Springer, 1993, pp 131–151.
176 Sigal LH: Early disseminated Lyme disease: cardiac manifestations. Am J Med 1995;98(suppl 4A):25–28.
177 Rubin DA, Sorbera C, Nikitin P, McAllister A, Wormser GP, Nadelman RB: Prospective evaluation of heart block complicating early Lyme disease. Pacing Clin Electrophysiol 1992;15:252–255.
178 Steere AC, Sikand VK, Meurice F, Parenti DL, Fikrig E, Schoen RT, Nowakowski J, Schmid CH, Laukamp S, Buscarino C, Krause DS: Vaccination against Lyme disease with recombinant *Borrelia burgdorferi* outer surface lipoprotein A with adjuvant. Lyme Disease Vaccine Study Group. N Engl J Med 1998;339:209–215.
179 Sigal LH, Zahradnik JM, Lavin P, Patella SJ, Bryant G, Haselby R, Hilton E, Kunkel M, Adler-Klein D, Doherty T, Evans J, Molloy PJ, Seidner AL, Sabetta JR, Simon HJ, Klempner MS, Mays J, Marks D, Malawista SE: A vaccine consisting of recombinant *Borrelia burgdorferi* outer-surface A to prevent Lyme disease. Recombinant Outer-Surface Protein A Lyme Disease Vaccine Study Consortium. N Engl J Med 1998;339:216–222.
180 Stanek G, Klein J, Bittner R, Glogar D: Isolation of *Borrelia burgdorferi* from the myocardium of a patient with longstanding cardiomyopathy. N Engl J Med 1990;322:249–252.
181 Marcus LC, Steere AC, Duray PH, Anderson AE, Mahoney EB: Fatal pancarditis in a patient with coexisting Lyme disease and babesiosis. Ann Intern Med 1985;103:374–376.
182 Reznick JW, Braunstein DB, Walsh RL, Smith CR, Wolfson PM, Gierke LW, Gorelkin L, Chandler FW: Lyme carditis: electrophysiologic and histopathologic study. Am J Med 1986;81:923–927.
183 Cox J, Krajden M: Cardiovascular manifestations of Lyme disease. Am Heart J 1991;122:1449–1455.
184 de Koning J, Hoogkamp-Korstanje JA, van der Linde MR, Crijns HJ: Demonstration of spirochetes in cardiac biopsies of patients with Lyme disease. J Infect Dis 1989;160:150–153.
185 van der Linde MR: Lyme carditis: clinical characteristics of 105 cases. Scand J Infect Dis 1991; 77(suppl):81–84.
186 McAlister HF, Klementowicz PT, Andrews C, Fisher JD, Feld M, Furman S: Lyme carditis: an important course of reversible heart block. Ann Intern Med 1989;110:339–345.
187 Pinto DS: Cardiac manifestations of Lyme disease. Med Clin North Am 2002;86:285–296.
188 Cary NR, Fox B, Wright DJ, Cutler SJ, Shapiro LM, Grace AA: Fatal Lyme carditis and endodermal heterotopia of the atrioventricular node. Postgrad Med J 1990;66:134–136.
189 Midttun M, Lebech AM, Hansen K, Videbaek J: Lyme carditis: a clinical presentation and long time follow-up. Scand J Infect Dis 1997;29:153–157.
190 Lardieri G, Salvi A, Camerini F, Cinco M, Trevisan G: Isolation of *Borrelia burgdorferi* from myocardium. Lancet 1993;342:490.
191 Gasser R, Dusleag J, Reisinger E, Stauber E, Feigl B, Pongratz S, Klein W, Furian C, Pierer K: Reversal by ceftriaxone of dilated cardiomyopathy *Borrelia burgdorferi* infection. Lancet 1992;339:1174–1175.
192 Sonnesyn SW, Diehl SC, Johnson RC, Kubo SH, Goodman JL: A prospective study of the seroprevalence of *Borrelia burgdorferi* infection in patients with severe heart failure. Am J Cardiol 1995;76: 97–100.
193 Sangha O, Phillips CB, Fleischman KE, Wang TJ, Fossel AH, Lew R, Liang MH, Shadick NA: Lack of cardiac manifestations among patients with previously treated Lyme disease. Ann Intern Med 1998; 128:346–353.
194 Steere AC, Schoen RT, Taylor E: The clinical evolution of Lyme arthritis. Ann Intern Med 1987;107: 725–731.

195 Krause PJ, McKay K, Thompson CA, Sikand VK, Lentz R, Lepore T, Closter L, Christianson D, Telford SR, Persing D, Radolf JD, Spielman A; Deer-Associated Infection Study Group: Disease-specific diagnosis of coinfecting tick-borne zoonoses: babesiosis, human granulocytic ehrlichiosis, and Lyme disease. Clin Infect Dis 2002;34:1184–1191.

196 Gans O, Landes E: Akrodermatitis atrophicans arthropathica. Hautarzt 1952;3:151–155.

197 Weber K: Erythema-chronicum migrans-Meningitis – eine bakterielle Infektionskrankheit? Münch Med Wochenschr 1974;116:1993–1998.

198 Bannwarth A: Chronische Lymphocytare Meningitis, entzündliche Polyneuritis und 'Rheumathismus'. Ein Beitrag zum Problem 'Allergie und Nervensystem' in zwei Teilen. Arch Psychiatr Nervenkr 1941;113:284–376.

199 Schaltenbrand G: Chronische aseptische Meningitis. Nervenarzt 1949;20:433–442.

200 Priem S, Munkelt K, Franz JK, Schneider U, Werner T, Burmester GR, Krause A: Epidemiology and therapy of Lyme arthritis and other manifestations of Lyme borreliosis in Germany: results of a nationwide survey. Z Rheumatol 2003;62:450–458.

201 van der Heijden IM, Wilbrink B, Rijpkema SG, Schouls LM, Heymans PH, van Embden JD, Breedveld FC, Tak PP: Detection of *Borrelia burgdorferi* sensu stricto by reverse line blot in the joints of Dutch patients with Lyme arthritis. Arthritis Rheum 1999;42:1473–1480.

202 Jaulhac B, Heller R, Limbach FX, Hansmann Y, Lipsker D, Monteil H, Sibilia J, Piemont Y: Direct molecular typing of *Borrelia burgdorferi* sensu lato species in synovial samples from patients with Lyme arthritis. J Clin Microbiol 2000;38:1895–1900.

203 Limbach FX, Jaulhac B, Puechal X, Monteil H, Kuntz JL, Piemont Y, Sibilia J: Treatment resistant Lyme arthritis caused by *Borrelia garinii*. Ann Rheum Dis 2001;60:284–286.

204 Vasiliu V, Herzer P, Rossler D, Lehnert G, Wilske B: Heterogeneity of *Borrelia burgdorferi* sensu lato demonstrated by an ospA-type-specific PCR in synovial fluid from patients with Lyme arthritis. Med Microbiol Immunol 1998;187:97–102.

205 Eiffert H, Karsten A, Thomssen R, Christen HJ: Characterization of *Borrelia burgdorferi* strains in Lyme arthritis. Scand J Infect Dis 1998;30:265–268.

206 Steere AC, Glickstein L: Elucidation of Lyme arthritis. Nat Rev Immunol 2004;4:143–152.

207 Puius YA, Kalish RA: Lyme arthritis: pathogenesis, clinical presentation, and management. Infect Dis Clin North Am 2008;22:289–300.

208 Guerau-de-Arellano M, Huber BT: Chemokines and Toll-like receptors in Lyme disease pathogenesis. Trends Mol Med 2005;11:114–120.

209 Coburn J, Fischer JR, Leong JM: Solving a sticky problem: new genetic approaches to host cell adhesion by the Lyme disease spirochete. Mol Microbiol 2005;57:1182–1195.

210 Hu LT, Eskildsen MA, Masgala C, Steere AC, Arner EC, Pratta MA, Grodzinsky AJ, Loening A, Perides G: Host metalloproteinases in Lyme arthritis. Arthritis Rheum 2001;44:1401–1410.

211 Behera AK, Hildebrand E, Scagliotti J, Steere AC, Hu LT: Induction of host matrix metalloproteinases by *Borrelia burgdorferi* differs in human and murine Lyme arthritis. Infect Immun 2005;73:126–134.

212 Johnston YE, Duray PH, Steere AC, Kashgarian M, Buza J, Malawista SE, Askenase PW: Lyme arthritis: spirochetes found in synovial microangiopathic lesions. Am J Pathol 1985;118:26–34.

213 Duray PH, Steere AC: The spectrum of organ and systems pathology in human Lyme disease. Zentralbl Bakteriol Mikrobiol Hyg [A] 1986;263:169–178.

214 Hollstrom E: Successful treatment of erythema chronicum migrans Afzelii. Acta Derm Venereol 1951;31:235–243.

215 Asbrink E, Olsson I: Clinical manifestations of erythema chronicum migrans Afzelius in 161 patients: a comparison with Lyme disease. Acta Derm Venereol 1985;65:43–52.

216 Herzer P: Joint manifestations of Lyme borreliosis in Europe. Scand J Infect Dis 1991;77(suppl):55–63.

217 Kryger P, Hansen K, Vinterberg H, Pedersen FK: Lyme borreliosis among Danish patients with arthritis. Scand J Rheumatol 1990;19:77–81.

218 Valesova M, Trnavsky K: Joint manifestations of Lyme borreliosis in Czechoslovakian patients. Z Rheumatol 1990;49:192–196.

219 Rees DH, Axford JS: Lyme arthritis. Ann Rheum Dis 1994;53:553–556.

220 Steere AC, Hardin JA, Ruddy S, Mummaw JG, Malawista SE: Lyme arthritis: correlation of serum and cryoglobulin IgM with activity, and serum IgG with remission. Arthritis Rheum 1979;22:471–483.

221 Hardin JA, Steere AC, Malawista SE: Immune complexes and the evolution of Lyme arthritis: dissemination and localization of abnormal C1q binding activity. N Engl J Med 1979;301:1358–1363.

222 Lawson JP, Steere AC: Lyme arthritis: radiologic findings. Radiology 1985;154:37–43.

223 Snydman DR, Schenkein DP, Berardi VP, Lastavica CC, Pariser KM: *Borrelia burgdorferi* in joint fluid in chronic Lyme arthritis. Ann Intern Med 1986;104:798–800.

224 Nocton JJ, Dressler F, Rutledge BJ, Rys PN, Persing DH, Steere AC: Detection of *Borrelia burgdorferi* DNA by polymerase chain reaction in synovial fluid from patients with Lyme arthritis. N Engl J Med 1994;330:229–234.

225 Strle F: Ocular manifestations of Lyme borreliosis. Acta Dermatovenerol Alp Panoncia Adriat 1994; 1–2:71–76.
226 Mikkila HO, Seppala IJ, Viljanen MK, Peltomaa MP, Karma A: The expanding clinical spectrum of ocular Lyme borreliosis. Ophthalmology 2000; 107:581–587.
227 Karma A, Seppala I, Mikkila H, Kaakkola S, Viljanen M, Tarkkanen A: Diagnosis and clinical characteristics of ocular Lyme borreliosis. Am J Ophthalmol 1995;119:127–135.
228 Mikkila H, Karma A, Viljanen M, Seppala I: The laboratory diagnosis of ocular Lyme borreliosis. Graefes Arch Clin Exp Ophthalmol 1999;237:225–230.
229 Colucciello M: Ocular Lyme borreliosis. N Engl J Med 2001;345:1350–1351.
230 Schonherr U, Strle F: Ocular manifestations; in Weber K, Burgdorfer W (eds): Aspects of Lyme Borreliosis. Heidelberg, Springer, 1993, pp 131–151.
231 Steere AC, Duray PH, Kauffmann DJ, Wormser GP: Unilateral blindness caused by infection with the Lyme disease spirochete, *Borrelia burgdorferi*. Ann Intern Med 1985;103:382–384.
232 Carvounis PE, Mehta AP, Geist CE: Orbital myositis associated with *Borrelia burgdorferi* (Lyme disease) infection. Ophthalmology 2004;111: 1023–1028.
233 Huppertz HI, Munchmeier D, Lieb W: Ocular manifestations in children and adolescents with Lyme arthritis. Br J Ophthalmol 1999;83:1149–1152.
234 de Boer JH, Luyendijk L, Rothova A, Kijlstra A: Analysis of ocular fluids for local antibody production in uveitis. Br J Ophthalmol 1995;79:610–616.
235 Preac-Mursic V, Pfister HW, Spiegel H, Burk R, Wilske B, Reinhardt S, Bohmer R: First isolation of *Borrelia burgdorferi* from an iris biopsy. J Clin Neuroophthalmol 1993;13:155–161.
236 Lohmann CP, Winkler von Mohrenfels C, Gabler B, Reischl U, Kochanowski B: Polymerase chain reaction (PCR) for microbiological diagnosis in refractory infectious keratitis: a clinical study in 16 patients. Klin Monatsbl Augenheilkd 2000;217:37–42.
237 Stanek G, Konrad K, Jung M, Ehringer H: Shulman syndrome, a scleroderma subtype caused by *Borrelia burgdorferi*? Lancet 1987;1:1490.
238 Granter SR, Barnhill RL, Hewins ME, Duray PH: Identification of *Borrelia burgdorferi* in diffuse fasciitis with peripheral eosinophilia: borrelial fasciitis. JAMA 1994;272:1283–1285.
239 Hashimoto Y, Takahashi H, Matsuo S, Hirai K, Takemori N, Nakao M, Miyamoto K, Iizuka H: Polymerase chain reaction of *Borrelia burgdorferi* flagellin gene in Shulman syndrome. Dermatology 1996;192:136–139.
240 Muller-Felber W, Reimers CD, de Koning J, Fischer P, Pilz A, Pongratz DE: Myositis in Lyme borreliosis: an immunohistochemical study of seven patients. J Neurol Sci 1993;118:207–212.
241 Reimers CD, de Koning J, Neubert U, Preac-Mursic V, Koster JG, Muller-Felber W, Pongratz DE, Duray PH: *Borrelia burgdorferi* myositis: report of eight patients. J Neurol 1993;240:278–283.
242 Holmgren AR, Matteson EL: Lyme myositis. Arthritis Rheum 2006;54:2697–2700.
243 Cadavid D, Bai Y, Dail D, Hurd M, Narayan K, Hodzic E, Barthold SW, Pachner AR: Infection and inflammation in skeletal muscle from nonhuman primates infected with different genospecies of the Lyme disease spirochete *Borrelia burgdorferi*. Infect Immun 2003;71:7087–7098.
244 Horowitz HW, Sanghera K, Goldberg N, Pechman D, Kamer R, Duray P, Weinstein A: Dermatomyositis associated with Lyme disease: case report and review of Lyme myositis. Clin Infect Dis 1994;18: 166–171.
245 Waton J, Pinault AL, Pouaha J, Truchetet F: Lyme disease could mimic dermatomyositis. Rev Med Interne 2007;28:343–345.
246 Schnarr S, Wahl A, Jurgens-Saathoff B, Mengel M, Kreipe HH, Zeidler H: Nodular fasciitis, erythema migrans, and oligoarthritis: manifestations of Lyme borreliosis caused by *Borrelia afzelii*. Scand J Rheumatol 2002;31:184–186.
247 Kramer N, Rickert RR, Brodkin RH, Rosenstein ED: Septal panniculitis as a manifestation of Lyme disease. Am J Med 1986;81:149–152.
248 Hassler D, Zorn J, Zoller L, Neuss M, Weyand C, Goronzy J, Born IA, Preac-Mursic V: Nodular panniculitis: a manifestation of Lyme borreliosis? Hautarzt 1992;43:134–138.
249 Viljanen MK, Oksi J, Salomaa P, Skurnik M, Peltonen R, Kalimo H: Cultivation of *Borrelia burgdorferi* from the blood and a subcutaneous lesion of a patient with relapsing febrile nodular nonsuppurative panniculitis. J Infect Dis 1992;165:596–597.
250 Oksi J, Mertsola J, Reunanen M, Marjamaki M, Viljanen MK: Subacute multiple-site osteomyelitis caused by *Borrelia burgdorferi*. Clin Infect Dis 1994;19:891–896.
251 Feder HM Jr, Johnson BJ, O'Connell S, Shapiro ED, Steere AC, Wormser GP; Ad Hoc International Lyme Disease Group, Agger WA, Artsob H, Auwaerter P, Dumler JS, Bakken JS, Bockenstedt LK, Green J, Dattwyler RJ, Munoz J, Nadelman RB, Schwartz I, Draper T, McSweegan E, Halperin JJ, Klempner MS, Krause PJ, Mead P, Morshed M, Porwancher R, Radolf JD, Smith RP Jr, Sood S, Weinstein A, Wong SJ, Zemel L: A critical appraisal of 'chronic Lyme disease'. N Engl J Med 2007;357:1422–1430.
252 Marques A: Chronic Lyme disease: a review. Infect Dis Clin North Am 2008;22:341–360.

253 Fraser DD, Kong LI, Miller FW: Molecular detection of persistent *Borrelia burgdorferi* in a man with dermatomyositis. Clin Exp Rheumatol 1992; 10:387–390.
254 Sartin JS, Oettel KR: A morphealike skin condition caused by *Borrelia burgdorferi* in an immunocompromised patient. Mayo Clin Proc 2006;81: 1259–1260.
255 Rodriguez M, Chou S, Fisher DC, De Girolami U, Amato AA, Marty FM: Lyme meningoradiculitis and myositis after allogeneic hematopoietic stem cell transplantation. Clin Infect Dis 2005;41:e112–e114.
256 Garcia-Monco JC, Frey HM, Villar BF, Golightly MG, Benach JL: Lyme disease concurrent with human immunodeficiency virus infection. Am J Med 1989;87:325–328.
257 Cordoliani F, Vignon-Pennamen MD, Assous MV, Vabres P, Dronne P, Rybojad M, Morel P: Atypical Lyme borreliosis in an HIV-infected man. Br J Dermatol 1997;137:437–439.
258 Dudle G, Opravil M, Luthy R, Weber R: Meningitis after acute *Borrelia burgdorferi* infection in HIV infection. Dtsch Med Wochenschr 1997;122:1178–1180.
259 Maraspin V, Lotrič-Furlan S, Cimperman J, Ružić-Sabljić E, Strle F: Erythema migrans in the immunocompromised host. Wien Klin Wochenschr 1999;111:923–932.
260 Furst B, Glatz M, Kerl H, Mullegger RR: The impact of immunosuppression on erythema migrans: a retrospective study of clinical presentation, response to treatment and production of *Borrelia* antibodies in 33 patients. Clin Exp Dermatol 2006; 31:509–514.
261 Maraspin V, Cimperman J, Lotrič-Furlan S, Logar M, Ružić-Sabljić E, Strle F: Erythema migrans in solid-organ transplant recipients. Clin Infect Dis 2006;42:1751–1754.
262 Millner M, Schimek MG, Spork D, Schnizer M, Stanek G: Lyme borreliosis in children: a controlled clinical study based on ELISA values. Eur J Pediatr 1989;148:527–530.
263 Barbour AG: Isolation and cultivation of Lyme disease spirochetes. Yale J Biol Med 1984;57:521–525.
264 Preac-Mursic V, Wilske B, Reinhardt S: Culture of *Borrelia burgdorferi* on six solid media. Eur J Clin Microbiol Infect Dis 1991;10:1076–1079.
265 Marlovits S, Khanakah G, Striessnig G, Vécsei V, Stanek G: Emergence of Lyme arthritis after autologous chondrocyte transplantation. Arthritis Rheum 2004;50:259–264.
266 Aberer E, Bergmann AR, Derler AM, Schmidt B: Course of *Borrelia burgdorferi* DNA shedding in urine after treatment. Acta Derm Venereol 2007; 87:39–42.
267 Rauter C, Mueller M, Diterich I, Zeller S, Hassler D, Meergans T, Hartung T: Critical evaluation of urine-based PCR assay for diagnosis of Lyme borreliosis. Clin Diagn Lab Immunol 2005;12:910–917.
268 Robertson J, Guy E, Andrews N, Wilske B, Anda P, Granström M, Hauser U, Moosmann Y, Sambri V, Schellekens J, Stanek G, Gray J: A European multicenter study of immunoblotting in serodiagnosis of Lyme borreliosis. J Clin Microbiol 2000;38: 2097–2102.
269 Hauser U, Lehnert G, Wilske B: Validity of interpretation criteria for standardized Western blots (immunoblots) for serodiagnosis of Lyme borreliosis based on sera collected throughout Europe. J Clin Microbiol 1999;37:2241–2247.
270 Wilske B, Zöller L, Brade V, Eiffert H, Göbel UB, Stanek G: MiQ (Quality Standards for the Microbiological Diagnosis of Infectious Diseases) 12 2000: Lyme Borreliosis. Munich/Jena, Urban & Fischer Verlag, 2000.
271 Wilske B, Habermann C, Fingerle V, Hillenbrand B, Jauris-Heipke S, Lehnert G, Pradel I, Rössler D, Schulte-Spechtel U: An improved recombinant IgG immunoblot for serodiagnosis of Lyme borreliosis. Med Microbiol Immunol 1999;188:139–144.
272 Steere AC, McHugh G, Damle N, Sikand VK: Prospective study of serologic tests for Lyme disease. Clin Infect Dis 2008;47:188–195.
273 Cetin E, Sotoudeh M, Auer H, Stanek G: Paradigm Burgenland: risk of *Borrelia burgdorferi* sensu lato infection indicated by variable seroprevalence rates in hunters. Wien Klin Wochenschr 2006;118: 677–681.
274 Barbour AG, Jasinskas A, Kayala MA, Davies DH, Steere AC, Baldi P, Felgner PL: A genome-wide proteome array reveals a limited set of immunogens in natural infections of humans and white-footed mice with *Borrelia burgdorferi*. Infect Immun 2008;76:3374–3389.

Franc Strle
Department of Infectious Diseases, University Medical Center Ljubljana
Japljeva 2
SI–1525 Ljubljana (Slovenia)
Tel. +386 1 522 2110, Fax +386 1 522 2456, E-Mail franc.strle@kclj.si

Lipsker D, Jaulhac B (eds): Lyme Borreliosis.
Curr Probl Dermatol. Basel, Karger, 2009, vol 37, pp 111–129

Treatment and Prevention of Lyme Disease

Yves Hansmann

Service des Maladies Infectieuses et Tropicales, Hôpitaux Universitaires de Strasbourg, et
Faculté de Médecine de Strasbourg, Université Louis Pasteur, Strasbourg, France

Abstract
Randomized controlled trials have ascertained the efficiency of antibiotics in treating erythema migrans, the hallmark of early stage Lyme borreliosis. Oral amoxicillin and doxycycline are first-line treatment options, though phenoxymethylpenicillin, cefuroxime axetil and azithromycin are alternative second-line options. Treatments for secondary and tertiary Lyme borreliosis are more poorly documented, and antibiotics are not always effective. This is due to the unique pathophysiology of late Lyme borreliosis, which involves not only bacterial infection, but also immunological response. Since there is no completely reliable method of diagnosis, it is difficult to choose the proper treatment and to evaluate treatment efficacy. However, numerous studies have shown that ceftriaxone and doxycycline are the 2 most efficient antibiotics, particularly in Lyme arthritis and in neuroborreliosis. In late Lyme borreliosis, these antibiotics are less efficient, and different treatment schemes with variations in dosage or duration did not produce convincing results.

The treatment of Lyme disease varies according to the clinical stage. For each stage, the pathophysiology differs, and therefore the antibiotherapy has to be adapted to the clinical signs. Recently published guidelines and recommendations follow this strategy, in order to help choose the best antibiotics for each clinical situation [1–4].

During the first stage of the infection, the main clinical sign, erythema migrans, is due to the progression of *Borrelia* in the skin. At this stage, many antibiotics are effective. Three families of antibiotics are frequently used: β-lactams (especially amoxicillin and ceftriaxone) and tetracyclines (especially doxycycline), and, as a second choice, macrolides, which are probably less efficient. In the next stage, hematogenous spread occurs and the bacteria can be found in the blood, and subsequently in the synovial fluid (in cases of arthritis) or in the cerebrospinal fluid (CSF; in cases of meningitis). To be effective, the treatment must not only have bactericidal activity, but must also diffuse correctly in these 2 fluids. For example, in neuroborreliosis, higher dosages of β-lactams are needed for sufficient diffusion into the CSF. Finally, the late stage of the disease is characterized by difficulty in identifying *Borrelia* in various tissues, so the main mechanism in this phase could be an immunological reaction to fragments of the bacteria acting as antigens. These immunologically based mechanisms are one possible explanation for the low efficacy of antibiotic treatment in a lot of patients with advanced Lyme disease [5].

Historically, the first time that the presence of *Borrelia* was correlated with the clinical symptoms, antibiotics were tested on their ability to cure patients with Lyme diseases. In the early stage, the antibiotics were effective and the symptoms regressed. The first reported cases were rapidly followed by larger studies that confirmed these results. However, there were only a few studies using rigorous scientific methodology. Many studies were retrospective or without real randomization, and neither controlled, nor comparative. Therefore, a lot of questions remained.

On the other hand, physicians quickly noticed that some patients with Lyme disease did not respond to the antibiotic treatment. Thus, some doubt remained about the real efficacy of antibiotics, as well as the responsibility of *Borrelia* in some manifestations of the disease (especially in the later stages); this raised a question about the validity of the diagnostic criteria of Lyme disease. There is still no treatment that can guarantee the regression of clinical symptoms after completing an antibiotic treatment in all stages of Lyme disease. So, it seems quite important to highlight prevention, and to inform all subjects living in highly endemic areas for Lyme disease to avoid tick bites. No repellents prevent all tick bites. However, knowing the pathophysiology of the transmission of *Borrelia* during a tick bite helps to prevent infection. *Borrelia* needs several hours for transition from the gut of ticks to their salivary glands. So, if the ticks are removed rapidly (within some hours), the risk of *Borrelia* transmission is low, though this is less certain in Europe than in North America.

In vitro Data

Several antibiotics have good in vitro activity against *Borrelia*. Among β-lactams, the best in vitro activity is obtained with parenteral third-generation cephalosporins. Amoxicillin and oral second- and third-generation cephalosporins also have good activity [6, 7]. Ureidopenicillins and carbapenems have shown interesting properties, but penicillin seems less efficient in vitro [7, 8]. Tetracyclines have activity equivalent to amoxicillin, and sometimes even to ceftriaxone or cefotaxime [6, 7, 9].

There are many differences within the family of macrolide antibiotics. The new telithromycin is the only one that has shown better in vitro activity than ceftriaxone [10]. Clarithromycin has superior activity compared to tetracyclines [11]. Other macrolides have sufficiently good activity to suggest that they could be useful in vivo: azithromycin, erythromycin, roxithromycin, dirithromycin and quinupristin-dalfopristin [10, 12, 13]. Trimethoprim is more difficult to test in vitro, but seems to have some activity against *Borrelia* [14]. Most of these results have been confirmed on different strains of *Borrelia*, *B. burgdorferi* sensu stricto and *B. afzelii*, isolated in Europe and the Far East [9, 15]. Other antibiotics did not show any activity against *Borrelia*: amikacin, aztreonam, vancomycin, fusidic acid and fluoroquinolones [6, 8, 12]. The in vitro test does not predict the risk of acquired resistance to most of the antibiotics, except for erythromycin under specific conditions, like a heavy inoculum [16, 17].

Pharmacological data are rarely used for treating borreliosis. However, 2 properties are important: the diffusion of antibiotics in CSF for neuroborreliosis, and the intracellular penetration for all forms of borreliosis.

β-Lactams are considered to have rather poor CSF penetration. High dosages of this family of antibiotics are often used to treat neuromeningeal infections. For tetracyclines, there are not much data about diffusion into CSF, and though their use has been validated in clinical studies, their diffusion into CSF appears to be relatively poor. The mean intrathecal concentrations were 0.6 mg/l in patients treated with 100 mg of doxycycline twice a day and 1.1 mg/l in patients treated with 200 mg twice a day. The minimal inhibitory concentration of doxycycline for *Borrelia* ranges between 0.6 and 0.7 mg/l, so theoretically the higher dosage should be more effective [18]. This has not been confirmed in clinical studies, however.

On the other hand, the intracellular penetration of doxycycline is superior to that of the β-lactams. This data could be important from a physiopathological point of view, because of the possibility of the intracellular presence of *Borrelia*. However, it has still not been shown that doxycycline is more effective than β-lactams in borreliosis, whatever the stage of the infection.

Some experimental animal models have confirmed the in vitro results, including the high activity of β-lactams and doxycycline in borreliosis. These studies have also confirmed some advantages for using macrolides and everninomycin [7, 11, 19–22].

The animal models can also help identify the best duration of treatment. For example, in *B. burgdorferi*-infected mice, a 1-day treatment with ceftriaxone showed the same activity as a 5-day treatment [23].

Primary (Early Localized) Lyme Borreliosis

During the early stage of the infection, the first objective of treatment is to make erythema migrans disappear. However, in most of the cases, the skin heals spontaneously even without antibiotic treatment. So another objective, actually the main one, is to prevent the dissemination of the disease, which could lead to the involvement of other organ systems and to the late manifestations of the disease. Obviously, an essential criteria when evaluating drug effectiveness should be the absence of the late manifestation of the disease. β-Lactams, tetracyclines and macrolides were tested for effective treatment of erythema migrans in clinical studies, which were sometimes controlled, randomized or double-blinded. Most of the studies were conducted in

North America, though some of them were conducted in Europe, where species diversity is more important. The results did not differ significantly according to the geographic area, suggesting that most of the different species of *Borrelia* (*B. burgdorferi, B. afzelii, B. garinii*) respond in the same manner to antibiotics. This clinical result was confirmed by in vitro studies [15].

The antibiotics tested initially were phenoxymethylpenicillin, doxycycline and erythromycin [24]. Efficacy of these antibiotics was higher for doxycycline (absence of neurological complications) compared to penicillin. Erythromycin was the least efficient of the 3 tested antibiotics, with an increased risk of neurological complications and a slower resolution of erythema migrans.

Among the β-lactams, phenoxymethylpenicillin was initially the antibiotic used most often to treat erythema migrans [25–29]. Amoxicillin showed equivalent activity to phenoxymethylpenicillin. The addition of probenecid does not seem to improve the clinical response [30, 31]. Only 1 study has compared amoxicillin without probenecid (3 × 500 mg/day) to azithromycin (3 × 500 mg/day). In this study, more azithromycin recipients (16%) than amoxicillin recipients (4%) had relapses [32].

The dosage of amoxicillin, in most cases, is 3 × 500 mg per day for adults and 50 mg/kg/day for children. Not everybody agrees with this, because of concern about underdosage in adults. Some authors propose increasing the dosage of amoxicillin if probenecid is not associated with it [3].

Two other β-lactams have been found to be equivalent to amoxicillin, but they offer no significant advantage: ceftriaxone, which requires parenteral administration, and cefuroxime axetil, which has a larger spectrum than amoxicillin and is more expensive [26, 33, 34].

In the studies, the duration of treatment was 10, 14 or 21 days [24, 25, 34, 35], though no duration was found to be clearly superior. After a 10-day treatment course, some studies showed more long-term complications [24, 26]. One comparative study showed equivalence whatever the duration of treatment, though there was 1 failure in the group of patients treated for 10 days compared to no failures in the group of patients treated longer, but this difference was not significant [34].

In all the therapeutic studies, tetracycline has shown similar activity to amoxicillin, and can thus be considered as another first-line option. The first studies using tetracycline showed equivalence to phenoxymethylpenicillin. Erythema migrans was cured more rapidly in patients treated with doxycycline compared to erythromycin [24].

Further studies compared doxycycline with several other antibiotics: phenoxymethylpenicillin, azithromycin, amoxicillin and cefuroxime axetil. In most cases, the activity of doxycycline was at least as efficient as the other antibiotics [27, 30, 31, 33–39]. Minocycline was used in only 1 study, and had the same efficacy as phenoxymethylpenicillin [29]. The recommended dosage of doxycycline is 200 mg per day (once or twice) for 2 weeks.

The first macrolide to be tested was erythromycin; results showed that it was inferior to both phenoxymethylpenicillin and doxycycline [24]. Azithromycin, a long half-

Table 1. Choice of antibiotic treatment in early localized or primary borreliosis (erythema migrans)

	Antibiotic	Dosage	Duration of treatment, days
Adults			
First-line choice	amoxicillin	3 × 500 or 3 × 1,000 mg/day	14–21
	doxycycline	200 mg/day	14–21
Second-line choice	cefuroxime axetil	2 × 500 mg/day	14–21
Third-line choice	azithromycin	500 mg first day, 250 mg following days	7–10
Children			
Less than 8 years	amoxicillin	50 mg/kg/day	14–21
More than 8 years	adult dosage		
Second-line choice	cefuroxime axetil	30 mg/kg/day	7–10

life elimination macrolide with excellent intracellular diffusion, showed globally comparable results to penicillin and doxycycline in terms of resolution of clinical symptoms and complications occurring after erythema migrans [27, 28, 31, 32, 37–39].

In children, 3 studies showed similar efficacies of phenoxymethylpenicillin (100,000 U/kg/day, 14 days), cefuroxime axetil (20 or 30 mg/kg/day, 14–20 days), azithromycin (20 mg/kg/day on the first day, 10 mg/kg/day over the following 4 days) and amoxicillin (50 mg/kg/day) [40–42]. Treatment recommendations for erythema migrans are shown in table 1. For pregnant or breast-feeding women, the treatment is the same, except for tetracyclines which are not recommended. In cases with an allergy to β-lactams, only macrolides can be used.

Secondary and Tertiary (Early Disseminated and Late) Lyme Borreliosis

Secondary Lyme borreliosis corresponds to the manifestations occurring during and after dissemination of *Borrelia* in the blood. Articular and neurological tissues, and less frequently the heart, the skin and the eye, are the principal targets of *Borrelia*.

An epidemiological study performed in eastern France from 2001 to 2003 [43] found that disseminated and late infections (secondary and tertiary) represent 37.3% of all of the diagnosed cases of Lyme diseases.

During the secondary stage, clinical manifestations are directly related to the presence of *Borrelia*. Without treatment, the disease progresses and can cause long-term complications. If this happens, the disease enters a new stage (called tertiary or late Lyme disease) where some clinical manifestations might not be due to *Borrelia*, but could possibly be explained by immunological modifications [44–47]. The precise mechanisms are not known, but the release of bacterial antigens, characterized by their similarity to articular or neurological antigens ('molecular mimicry'), could be the cause of the clinical manifestations. Thus, we can understand why antibiotics are less efficient in tertiary Lyme disease, but still remain the only treatment that can be potentially curative.

Another problem with secondary Lyme disease that remains is the difficulty in diagnosing the disease at this stage; this difficulty directly affects evaluation of its treatment. Accurate diagnosis requires several clinical and biological or microbiological criteria [48]. Direct identification of *Borrelia* remains exceptional. Culture of the infected tissue requires specific medium; however, its sensitivity is low. Molecular diagnosis, like PCR, allows more frequent identification of *Borrelia*, but it involves tissue samples. So, in most situations, the diagnosis is based on the clinical manifestations and on the detection of specific antibodies. If the clinical manifestations are unspecific, the presence of *Borrelia* antibodies is insufficient to confirm diagnosis. So, in clinical practice, antibiotics are often given to patients even if the diagnosis has not been definitely confirmed. However, this problem is also frequently encountered in a lot of therapeutic studies. Unrestrictive criteria allow many patients who are not infected with *Borrelia* to be included in studies. The consequence is that the response to treatment becomes difficult to evaluate. On the other hand, a diagnosis of neuroborreliosis according to classical diagnostic criteria requires the presence of meningitis, yet most of authors agree that some cases of neuroborreliosis affect only the peripheral nervous system, so no CSF effect can be found. Even though this form of peripheral neuropathy is due to borreliosis, it does not comply with the diagnostic criteria, and therefore cannot be included in clinical studies to test the efficacy of antibiotics. For these forms of neuroborreliosis, we have no evidence-based guidance to determine the treatment.

In real-life clinical practice, the physician often prescribes antibiotics to a patient because, even if the diagnosis is not confirmed, it cannot be excluded. A study conducted in the USA in 1994 to evaluate the toxicity of ceftriaxone used to treat Lyme disease showed that only 2% of the patients responded to the EUCALB (European Union Concerted Action on Lyme Borreliosis) diagnostic criteria [49]. In another therapeutic study, the consequences of overdiagnosis and overtreatment were evaluated. Even though only 21% of the patients met the criteria for Lyme disease, these patients relied heavily on medical assistance and were subjected to high antibiotic toxicity. This raises questions about the wisdom of prescribing antibiotics to a large number of patients without any certainty of the diagnosis of borreliosis [50]. On the other hand, Donta [51] showed in 1997 that the prescription of doxycycline for patients with articular or neurological manifestations led to significant improvement in 61% of the patients, whatever the results of *Borrelia* serological testing had been.

Finally, for several reasons the late manifestations of borreliosis are probably the most difficult to be efficiently treated with antibiotics. Indeed, some clinical manifestations are probably not directly due to bacterial proliferation, and the difficulty in establishing a diagnosis with certainty leads to difficulty in evaluating the response to antibiotic treatment.

Which Antibiotics Should Be Used for Secondary or Tertiary Lyme Arthritis or Neuroborreliosis?

Since the 1980s, some clinical studies have validated different treatment options. These studies have shown the superiority of antibiotics compared to a placebo in eliminating the clinical manifestations in second stage borreliosis. Several clinical studies have tested β-lactams and tetracyclines during this stage in patients with articular manifestations, neurological manifestations or both. These studies have helped validate the use of these treatments in secondary Lyme disease. In most of these studies, no significant difference between the different families of antibiotics was found, whatever the manifestation of borreliosis. However, we have to consider that:

- A multitude of variables make these studies difficult to interpret and limit our ability to establish evidence-based recommendations: diagnostic criteria are not very specific for Lyme arthritis, or can be too restrictive for neuroborreliosis (CSF results are necessary and not always tested in therapeutic studies); the large number of treatment modalities (choice of antibiotic, dosage, duration of treatment, association of several antibiotics, multiple antibiotic schemes); and the difficulty in defining healing criteria (improvements in clinical signs, absence of microbiological criteria, duration of follow-up).
- The main difference between treating articular or neurological borreliosis is the necessity of significant antibiotic diffusion into the CSF for neurological manifestations, meaning that for each indication, a specific treatment should be proposed.

Treatment of Lyme Arthritis

For articular manifestations during secondary Lyme borreliosis, several antibiotics have proven to be efficient: penicillin, ceftriaxone and doxycycline [52–59]. Penicillin was the first antibiotic tested, but it sometimes leads to the persistence of musculoskeletal manifestations [52], especially if administered intramuscularly. Efficacy is best when it is used intravenously at a high dosage [53] for at least 10 days. Many studies used 3 weeks of treatment. Amoxicillin associated with probenecid is effective in treating Lyme arthritis. Since amoxicillin has always been tested in association with probenecid during the comparative clinical studies, it is difficult to know exactly what is the best dosage of this antibiotic for treating secondary borreliosis when used without probenecid. Third-generation cephalosporins are at least as efficient as penicillin. Of these, the most frequently used is ceftriaxone because of its simple once daily administration. The efficacy of ceftriaxone in Lyme arthritis is either equivalent to penicillin or better. If oral treatment of Lyme arthritis fails, a second-line treatment with ceftriaxone can be efficient [60]. Ceftriaxone can also be used in children [57, 61]. Cefotaxime is rarely used, even though the efficacy is the same in Lyme arthritis, because administration requires 3 daily injections [62, 63]. Cefixime, an oral cephalosporin, showed lack of efficacy in Lyme arthritis with more relapses after treatment than ceftriaxone [64]. Doxycycline is also effective in Lyme arthritis. Two studies suggested that a 2-week treatment with doxycycline, amoxicillin or ceftriaxone in Lyme arthritis leads to a good resolution of symptoms, without relapse within a 40-week follow-up [65, 66]. Given for 21 days at 200 mg/day, doxycycline has shown equivalent effectiveness to ceftriaxone and to amoxicillin plus probenecid [60, 67]. Doxycycline cannot be used in children.

In conclusion, doxycycline and ceftriaxone are the most efficient antibiotics for Lyme arthritis. Since doxycycline is less expensive than ceftriaxone, it can be used as a first-line treatment for articular borreliosis (table 2).

Treatment of Neuroborreliosis

For neuroborreliosis, most of the clinical trials included different types of manifestations: radiculitis (with or without meningitis), facial palsy (that has to be considered as a special form of radiculitis), peripheral neuropathy or central nervous system involvement. High-dosage intravenous penicillin is an effective treatment for neuroborreliosis [52]. For amoxicillin, the use of probenecid, which prolongs its half-life, could hinder the diffusion of amoxicillin into the CSF [68, 69]. Ceftriaxone showed equivalence or a better efficacy at 2 g/day than penicillin. Increasing the dosage to 4 g/day showed no additional benefit [55, 61]. Ceftriaxone was effective in cases of neuroborreliosis where penicillin had failed [54–56], and can also be used in children with neurological involvement [57, 61]. It is also effective for meningoradiculitis, even if the central nervous system is involved [70]. Among patients with Lyme encephalopathy, characterized by loss of memory, ceftriaxone is able to improve the clinical signs in some, but not all, cases [71]. This superiority could be explained by the relatively good diffusion of ceftriaxone into the central nervous system. Cefotaxime has also been compared to penicillin; however, despite its good activity, this antibiotic has no real advantage over ceftriaxone which is much easier to administer, especially in ambulatory patients [62, 63].

The question of the use of doxycycline for neuroborreliosis has not been totally solved. Several studies seem to show that its efficacy (200 mg/day, 3 weeks) in neuroborreliosis could be equivalent to ceftriaxone and high-dosage intravenous penicillin [72–74]. However, in other studies, neurological complications occurred after doxycycline treatment [60, 67], perhaps because doxycycline diffuses poorly into the CSF. Only when its dosage was increased to 400 mg/day, in order to improve the CSF diffusion, was it found to be equivalent to ceftriaxone [58].

Table 2. Choice of antibiotic treatment in borreliosis (except isolated erythema migrans) according to the clinical stage of the disease

	First-line treatment	Alternative treatment	Other possibilities[1]
Disseminated early forms (multiple erythema migrans[2])	ceftriaxone 2 g/day 14 days or doxycycline 200 mg/day 14–21 days		
Borrelial lymphocytoma	amoxicillin 1.5–3 g/day (B-III) or doxycycline 200 mg/day 14–21 days (B-III)		
ACA	ceftriaxone 2 g/day or doxycycline 200 mg/day 30 days (B-II)		penicillin G or amoxicillin 30 days (B-II)
Neuroborreliosis	ceftriaxone 2 g or 50–75 mg/kg/day 14–28 days (B-I)	doxycycline 200 mg/day[3] 14–21 days (B-II)	intravenous penicillin G 400,000–500,000 U/day (B-II)
Lyme arthritis	doxycycline[4] 200 mg/day 14–21 days (B-I)	ceftriaxone 2 g/day 14–28 days (B-I)	amoxicillin (+ probenecid) 4 × 500 mg/day 30 days? (B-II)
Lyme carditis	ceftriaxone 2 g/day or doxycycline 200 mg/day 14–21 days (B-III)		
Ocular borreliosis	ceftriaxone 2 g/day 14–21 days (B-III)	doxycycline 200 mg/day (B-III)	

ACA = Acrodermatitis chronica atrophicans. Strength of recommendation: A = strongly in favor, B = moderately in favor, C = optional, D = moderately against, E = strongly against. Quality of evidence: I = evidence from ≥1 properly randomized, controlled trial; II = evidence from ≥1 well-designed clinical trial, without randomization, from cohort or case-controlled analytic studies (preferably from >1 center), from multiple time series studies, or from dramatic results from uncontrolled experiments; III = evidence from opinions of respected authorities, based on clinical experience, descriptive studies, or reports of expert committees.

[1] Evaluated, but no clinical evidence of equivalent efficacy with first-line treatments, so these options should not be used first.

[2] Only few data are available; in so far as this stage corresponds to a hematogenous dissemination, treatment options have to address the risk of articular or neurological localization.

[3] No clinically proven benefit for increasing the dosage to 400 mg/day.

[4] Pharmaco-economical benefit of doxycycline versus ceftriaxone.

Facial palsy is one of the most frequent manifestations in neuroborreliosis, for which some specific recommendations exist. Although it may persist for a long time, facial palsy generally has a good prognosis [75]. Both ceftriaxone and doxycycline treatments have shown good activity in treating facial palsy, though resolution occurs slowly [74, 75]. The Infectious Disease Society of America recommends the use of amoxicillin in absence of meningitis [2, 76]. However, there is only a descriptive non-comparative study supporting this recommendation. So, the use of ceftriaxone or doxycycline, by analogy with the recommendations for other forms of neuroborreliosis (including peripheral neuropathy without meningitis), should be considered until more data can justify the use of oral amoxicillin [1].

In conclusion, 2 g/day of ceftriaxone remains the reference treatment for meningoradiculitis in neuroborreliosis. As for Lyme arthritis, the optimal duration of treatment is not clearly established, and the response seems better if the treatment is started rapidly, less than 3 months after the onset of the clinical manifestations [77, 78]. Doxycycline can be used as an alternative treatment (table 2).

Post-Lyme Disease and Late-Stage Borreliosis

All the therapeutic studies in secondary Lyme borreliosis (neuroborreliosis and Lyme arthritis) showed that a complete response to treatment is not obtained for all patients, even if ceftriaxone or doxycycline are used. Some authors have highlighted the problem of the patients that did not respond to several antibiotic treatments, and/or studied the second-line treatment after failure of a first-line antibiotic. In all the studies, a certain number of patients remained symptomatic, whatever treatment they received. This points out two sorts of problems: first, the risk of a false diagnosis in patients without criteria for borreliosis, a very frequent situation in clinical practice, as well as in clinical studies; second, the possibility of developing a late form of borreliosis or even the so-called 'post-Lyme disease'. The difference between the late form of borreliosis and post-Lyme disease could be the persistence of *Borrelia* (or at least antigens) in the so-called 'late form', suggesting that the clinical manifestations are directly related to the presence of bacteria. From a therapeutic point of view, these 2 stages of the disease are characterized by the often poor response to antibiotherapy.

There are 2 types of clinical studies: (1) studies that concern patients with clinical manifestations that have evolved over several months, sometimes for more than 1 year, and who have never been treated with effective antibiotics for borreliosis; (2) studies including patients who have had clinical manifestations for more than 1 year and who have already been treated.

For the first type of patients, it appears that the older the clinical manifestations, the more difficult it is to cure borreliosis. Different lines of long-duration treatments have been tested: first-line treatment with tetracyclines or oral amoxicillin associated with probenecid, followed by administration of ceftriaxone or benzathine penicillin [60, 79], or prolongation of oral antibiotic treatment after initial parenteral treatment or an increase in the dosage of ceftriaxone [55, 57]. Generally, there was no clinically evident benefit, but the evaluation of efficacy also depends on the duration of the follow-up: relapses, which occur several months after initial antibiotic treatment, are usually considered to be failures. Only a 28-day ceftriaxone (2 g/day) treatment gave better results than a 14-day treatment, but without reaching a significant statistical difference in a non-randomized study [80].

For the second type of patients, a descriptive study showed that after a new treatment, clinical signs were resolved in 42% of the patients, 36% of the patients had improvement followed by recurrence and 22% had no response at all [50]. However, in this study, many of the treated and evaluated patients did not have all the criteria required for the diagnosis of Lyme borreliosis. Several randomized studies have evaluated the efficacy of ceftriaxone (3 weeks) versus prolonged therapy with oral antibiotics, and ceftriaxone (30 days) followed by 6 weeks of oral treatment versus placebo, without any benefit for patients receiving antibiotics [81–83]. The persistence of a positive serology is not associated with the absence of response to treatment in these studies.

In clinical practice, the situation where a patient with secondary borreliosis did not respond to a first-line antibiotic is relatively frequent. If the diagnosis is based on solid criteria, it seems reasonable to propose an alternative treatment (ceftriaxone if the first-line treatment was doxycycline, or doxycycline if the first-line treatment was ceftriaxone). This proposition has to take into account the possibility of delayed improvement, occurring only some weeks after the treatment.

What Place for Other Antibiotics?

Other antibiotics have been tested during late Lyme borreliosis, especially macrolides. Clarithromycin (500 mg twice a day), azithromycin (250 or 500 mg/day), erythromycin (500 mg, 3 times a day) sometimes associated with hydroxychloroquine (200 mg, twice a day) have been proposed, especially in long-term chronic borreliosis. In a descriptive study, after 3 months of treatment, 80% of these patients had 50% improvement in their clinical signs; the results were even better if hydroxychloroquine was added. However, these results should be confirmed in randomized studies, and are not yet sufficient to justify macrolide prescription for treatment of late borreliosis [84].

Treatment for Other Manifestations of Lyme Disease

Usually, for borrelial lymphocytoma, the same treatment regimens are used as for erythema migrans. However, complete recovery of borrelial lymphocytoma is slow, with complete regression occurring in 1–12 weeks.

Only non-randomized studies were conducted in patients with acrodermatitis chronica atrophicans (ACA). These studies suggested that prolonged therapy (at least 30 days) is more efficient if using penicillin, ceftriaxone or doxycycline. However, in 47% of treated patients, cutaneous manifestations persist [85, 86] in dependence upon the stage of ACA, with a better prognosis for the early inflammatory stage than the late atrophic. If clinical signs are associated with neurological involvement, treatment with penicillin, cefuroxime axetil followed by doxycycline, or doxycycline alone over 3 weeks showed a good efficacy, not only on the cutaneous manifestations, but also on the neurological manifestations that can be associated with ACA (85% improvement 6 months after the beginning of treatment). However, the electromyographic abnormalities were not influenced by the treatment [87].

In cardiac or other tissue involvement during borreliosis, no study has shown an advantage for any kind of treatment. So, it appears that the classically validated treatments in early disseminated forms of borreliosis should also be used: ceftriaxone or doxycycline.

For symptomatic patients, or patients with second- or third-degree atrioventricular block, hospitalization and continuous cardiac monitoring is recommended. A temporary pacemaker can be required. First-line antibiotherapy with ceftriaxone seems preferable in severe disease, but oral regimens can be proposed for outpatient treatment. A duration of 14–21 days is required.

For other forms of secondary (early disseminated) borreliosis, the same treatment regimens as for Lyme arthritis or for neuroborreliosis are usually recommended, without any study that can support this choice. If the eyes are involved, ceftriaxone treatment should be proposed in the first-line because of the poor diffusion of doxycycline in the aqueous humor.

Conclusions

Early borreliosis generally has an excellent prognosis, with a good response to antibiotherapy and no recurrence after long-term follow-up [88]. Oral amoxicillin or oral doxycycline are first-line options and are adequate to cure patients with erythema migrans. In secondary (early disseminated) borreliosis, oral β-lactam treatment may fail, suggesting that the use of ceftriaxone or tetracyclines is more effective, though no clinical study has proven this. Pharmacological data encourages the use of ceftriaxone in patients with neuroborreliosis, whereas pharmaco-economical studies support the use of doxycycline. In late borreliosis, antibiotics are poorly efficient, except for some situations, e.g. the inflammatory stage of ACA. At this stage, there is no obvious benefit for prolonged therapy, though further investigations are needed.

Prevention of Borreliosis

Borreliosis is a very frequent infection in areas where its vectors are present. There are several different strategies to prevent Lyme disease: actions against its reservoir, actions against its vector or against the presence of *Borrelia* in the vector, prevention of tick bites, prevention of the disease by stimulating the immune system in humans and finally prophylaxis after tick bites.

Among the different strategies that can be implemented to prevent Lyme disease, the best ones to rely on are preventing human tick bites and vaccination.

This strategy remains the cornerstone of the prevention of Lyme disease.

The first stage of this strategy is to prevent the contact between ticks and humans that occurs when people go into the tick's biotope. Repellents that prevent mosquito bites do so by disturbing the arthropods' ability to locate their targets. Most of these repellents are tested for their ability to repel mosquitoes, and they might not be as effective against ticks. Some studies suggest that repellents, especially those containing DEET (N,N-diethyl-3-methylbenzamide), could effectively decrease the risk of tick bites. However, to be effective, a certain number of rules must be followed: repellents must be regularly applied on the skin, they must be applied on all of the exposed skin and the contraindications should be respected, especially in young children and pregnant women [89].

Among the numerous repellents, the products containing DEET are most often used. Their activity, proven against mosquitoes, has also been proven against ticks [90]. To be efficient they must be at least 30 or 35% DEET, and remain efficient for 4–5 h. They cannot be used at this dosage by children or pregnant women (risk of neurotoxicity and skin toxicity). At a lower dosage, DEET can be attractive for ticks. Other repellents (picaridin and N-butyl,N-acetyl-3ethylaminopropionate or EBAAP) can also be used. For EBAAP, protection is limited to 4 h. Picaridin is recommended by the World Health Organization against arthropod bites [91], but has not been tested against *Ixodes*. There are also some natural repellents that are effective against ticks. Citronella and *p*-menthane-3-8-diol both repel ticks for 2 to 4 h [92, 93]. Soya oil has a short-duration activity [94], and other natural products have been tested with less or more repellent activity [95]. Impregnation of clothes with repellents is a complementary strategy. DEET can also be useful, and its efficacy may then last for 4 to 6 weeks. Permethrin is an insecticide and a repellent. When used on clothes, it is to be considered more efficient against ticks than DEET, and it is effective for 6 weeks (up to 6 months if it is applied by immersion). Permethrin on clothes resists removal by washing or ironing. A recent study suggested that *I. ricinus* may be more attracted to light-colored than dark-colored clothing [95].

After a tick's initial contact with a human, *Borrelia* is transferred from the gut of *Ixodes* to its salivary glands. This property of *Borrelia* cycle may help preventing Lyme disease. Indeed, thanks to this approximately 24-hour delay in the migration of the bacteria, the rapid withdrawal of ticks after each walk, trek or outdoor activity can be considered an efficient measure of prevention. However, some reports suggest that transmission may be faster in Europe.

Tick removal techniques are not clearly defined. It seems preferable that the whole tick be removed by grasping it as close to the skin as possible, though awkward attempts may leave tick mouth parts in the skin. To minimize the risk of breaking the tick, specific instruments are recommended, like fine-tip forceps used with vertical traction without twisting. Specific hooks are also suitable, but need a twisting gesture to remove the tick. The use of these instruments limits the risk of applying pressure to the tick, and thus the risk of salivary regurgitation. However, if a mouth part remains in the skin, it should not be removed. The risk of skin damage is greater than the risk of transmission of *Borrelia,* which is only initially present in the gut of ticks. The use of chemical methods (alcohol, oil, etc.) is not recommended because of their ineffectiveness, the increased delay and because they induce regurgitation. Immediate removal of the tick remains an important step against transmission of *Borrelia.*

Prevention of Lyme Disease by Specific Immunization

There is currently no vaccination available against Lyme disease. A few years ago, a vaccine was commercialized in the USA, but it was taken out of service because of commercial reasons and concerns about its toxicity. It was estimated to protect between 70 and 80% of vaccinated subjects in North America, but it was never recommended in Europe where it was expected to be less effective because of the broader diversity of *Borrelia* species. However, this prevention strategy still holds promise and is being explored by several research centers.

Antibiotic Prophylaxis after Tick Bites [96]

Only 1 randomized controlled study tested the use of a single dose of 200 mg of doxycycline administered within 72 h after a tick bite as a primary prophylaxis [97]. This study showed a decrease in the frequency of erythema migrans in the group of patients treated with doxycycline. However, in this study there was no evaluation of the long-term complications of borreliosis. Another study, performed in Russia, evaluated the risk of transmission of *Borrelia* in humans bitten by infected ticks, with or without doxycycline (200 mg/day over 5 days). Infection occurred in 12.3% of non-treated patients and in 0.8% of treated patients [98]. The strategy of treating patients after a tick bite is recommended by the IDSA if: (1) the attached tick can be reliably identified as an adult or nymphal *I. scapularis* tick that is estimated to have been attached for 36 h on the basis of the degree of engorgement of the tick with blood or of certainty about the time of exposure to the tick, (2) prophylaxis can be started within 72 h of the time that the tick was removed, (3) ecological information indicates that the local rate of infection of these ticks with *B. burgdorferi* is ≥20%, and (4) doxycycline treatment is not contraindicated [2].

The problem that remains is identifying such risk factors in daily practice for all physicians. This treatment could be proposed to some patients, especially in highly endemic areas for Lyme disease.

Other works studied the efficacy of antibiotic prophylaxis after tick bites [99–101]. A meta-analysis of 3 of these studies showed that after a tick bite, there was no benefit from taking oral G penicillin, amoxicillin or doxycycline for 3 or 10 days [102].

For children and pregnant women, there are no recommendations. Some authors propose a systematic treatment. They argue that there is a risk of a severe form of the disease for the fetus and for the children less than 3 years old [103–105]. Generally, the treatment used in these circumstances is the same as for curative treatment of erythema migrans: amoxicillin. No overall study has been done to evaluate the efficacy of this systematic treatment [106–110].

In an American study, the risk of developing Lyme disease after a tick bite by an engorged *I. scapularis* (estimated to have been attached for 72 h) was 20% [111].

References

1 Halperin JJ, Shapiro ED, Logigian E, Belman AL, Dotevall L, Wormser GP, Krupp L, Gronseth G, Bever CT: Practice parameter: treatment of nervous system Lyme disease (an evidence-based review): report of the Quality Standards Subcommittee of the American Academy of Neurology. Neurology 2007;69:91–102.

2 Wormser GP, Dattwyler RJ, Shapiro ED, Halperin JJ, Steere AC, Klempner MS, Krause PJ, Bakken JS, Strle F, Stanek G, Bockenstedt L, Fish D, Dumler JS, Nadelman RB: The clinical assessment, treatment and prevention of Lyme disease, human granulocytic anaplasmosis, and babesiosis: clinical practice guidelines by the Infectious Diseases Society of America. Clin Infect Dis 2006;43:1089–1134.

3 SPILF: Lyme borreliosis: diagnostic, therapeutic and preventive approaches. Short text (in French). Med Mal Infect 2007;37:187–193.

4 Hansmann Y: Treatment of Lyme borreliosis secondary and tertiary stages (in French). Med Mal Infect 2007;37:479–486.

5 Steere AC: Lyme disease. N Engl J Med 2001;345: 115–125.

6 Hunfeld KP, Kraiczy P, Wichelhaus TA, Schäfer V, Brade V: Colorimetric in vitro susceptibility of penicillins, cephalosporins, macrolides, streptogramins, tetracyclines, and aminoglycosides against *Borrelia burgdorferi* isolates. Int J Antimicrob Agents 2000;15:11–17.

7 Johnson RC, Kodner CB, Jurkovich PJ, Collins J: Comparative in vitro and in vivo susceptibilities of the Lyme disease spirochete *Borrelia burgdorferi* to cefuroxime and other antimicrobial agents. Antimicrob Agents Chemother 1999;34:2133–2136.

8 Hunfeld KP, Weigand J, Wichelhaus TA, Kekouh E, Kraiczy P, Brade V: In vitro activity of mezlocillin, meropenem, aztreonam, vancomycin, teicoplanin, ribostamycin and fusidic acid against *Borrelia burgdorferi*. Int J Antimicrob Agents 2001;17:203–208.

9 Muqing L, Toshiyuki M, Jianhui W, Masato K, Yasutake Y: In vitro and in vivo susceptibilities of Lyme disease *Borrelia* isolated in China. J Infect Chemother 2000;6:65–67.

10 Hunfeld KP, Wichelhaus TA, Rödel R, Acker G, Brade V, Kraiczy P: Comparison of in vitro activities of ketolides, macrolides, and an azalide against the spirochete *Borrelia burgdorferi*. Antimicrob Agents Chemother 2004;48:344–347.

11 Alder J, Mitten M, Jarvis K, Gupta P, Clement J: Efficacy of clarithromycin for treatment of experimental Lyme disease in vivo. Antimicrob Agents Chemother 1993;37:1329–1333.

12 Levin JM, Nelson JA, Segreti J, Harrison B, Benson CA, Strle F: In vitro susceptibility of *Borrelia burgdorferi* to 11 antimicrobial agents. Antimicrob Agents Chemother 1993;37:1444–1446.

13 Murgia R, Cinco M: Sensitivity of *Borrelia* and *Leptospira* to quinupristin-dalfopristin in vitro. New Microbiol 2001;24:193–196.

14 Reisinger EC, Wendelin I, Gasser R: In vitro activity of trimethoprim against *Borrelia burgdorferi*. Eur J Clin Microbiol Infect Dis 1997;16:458–460.

15 Ruzic-Sabljic E, Podreka T, Maraspin V, Strle F: Susceptibility of *Borrelia afzelii* strains to antimicrobial agents. Int J Antimicrob Agents 2005;25: 474–478.

16 Terekhova D, Sartakova ML, Wormser GP, Schwartz I, Cabello FC: Erythromycin resistance in *Borrelia burgdorferi*. Antimicrob Agents Chemother 2002; 46:3637–3640.

17 Hunfeld KP, Ruzic-Sabljic E, Norris DE, Kraiczy P, Strle F: In vitro susceptibility testing of *Borrelia burgdorferi* sensu lato isolates cultured from patients with erythema migrans before and after antimicrobial chemotherapy. Antimicrob Agents Chemother 2005;49:1294–1301.

18 Dotevall L, Hagberg L: Penetration of doxycycline into cerebrospinal fluid in patients treated for suspected Lyme neuroborreliosis. Antimicrob Agents Chemother 1989;33:1078–1080.

19 Kazragis RJ, Dever LL, Jorgensen JH, Barbour AG: In vivo activities of ceftriaxone and vancomycin against *Borrelia* spp. in the mouse brain and other sites. Antimicrob Agents Chemother 1996;40: 2632–2636.

20 Moody KD, Adams RL, Barthold SW: Effectiveness of antimicrobial treatment against *Borrelia burgdorferi* infection in mice. Antimicrob Agents Chemother 1994;38:1567–1572.

21 Pavia CS, Wormser GP, Nowakowski J, Cacciapuoti A: Efficacy of evernimicin (SCH27899) in vitro and in an animal model of Lyme disease. Antimicrob Agents Chemother 2001;45:936–937.

22 Li M, Masuzawa T, Wang J, Kawabata M, Yanagihara Y: In-vitro and in-vivo susceptibilities of Lyme disease *Borrelia* isolated in China. J Infect Chemother 2000;6:65–67.

23 Pavia C, Inchiosa MA, Wormser GP: Efficacy of short-course therapy for *Borrelia burgdorferi* infection in C3H mice. Antimicrob Agents Chemother 2002;46:132–134.

24 Steere AC, Hutchinson GJ, Rahn DW, Sigal LH, Craft JE, DeSanna ET, et al: Treatment of early manifestation of Lyme disease. Ann Intern Med 1993;99:22–26.

25 Aberer E, Kahofer P, Binder B, Kinaciyan P, Schauperl H, Berghold A: Comparison of a two- or three-week regimen and a review of treatment of erythema migrans with phenoxymethylpenicillin. Dermatology 2006;212:160–167.

26 Weber K, Preac-Mursic V, Wilske B, Thurmayr R, Neubert U, Scherwitz C: A randomized trial of ceftriaxone versus oral penicillin for the treatment of early European Lyme borreliosis. Infection 1990; 18:91–96.

27 Strle F, Ruzic E, Cimperman J: Erythema migrans: comparison of treatment with azithromycin, doxycycline and phenoxymethylpenicillin. J Antimicrob Chemother 1992;30:543–550.

28 Weber K, Wilkse B, Preac-Mursic V, Thurmayr R: Azithromycin versus penicillin V for the treatment of early Lyme borreliosis. Infection 1993;21:367–372.

29 Breier F, Kunz G, Klade H, Stanek G, Aberer E: Erythema migrans: three weeks treatment for prevention of late Lyme borreliosis. Infection 1996; 24:69–72.

30 Dattwyler RJ, Volkman DJ, Conaty SM, Platkin SP, Luft BJ: Amoxycillin plus probenecid versus doxycycline for treatment of erythema migrans borreliosis. Lancet 1990;336:1404–1406.

31 Massarotti EM, Luger SW, Rahn DW, Messner RP, Wong JB, Johnson JC, et al: Treatment of early Lyme disease. Am J Med 1992;92:396–403.

32 Luft BJ, Dattwyler RJ, Johnson RC, Luger SW, Bosler EM, Rahn DW, et al: Azithromycin compared with amoxicillin in the treatment of erythema migrans: a randomized, double blinded, controlled trial. Ann Intern Med 1996;124:785–791.

33 Nadelman RB, Luger SW, Frank E, Wisniewski M, Collins JJ, Wormser GP: Comparison of cefuroxime axetil and doxycycline in treatment of early Lyme disease. Ann Intern Med 1992;117:273–280.

34 Wormser GP, Ramanathan R, Nawakowski J, McKenna D, Holmgren D, Visintainer P, Dornbush R, Singh B, Nadelman RB: Duration of antibiotic therapy for early Lyme disease: a randomized, double blinded, controlled trial. Ann Intern Med 2003;138: 697–704.

35 Nawakowski J, Nadelman RB, Forseter G, McKenna D, Wormser GP: Doxycycline versus tetracycline therapy for Lyme disease associated with erythema migrans. J Am Acad Dermatol 1995;32:223–227.

36 Luger SW, Paparone P, Wormser GP, Nadelman RB, Grunwaldt E, Gomez G: Comparison of cefuroxime axetil and doxycycline in the treatment of early Lyme disease with erythema migrans. Antimicrob Agents Chemother 1995;39:661–667.

37 Strle F, Preac-Mursic V, Cimperman J, Ruzic E, Maraspin V, Jereb M: Azithromycin versus doxycycline for treatment of erythema migrans: clinical and microbiological findings. Infection 1993;21: 83–88.

38 Barsic B, Maretic T, Majerus L, Strugar J: Comparison of azithromycin and doxycycline in the treatment of erythema migrans. Infection 2000;28:153–156.

39 Strle F, Maraspin V, Lotric-Furlan S, Ruzic-Sabljic E, Cimperman J: Azithromycin and doxycycline for treatment of *Borrelia* culture positive erythema migrans. Infection 1996;24:64–68.

40 Arnez M, Radsel-Medvescek A, Pleterski-Rigler D, Ruzic-Sabljic E, Strle F: Comparison of cefuroxime-axetil and phenoxymethylpenicillin for the treatment of children with solitary erythema migrans. Wien Klin Wochenschr 1999;111:916–922.

41 Arnez M, Pleterski-Rigler D, Luznik-Bufon T, Ruzic-Sabljic E, Strle F: Solitary erythema migrans in children: comparison of treatment with azithromycin and phenoxymethylpenicillin. Wien Klin Wochenschr 2002;114:498–504.

42 Eppes SC, Childs JA: Comparative study of cefuroxime axetil versus amoxicillin in children with early Lyme disease. Pediatrics 2002;109:1173–1177.
43 Institut de veille sanitaire: La maladie de Lyme: données du réseau de surveillance de la maladie en Alsace. www.invs.sante.fr.
44 Steere AC, Gross D, Meyer AL, Huber BT: Auto-immune mechanism in antibiotic treatment-resistant Lyme arthritis. J Autoimmun 2001;16:263–268.
45 Singh SK, Girschick HJ: Lyme borreliosis: from infection to autoimmunity. Clin Microbiol Infect 2004;10:598–614.
46 Lengl-Janssen B, Strauss AF, Steere AC, Kamradt T: The T helper response in Lyme arthritis: differential recognition of *Borrelia burgdorferi* outer surface protein A in patients with treatment-resistant or treatment responsive Lyme arthritis. J Exp Med 1994;180:2069–2078.
47 Drouin EE, Glickstein LJ, Steere A: Molecular characterization of the $OspA_{161-175}$ T cell epitope associated with treatment resistant Lyme arthritis: differences among the three pathogenic species of *Borrelia burgdorferi* sensu lato. J Autoimmun 2004; 23:281–292.
48 European Union Concerted Action on Lyme Borreliosis: Diagnosis of Lyme borreliosis. www.eucalb.com.
49 Ettestad PJ, Campbell GL, Welbel SF, Genese CA, Spitalny KC, Marchetti CM, Dennis DT: Biliary complications in the treatment of unsubstantiated Lyme disease. J Infect Dis 1995;171:356–361.
50 Reid MC, Schoen RT, Evans J, Rosenberg JC, Horwitz RI: The consequences of overdiagnosis and overtreatment of Lyme disease: an observational study. Ann Intern Med 1998;128:354–362.
51 Donta ST: Tetracycline therapy for chronic Lyme disease. Clin Infect Dis 1997;25(suppl 1):S52–S56.
52 Steere AC, Pachner AR, Malawista SE: Neurologic abnormalities of Lyme disease: successful treatment with high-dose intravenous penicillin. Ann Intern Med 1983;99:767–772.
53 Steere AC, Green J, Schoen RT, Taylor E, Hutchinson GJ, Rahn DW, Malawista ME: Successful parenteral penicillin therapy of established Lyme arthritis. N Engl J Med 1985;312:869–874.
54 Dattwyler RJ, Halperin JJ, Pass H, Luft BJ: Ceftriaxone as effective therapy in refractory Lyme disease. J Infect Dis 1987;155:1322–1324.
55 Dattwyler RJ, Halperin JJ, Volkman DJ, Luft BJ: Treatment of late Lyme borreliosis – randomised comparison of ceftriaxone and penicillin. Lancet 1988;1:1191–1194.
56 Borg R, Dotevall L, Hagberg L, Maraspin V, Lotric-Furlan S, Cimperman J, Strle F: Intravenous ceftriaxone compared with oral doxycycline for the treatment of Lyme neuroborreliosis. Scand J Infect Dis 2005;37:449–454.
57 Eichenfield AH, Goldsmith DP, Benach JL, Ross AH, Loeb FX, Doughty RA, Athreya BH: Childhood arthritis: experience in an endemic area. J Pediatr 1986;109:753–758.
58 Borg R, Dotevall L, Hagberg L, Maraspin V, Lotric-Furlan S, Cimperman J, Strle F: Intravenous ceftriaxone compared with oral doxycycline for the treatment of Lyme neuroborreliosis. Scand J Infect Dis 2005;37:449–454.
59 Caperton EM, Heim-Dutoit KM, Matzke GM, Peterson PK, Johnson RC: Ceftriaxone therapy of chronic inflammatory arthritis: a double-blind placebo controlled trial. Arch Intern Med 1990;150: 1677–1682.
60 Steere AC, Levin RE, Molloy PJ, Kalish RA, Abraham JH, Liu NY, Schmid CH: Treatment of Lyme arthritis. Arthritis Rheum 1994;37:878–888.
61 Mulleger RR, Millner MM, Stanek G, Spork KD: Penicillin G sodium and ceftriaxone in the treatment of neuroborreliosis in children a prospective study. Infection 1991;19:279–283.
62 Pfister HW, Preac-Mursic V, Wilske B, Einhaupl KM: Cefotaxime vs. penicillin G for acute neurologic manifestations in Lyme borreliosis: a prospective randomized study. Arch Neurol 1989;46:1190–1194.
63 Pfister HW, Preac-Mursic V, Wilske B, Schielke E, Sorgel F, Einhaupl KM: Randomized comparison of ceftriaxone and cefotaxime in Lyme neuroborreliosis. J Infect Dis 1991;19:279–283.
64 Oksi J, Nikoskelainen J, Viljanen MK: Comparison of oral cefixime and intravenous ceftriaxone followed by oral amoxicillin in disseminated Lyme borreliosis. Eur J Clin Microbiol Infect Dis 1998;17: 715–719.
65 Renaud I, Cachin C, Gerster JC: Good outcomes of Lyme arthritis in 24 patients in an endemic area of Switzerland. Joint Bone Spine 2004;71:39–43.
66 Valesova H, Mailer J, Havlik J, Hulinska D, Hercogova J: Long-term results in patients with Lyme arthritis following treatment with ceftriaxone. Infection 1996;24:98–102.
67 Eckman MH, Steere AC, Kalish RA, Pauker SG: Cost effectiveness of oral as compared with intravenous antibiotic therapy for patients with early Lyme disease or Lyme arthritis. N Engl J Med 1997;337: 357–363.
68 Wormser GP, Nadelman RB, Dattwyler RJ, Dennis DT, Shapiro ED, Steere AC, Rush TJ, Rahn DW, Coyle PK, Persing DH, Fish D, Luft BJ: Practice guidelines for the treatment of Lyme disease. Clin Infect Dis 2000;31(suppl):S1–S14.

69 Fishman RA: Blood-brain and CSF barriers to penicillin and related organicacids. Arch Neurol 1966; 15:113–124.
70 Logigian EL, Kaplan RF, Steere AC: Chronic neurologic manifestations of Lyme disease. N Engl J Med 1990;323:1438–1444.
71 Logigian EL, Kaplan RF, Steere AC: Successful treatment of Lyme encephalopathy with intravenous ceftriaxone. J Infect Dis 1999;180:377–383.
72 Karlsson M, Hammers-Berggren S, Lindquist L, Stiernstedt G, Svenugsson B: Comparison of intravenous penicillin G and oral doxycycline for treatment of Lyme neuroborreliosis. Neurology 1994; 44:1203–1207.
73 Dattwyler RJ, Luft BJ, Kunkel MJ, Finkel MF, Wormser GP, Rush TJ, Grunwaldt E, Agger WA, Franklin M, Oswald D, Cockey L, Maladorno D: Ceftriaxone compared with doxycycline for the treatment of acute disseminated Lyme borreliosis. N Engl J Med 1997;337:289–294.
74 Dotevall L, Hagberg L: Successful oral doxycycline treatment of Lyme disease-associated facial palsy and meningitis. Clin Infect Dis 1999;28:569–574.
75 Thorstrand C, Belfrage E, Bennet R, Malmborg P, Eriksson M: Successful treatment of neuroborreliosis with ten day regimens. Pediatr Infect Dis 2002; 21:1142–1145.
76 Clark JR, Carlson RD, Sasaki CT, Pachner AR, Steere AC: Facial paralysis in Lyme disease. Laryngoscope 1985;95:1341–1345.
77 Rohacova H, Hancil J, Hulinska D, Mailer H, Havlik J: Ceftriaxone in the treatment of Lyme neuroborreliosis. Infection 1996;24:88–90.
78 Kaiser R: Clinical courses of acute and chronic neuroborreliosis following treatment with ceftriaxone (in German). Nervenarzt 2004;75:553–557.
79 Cimmino MA, Accardo S: Long term treatment of chronic Lyme arthritis with benzathine penicillin. Ann Rheum Dis 1992;51:1007–1008.
80 Dattwyler RJ, Wormser GP, Rush TJ, Finkel MF, Schoen RT, Grunwaldt E, Franklin M, Hilton E, Bryant GL, Agger WA, Maladorno D: A comparison of two treatment regimens of ceftriaxone in late Lyme disease. Wien Klin Wochenschr 2005;117:393–397.
81 Kaplan RF, Trevino RP, Johnson GM, Levy L, Dornbush R, Hu LT, Evans J, Weinstein A, Schmid CH, Klempner MS: Cognitive function in post-treatment Lyme disease: do additional antibiotics help? Neurology 2003;60:1916–1922.
82 Klempner MS, Hu LD, Evans J, Schmid CH, Johnson GM, Trevino RP, Norton D, Levy L, Wall D, McCall J, Kosinski M, Weinstein A: Two controlled trials of antibiotic treatment in patients with persistent symptoms and a history of Lyme disease. N Engl J Med 2001;345:85–92.
83 Krupp LB, Hyman LG, Grimson R, Coyle PK, Melville P, Ahnn S, Dattwyler R, Chandler B: Study and Treatment of Post-Lyme Disease (STOP-LD): a randomized double masked clinical trial. Neurology 2003;60:1923–1930.
84 Donta ST: Macrolide therapy of chronic Lyme disease. Med Sci Monit 2003;9:136–142.
85 Aberer E, Breier F, Stanek G, Schmidt B: Success and failure in the treatment of acrodermatitis chronica atrophicans. Infection 1996;24:85–87.
86 Weber K, Preac-Mursic V, Neubert U, Thurmayr R, Herzzr P, Wilske B, Schierz G, Marget W: Antibiotic therapy of early European Lyme borreliosis and acrodermatitis chronica atrophicans. Ann NY Acad Sci 1988;539:324–345.
87 Kindstrand E, Nilsson BY, Hovmark A, Pirskanen R, Asbrink E: Peripheral neuropathy in acrodermatitis chronica atrophicans – effect of treatment. Acta Neurol Scand 2002;106:253–257.
88 Lipsker D, Antoni-Bach N, Hansmann Y, Jaulhac B: Long term prognosis of patients treated for erythema migrans in France. Br J Dermatol 2002;146: 872–876.
89 Boulanger N: What primary prevention should be used to prevent Lyme disease? Med Mal Infect 2007; 37:456–462.
90 Carroll JF, Klun JA, Debboun M: Repellency of DEET and SS220 applied to skin involves olfactory sensing by two species of ticks. Med Vet Entomol 2005;19:101–106.
91 WHO Committee to Advise on Tropical Medicine and Travel (CATMAT): Statement on personal protective measures to prevent arthropod bites. Can Commun Dis Rep 2005;31:1–18.
92 Throsell W, Mikiver A, Tunon H: Repelling properties of some plant material on tick Ixodes ricinus. Phytomedicine 2006;13:132–134.
93 Gardulf A, Wohlfart A, Gustafson R: A prospective cross-over field trial shows protection of lemon eucalyptus extract against tick bites. J Med Entomol 2004;41:1064–1067.
94 Fradin MS, Day JF: Comparative efficacy of insect repellents against mosquito bites. N Engl J Med 2002;347:13–18.
95 Sternberg L, Berglund J: Detecting ticks on light versus dark clothing. Scand J Infect Dis 2005;37: 361–364.
96 Patey O: Lyme disease: prophylaxis after tick bite. Med Mal Infect 2007;37:446–455.
97 Nadelman RB, Nowakowski J, Fish D, et al: Prophylaxis with single dose doxycycline for the prevention of Lyme disease after an *Ixodes scapularis* tick bite. N Engl J Med 2001;345:79–84.
98 Korenberg EI, Vorobyeva NN, Moskvitina HG, Gorban LY: Prevention of borreliosis in persons bitten by infected ticks. Infection 1996;24:187–189.

99 Wormser GP: Controversies in the use of antimicrobial for the prevention and treatment of Lyme disease (letter). N Engl J Med 2001;345:1349.
100 Magid D, Schwartz B, Craft J, Schwartz JS: Prevention of Lyme disease after tick bites. N Engl J Med 1992;327:534–541.
101 Dennis DT, Meltzer MI: Antibiotic prophylaxis after tick bites. Lancet 1997;350:1191–1192.
102 Warshafsky S, Nowakowski J, Nadelman RB, Kamer RS, Peterson SJ, Wormser GP: Efficacy of antibiotic prophylaxis for prevention of Lyme disease. J Gen Intern Med 196;11:329–333.
103 Centers for Disease Control: Update: Lyme disease and cases occurring during pregnancy – United States. MMWR Morbid Mortal Wkly Rep 1985;34: 376–378, 383–384.
104 Markowitz LE, Steere AC, Benach JL, Stade JD, Broome CV: Lyme disease during pregnancy. JAMA 1986;255:3394–3396.
105 Schlesinger PA, Duray PH, Burke BA, Steere AC, Stillman MT: Maternal-fetal transmission of the Lyme disease spirochete, *Borrelia burgdorferi*. Ann Intern Med 1985;103:67–69.
106 Strobino BA, Williams CL, Abid S, Chalson R, Spierling P: Lyme disease and pregnancy outcome: a prospective study of two thousand prenatal patients. Am J Obstet Gynecol 1993;169:367–374.
107 Maraspin V, Cimperman J, Lotric-Furlan S, Pleterski-Riegler D, Strle F: Treatment of erythema migrans in pregnancy. Clin Infect Dis 1996;22:788–793.
108 Williams CL, Strobino BA, Weinstein A, Spierling P, Medici F: Maternal Lyme disease and congenital malformations: a cord blood serosurvey in endemic and control areas. Paediatr Perinat Epidemiol 1995;9:320–330.
109 Strobino BA, Abid S, Gewitz M: Maternal Lyme disease and congenital heart disease: a case-control study in an endemic area. Am J Obstet Gynecol 1999;180:711–716.
110 Maraspin V, Cimperman J, Lotric-Furlan S, Pleterski-Riegler D, Strle F: Erythema migrans in pregnancy. Wien Klin Wochenschr 1999;111:933–940.
111 Sood SK, Salzman MB, Johnson BJ, Happ CM, Feig K, Carmody L, Rubin LG, Hilton E, Piesman J: Duration of tick attachment as a predictor of the risk of Lyme disease in an area in which Lyme disease is endemic. J Infect Dis 1997;175:996–999.

Yves Hansmann
Service des Maladies Infectieuses et Tropicales, Hôpitaux Universitaires de Strasbourg
1, place de l'hôpital
FR–67091 Strasbourg Cedex (France)
Tel. +33 3 88 11 53 51, Fax +33 3 88 11 64 64, E-Mail yves.hansmann@chru-strasbourg.fr

Lipsker D, Jaulhac B (eds): Lyme Borreliosis.
Curr Probl Dermatol. Basel, Karger, 2009, vol 37, pp 130–154

Other Tick-Borne Diseases in Europe

Idir Bitam · Didier Raoult

Unité des Rickettsies CNRS-IRD UMR 6236, Faculté de Médecine, Université de la Méditerranée, Marseille, France

Abstract

Ticks are obligate blood-sucking arthropods that transmit pathogens while feeding, and in Europe, more vector-borne diseases are transmitted to humans by ticks than by any other agent. In addition to neurotoxins, ticks can transmit bacteria (e.g. rickettsiae, spirochetes) viruses and protozoa. Some tick-borne diseases, such as Lyme disease and ehrlichiosis, can cause severe or fatal illnesses. Here, we examine tick-borne diseases other than Lyme disease that are found in Europe; namely: anaplasmosis, relapsing fever, tularemia, tick-borne encephalitis, tick-borne babesiosis and tick-borne rickettsiosis. Each disease is broken down into a description, epidemiology, signs and symptoms, diagnosis and treatment, providing clear overviews of each disease course and the interventions required. Furthermore, in the section concerning tick-borne rickettsiosis, a clear summary of the *Rickettsia conorii* complex and its role in the disease is provided.

In Europe, more vector-borne diseases are transmitted to humans by ticks than by any other agent [1]. In addition to neurotoxins, ticks can transmit bacteria (e.g. rickettsiae, spirochetes) viruses and protozoa [2]. Some tick-borne diseases, such as Lyme disease [3, 4] and ehrlichiosis, can cause severe or fatal illnesses [5, 6]. Cardiopulmonary complications associated with tick-borne diseases are particularly serious and may be life-threatening [5, 7]. Many species of ticks that have been found over a very wide geographic distribution [8, 9] may transmit diseases to humans (table 1). Ticks are obligate blood-sucking arthropods that transmit pathogens while feeding [9]. Large reservoirs of ticks feed on the rodents and small mammals that inhabit wooded areas, gardens and parklands [10, 11]. Nevertheless, outbreaks of tick-borne diseases are not confined to rural areas. Successful management of tick-borne diseases depends on a high index of suspicion and an awareness of their geographic epidemiology and clinical features [3, 12]. Tick-borne diseases have protean manifestations. Patients at risk of tick bites may harbor 2 or more concurrent tick-borne infections [13]. The diagnosis of a tick-borne disease is most often based on a constellation of clinical signs and a history of outdoor pursuits, skin rashes or tick bites [3, 9, 14].

Table 1. Causative agents and vectors of tick-borne diseases in Europe

Disease	Causative agents	Vectors
Lyme disease	*Borrelia burgdorferi* s.l.	*Ixodes ricinus*
Anaplasmosis	*Anaplasma phagocytophilum*	*Ixodes ricinus*
Relapsing fever	*Anaplasma marginale*	
	Borrelia duttonii	*Ornithodoros moubata*
	Borrelia crocidurae	*Ornithodoros sonrai*
	Borrelia hispanica	*Ornithodoros erraticus*
Tularemia	*Francisella tularensis*	*Ixodes ricinus* *Dermacentor reticulatus* *Dermacentor variabilis*
Tick-borne encephalitis	TBEV	*Ixodes* ticks
Rickettsiosis	*Rickettsia conorii conorii* *Rickettsia conorii israelensis* *Rickettsia conorii caspia*	*Rhipicephalus sanguineus*
	Rickettsia sibirica mongolitimonae	*Hyalomma anatolicum excavatum* *Rhipicephalus pusillus*
	Rickettsia slovaca	*Dermacentor* sp.
	Rickettsia aeschlimannii	*Hyalomma* sp.
	Rickettsia massiliae	*Rhipicephalus sanguineus* *Rhipicephalus turanicus*
	Rickettsia helvetica	*Ixodes ricinus*
	Rickettsia raoultii	*Dermacentor nuttalli* *Dermacentor silvarum* *Dermacentor reticulatus* *Rhipicephalus pumilio*

TBEV = Tick-borne encephalitis virus.

Anaplasmosis

Introduction

The genus *Anaplasma* (Rickettsiales: Anaplasmataceae) includes several pathogens such as *A. marginale* and *A. phagocytophilum* that have an impact on human and animal health [15]. *A. phagocytophilum* belong to the order Rickettsiales and are obligate intracellular bacteria. They have long been known to cause tick-borne fever in ungulates, and have been identified more recently as the causative agent of the emerging disease human granulocytic anaplasmosis (HGA). *A. marginale* can be transmitted mechanically among cattle by the blood-contaminated mouthparts of biting flies; it is transmitted biologically by ticks [16]. About 20 tick species have been shown to transmit anaplasmosis, although field evidence indicating that the tick is the principal disease vector is lacking [17]. *A. phagocytophilum* is transstadially and not transovarially transmitted by tick vector *Ixodes ricinus* in Europe [18]. The geographic occurrence of endemic cycles of *A. phagocytophilum* correlates with the geographic occurrence of tick vectors [19]. Thus, the natural maintenance of *A. phagocytophilum* is dependent on horizontal transmission involving either acutely or persistently infected mammals and ticks.

Epidemiology

Although 5 Anaplasmataceae members, including *A. phagocytophilum,* infect humans, it is this particular bacteria that infects granulocytes and causes HGA [15]. The agent of human granulocytic anaplasmosis is a tick-borne pathogen, which is not frequently found in Europe. The disease occurs year-round with most of the infections occurring during May through August. *A. phagocytophilum* is found in *I. ricinus* [20]. The first case of clinically recognized human granulocytic anaplasmosis was described in the USA in 1994 [21]. Soon after, the disease emerged in Europe in 1997, in Slovenia [22]. Thereafter, seroepidemiologic surveys have found a prevalence of antibodies in a range of 0–2.9% in blood donors, in 1.5% of patients who live in *I. ricinus*-exposed areas, in 8.6% of tick-exposed individuals in southern Europe [23, 24] and in 1.5–24.4% of tick-exposed people throughout northern and central Europe [25].

Several clinical cases have been reported in Europe, including Slovenia [26, 27], The Netherlands [28], Spain [29], Sweden [30], Croatia [31], Poland [32] and France [33]. More recently, a study carried out in southern Europe characterized *A. phagocytophilum* infections in humans. *A. phagocytophilum* is maintained in cattle, donkeys, deer and birds, and is most likely transmitted by several ticks species in southern Europe [16]. The presence of concurrent infections in cattle and deer suggests that these pathogens may multiply in the same reservoir host, and illustrates the complexity of the epidemiology of bovine and human anaplasmosis in southern Europe.

Signs and Symptoms

The diseases of ruminants such as cattle, sheep and goats ('pasture fever' or 'tick-borne fever' [18]) and humans (HGA) appear most commonly as an undifferentiated febrile illness occurring in spring or summer [34]. The incubation period following the tick-bite is 7–10 days. Symptoms include high fever, rigors, generalized myalgia, severe headaches and malaise [32, 35]. Anorexia, arthralgia, nausea and a nonproductive cough are frequent. Leucopenia and thrombocytopenia are often seen, and less frequently anemia. The disease may be severe, particularly in the elderly, when there is concomitant chronic illnesses and a lack of/delayed specific antibiotic treatment [35]. The case fatality rate is low for HGA (0.7%) in the USA, but is not described for Europe.

It is related to complicating opportunistic infections, although poor outcomes are also associated with antecedent medical conditions, such as diabetes mellitus [35].

Laboratory Findings

Laboratory confirmation of HGA is based on several tests that are not widely available for routine use at present [36]. *Anaplasma* sp. are Gram-negative and not motile; these bacteria are small (often pleomorphic or coccoid) cells ranging from 0.3 to 0.4 μm in diameter, and they are found in cytoplasmic inclusion bodies (morula) in mature or immature hematopoietic mammalian cells. As for in vitro cultivation diagnosis, there are only a small number of practicing laboratories because this technique requires the application of antibiotic-free cell culture methods, not available in clinical laboratories. Although both pathogens are able to grow in several different cell lines, HGA is most often isolated by inoculation of mononuclear leukocytes from density gradients into the DH82 canine histiocytic cell line [37]. Prior doxycycline treatment diminishes the sensitivity of culture to a greater degree than it does for PCR or blood smear examination [38].

Indirect immunofluorescence assay remains the most widely available test. A 4-fold rise or fall in the antibody titer, with a minimum peak of 1:64 and a single serum antibody titer greater than or equal to 1:128, is necessary for the diagnosis. However, limitations include a delay in seroconversion (early sera will often return negative), as well as possible false-positive detection due to cross-reacting bacteria [24].

PCR performed using EDTA or citrate anticoagulated blood is rapidly becoming the diagnostic test of choice at or shortly after presentation. PCR obviates the need for culture. PCR detection sensitivity is relatively high; it is reported to range between 67 and 90% [35, 39]. Recent advances in molecular methods promise even greater analytical sensitivity, and multiplex testing that could identify several agents of anaplasmosis from a single test has been described elsewhere [40].

Treatment

Although no clinical trials have been conducted, empirical data show that all forms of ehrlichiosis respond to tetracyclines [41]. When the antibiotic susceptibilities of 8 strains of *A. phagocytophilum* were recently tested in vitro, doxycycline and rifampin were the most active drugs [42]. However, levofloxacin was also active [36]. Doxycycline therapy is highly efficacious, relapse after therapy has never been reported [41], and it can be used to treat both infections in adults and children. For children <8 years of age who are not seriously ill, the recommended approach is doxycycline treatment for 3 days after the patient's fever has abated [20].

Relapsing Fever

Introduction

Relapsing fever, an infectious disease with a sudden onset of high fever with septicemic signs and symptoms, is characterized by the occurrence of 1 or more spells of fever after the subsidence of the primary febrile attack [43]. Endemic tick-borne relapsing fever (TBRF) is due to at least 16 distinctive *Borrelia* species harbored in soft ticks of the genus *Ornithodoros (Alectorobius)* [44]. Clinically, the manifestations of louse-borne relapsing fever and TBRF are quite similar. TBRF is a serious disease with, if untreated, a mortality rate of up to 5%. TBRF acquired during pregnancy poses a high risk of pregnancy loss, up to 50%.

Neurological symptoms have been reported for 9% of the patients with TBRF. Such findings were reported previously among TBRF patients in Senegal and TBRF patients returning from Senegal to Europe. Tetracycline or doxycycline effectively eliminates the spirochetemia [45].

Epidemiology and Transmission

TBRF is a zoonotic disease transmitted worldwide by soft body ticks of the genus *Ornithodoros*. The disease was mentioned in 1857 by Livingston, who described a recurrent febrile illness among African natives who were exposed to ticks [46]. The causative link with ticks was reported in 1905 by Dutton and Todd, who demonstrated spirochetes in *Ornithodoros moubata* in East Africa [47]. *Ornithodoros* ticks are included in the soft tick family Argasidae [48].

These arthropods are hematophagous at all growing stages. Ticks are infected during a blood meal on a spirochetemic vertebrate. *Borrelia* then spread to all tissues of the tick, including the ovaries (responsible for transmission between the different tick developmental stages and between generations), salivary glands and excretory organs. Vertebrates and humans become infected during a blood meal through contamination of the feeding site by salivary and/or coxal secretions [48]. The soft body tick feeds for a short time only (usually less than half an hour), then returns to the earth or the floor/walls of the house. In Africa, humans are believed to be the only reservoir for *B. duttonii* transmitted by *O. moubata*, which is unlike the situation for *B. crocidurae* and *B. tillae* by *O. zumpti*, where rodents and other insectivores are reservoirs [49].

Six TBRF borrelioses are known to occur in Europe or close to its boundaries. At present, the greatest endemic risk in Europe lies in the Iberian peninsula, particularly in the Mediterranean part [46]. Twenty-two species of *Ornithodoros* have been reported in humans, and 12 species are frequently found [50]. Transmission of TBRF has also occurred through transfusion or laboratory contamination, and during pregnancy [48]. A few cases of relapsing fever are diagnosed every year in France in travelers from disease-endemic countries [51] (http://www.pasteur.fr/sante/clre/cadrecnr/borrelia-index.html).

Relapsing fever-associated *Borrelia* species have been named on the basis of the cospeciation concept, taking into account the geographic endemicity of the vectors. Some of these organisms have a worldwide distribution, e.g. *B. recurrentis* is transmitted by human body lice [52], while other species are geographically restricted. The specificity of the association between *Borrelia* species and vectors has been questioned as *B. duttonii*, *B. crocidurae* and *B. hispanica*, which are naturally transmitted in nature by *O. moubata*, *O. sonrai* (formerly *O. erraticus sonrai*) and *O. erraticus* (formerly *O. erraticus erraticus*), respectively, could be experimentally adapted to lice [52]. *B. hispanica* is found in Spain, Portugal, Cyprus, Greece and North Africa. This species has been isolated in *O. erraticus*, an endophilic tick commonly found under meso-Mediterranean vegetation in south-western Europe. This tick species usually lives in the burrows of wild rodents, its natural host. In Spain and Portugal, however, it has adapted to bite domestic pigs that are continuously grazed and sometimes kept in overnight in large burrows or inside old buildings, and the tick has adapted to live in these habitats [50, 53]. Humans may be bitten, and hence relapsing fever was sporadically reported in countries such as Spain during the 20th century, probably with an underestimated incidence [48, 53]. The disease caused by *B. hispanica* is one of the less severe TBRF, and presents with neurological signs in less than 5% of cases [48].

Signs and Symptoms

The disease is transmitted either by tick saliva during feeding or in coxal fluid excreted during feeding [54]. TBRF begins between 4 and 14 days after the tick bite, with an acute onset of high fever, chills, constitutional symptoms and iritis [55, 56]. The clinical characterization is recurrent episodes of fever and spirochetemia [57]. Severity of the symptoms varies according to the infecting species of *Borrelia*. The average inoculation period is 1 week. Influenza-like symptoms, arthralgia (possibly severe), dizziness, nausea and vomiting are common. Fever is usually high (greater than 40°C), irregular in pattern and sometimes associated with delirium. Most patients have splenomegaly and meningeal signs may be present. Other complications can include epistaxis, hemoptysis, iridocyclitis, coma, cranial nerve palsy, pneumonitis, myocarditis and rupture of the spleen [58].

The first cases to be recognized among pregnant women have been fulminant and, if untreated, led to death within 36–48 h. Even when treatment was available, these patients had preterm deliveries or spontaneous abortions [57].

Diagnosis

Diagnosis is usually made during the primary attack, by observation of spirochetemia on thin or thick blood smears with dark-field microscopy or with conventional microscopy after Giemsa, Wright or Diff-Quick® staining [46]. Thick blood smears provide 20 times the sensitivity of thin blood smears. Quantitative buffy coat fluorescence analysis has also been described as a very sensitive and specific technique for detecting *Borrelia* in blood [43]. Mouse inoculation has been used for a long time for the isolation of TBRF *Borrelia*, but some of the TBRF *Borrelia* species can be cultured on axenic medium. Kelly's medium serves as the basis for Barbour-Stoenner-Kelly medium, which has been used for the cultivation of Lyme disease spirochetes as well as for the recent successes with TBRF *Borrelia* [59]. These TBRF *Borrelia* species have fastidious culture requirements, although cultivation of a strain of *B. duttonii* and *B. crocidurae* was reported by Cutler et al. [60]. In contrast, *B. hermsii*, *B. turicatae* and *B. parkeri* are easily cultivable [61]. Molecular methods are being used with increasing frequency, and offer the possibility of species identification [46]. To date, specific serological assays are not available for most of the known TBRF because of the lack of available antigens. If they were available, they could be useful when the blood smear is negative and PCR is unavailable.

Treatment

The treatment of choice is doxycycline (100 mg orally, twice a day, for 5 to 10 days). Alternative therapy includes erythromycin (500 mg orally 4 times per day, for 5 to 10 days). Therapy may lead to a Jarisch-Herxheimer reaction (i.e. generalized malaise, headache, fever, sweating, rigors, seizures or stroke), especially if given during the late febrile stage. Administering acetaminophen 2 h before and after antibiotic administration may lessen the severity of the reaction. Steroids and nonsteroidal anti-inflammatory drugs do not prevent or modify the cardiopulmonary disturbances of the reaction [62].

Tularemia

Introduction

Tularemia (also known as rabbit fever) is an infectious disease caused by the small, pleomorphic, heat-labile, Gram-negative, rod-shaped bacterium *Francisella tularensis*. The subspecies *holarctica* is the only subspecies found in Europe, but it is spread over the whole northern hemisphere [63]. In humans or in rabbits, strains belonging to subspecies *F. tularensis* cause the most severe form of the disease, but strains belonging to all subspecies are highly virulent in mice. The aggressive features of subspecies *F. tularensis* have been an important basis for the designation of *F. tularensis* as 1 of 6 category A agents, i.e. agents that would have a great adverse impact on public health if used for bioterrorism [64]. The microorganism is a facultative intracellular pathogen affecting a wide range of animal species.

Epidemiology

Three subspecies are known: *F. tularensis* subsp. *tularensis* occurring in North America and Europe; *F. tularensis* subsp. *palaearctica (holarctica)* occurring in Europe [65], Asia and to a minor extent in North America; and *F. tularensis* subsp. *mediasiatica*, found only in the Central Asian region. *F. tularensis* subsp. *tularensis* is highly virulent for mammals and causes severe illness in humans [66]. Tularemia outbreaks have been commonly reported in some areas of Europe, such as in Sweden, Finland, Spain and Kosovo [67, 68]. In 2000, 270 cases in Sweden and 327 cases in Kosovo were reported [67, 68]. In some endemic regions, outbreaks occur frequently, whereas adjacent parts of the same country may be completely free of the disease [67].

The disease has been reported in many countries in the northern hemisphere, but, for unknown reasons, never in the southern hemisphere [69]. Usually, cases are reported during the summer, from June to September. The most common route is through microlesions in the skin of hunters who have skinned infected rabbits. In the summer, human transmission occurs also via ticks and deer flies. The tick vectors include *I. ricinus* and *Dermacentor variabilis. D. reticulatus* was also found positive for *F. tularensis* from Portugal [70], as were horse flies. Although less common, consumption of undercooked infected meat and contaminated water can also lead to infection [71]. In particular, increases in rodent tularemia appear to be closely linked to epidemic outbreaks of human tularemia [69].

Signs and Symptoms

After an incubation period of 3–5 days (range 1–25 days), 7 clinical forms – according to route of inoculation (skin, mucous membranes, gastrointestinal tract, eyes, respiratory tract), dose of the inoculum and virulence of the organism (types A or B) – can be identified [72, 73] (table 2).

The different presentations include pneumonic, ulceroglandular, typhoidal, glandular, oculoglandular, oropharyngeal and septicemic. After inoculation, *F. tularensis* is ingested by and multiplies within macrophages.

Usually, whatever the clinical form, the onset of tularemia is abrupt, with fever, chills, myalgia, arthralgia, headache, coryza, sore throat, and sometimes pulse-temperature dissociation, nausea, vomiting and diarrhea [74].

Table 2. Summary of clinical and biological description of tularemia

Clinical features
Incubation period: 3–5 days
Ulceroglandular tularemia (most common form: 75–85%)
Local papule at the site of inoculation associated with fever and aches
Papule pruritic ulcer → enlarges to pustule ulcer → ruptures to painful indolent ulcer, which may be covered by an eschar
Tender enlargement of >1 regional lymph node, which may become fluctuant and rupture releasing caseous material
Serological diagnosis and PCR on cutaneous biopsy or adenopathies
Glandular tularemia
Lymphadenopathy and fever
No ulcer
Serological diagnosis and PCR on lymph nodes
Oculoglandular tularemia
Purulent conjunctivitis, chemosis, conjunctival nodules or ulceration, periorbital edema
Tender preauricular or cervical lymphadenopathy
Serological diagnosis and PCR
Tularemia pneumonia (primary and secondary pneumonia)
Inhalational exposure presents as an acute flu-like illness
Progression to severe pneumonia with bloody sputum, respiratory failure and death if appropriate treatment is not started
Chest radiography: peribronchial infiltrates, bronchopneumonia, pleural effusions and hilar lymphadenopathy
Serological diagnosis
Oropharyngeal tularemia
Stomatitis, exudative pharyngitis or tonsillitis with painful mucosal ulceration
Retropharyngeal abscess or suppuration of regional lymph nodes
Serological diagnosis
Typhoidal tularemia
Acute flu-like illness
Diarrhea, vomiting, headache, chills, rigors, myalgia, arthralgia, weight loss, prostration
No indication of inoculation site
No anatomic localization of infection
Serological diagnosis
Tularemia sepsis
Nonspecific signs of confusion
Septic shock, disseminated intravascular coagulation and hemorrhage, acute respiratory distress syndrome, organ failure and coma
Diagnosis
Confirmatory tests for identification of *F. tularensis*
Isolation of *F. tularensis* from a clinical specimen
Demonstration of a specific antibody response in serially obtained sera
PCR
For probable case
A single high titer
Detection of *F. tularensis* in a clinical specimen by fluorescent assay

Table 2 (continued)

Treatment
Private room placement for patients with pneumonia is NOT necessary
Treatment of choice: streptomycin or gentamicin (10 days)
Quinolones are an effective alternative (10–14 days)
Tetracyclines and chloramphenicol are associated with a high relapse rate (therapy at least 14–21 days)
Combination of aminoglycosides and fluoroquinolones in severe cases
Post-exposure prophylaxis
Streptomycin, gentamicin, doxycycline or ciprofloxacin (14 days)
Vaccination is NOT recommended for post-exposure prophylaxis

Diagnosis

Tularemia should be suspected if the patient has been exposed to rabbits, wild rodents, or ticks, or has characteristic symptoms, such a primary pustular lesion on an extremity. Isolation of the organism from skin lesions, lymph nodes or sputum is diagnostic, but dangerous because the organism can be highly infectious. This bacteria is considered as a potential biologic weapon. PCR after inactivation of the bacteria could be therefore an efficient and safe diagnostic method. Extreme caution should be maintained when handling infected tissues or culture media. Acute and convalescent titers also can confirm the diagnosis. Leukocytosis is common, but the white blood cell count may be normal. Abnormal chest radiographic findings (i.e. a triad of oval opacities, hilar adenopathy and pleural effusions) are more likely with tularemia than in other tick-borne diseases [75, 76].

Rapid methods for the identification of *F. tularensis,* such as the immunofluorescence assay and the enzyme-linked immunosorbent assay for the detection of antigens and the RNA hybridization assay, have been tried, but have so far not been included in routine diagnostics [77]. The use of PCR for the direct diagnosis of ulceroglandular tularemia is thus highly promising, and more work on the conditions that might influence the assay seems to be warranted.

Treatment

Many guidelines have been published for treatments and prophylaxis of tularemia [72, 78]. Treatment should begin before confirmatory laboratory tests are obtained. If available, the treatment of choice for tularemia is streptomycin (0.5 g intramuscularly every 12 h until the patient's body temperature is normal; thereafter, 0.5 g per day for 5 days). Gentamicin (3–5 mg/kg/day, intramuscularly or intravenously, in 3 divided doses for 7 to 14 days) is also effective [72]. If renal disease is present, the dose of gentamicin needs to be reduced. Chloramphenicol or tetracyclines have also been used, but relapses occasionally occur with these medications, and they may not prevent node suppuration [79].

Tick-Borne Encephalitis

Introduction

Tick-borne encephalitis (TBE) is caused by an RNA virus belonging to the *Flavivirus* genus. The species tick-borne encephalitis virus (TBEV) includes 3 subtypes (European, Far-Eastern and Siberian) based on the sequencing and geographic data [80, 81].

Epidemiology

Ixodes ticks that transmit TBEV in European climates complete their development cycle within 3 years, and the infection is transmissible even in the nymph phase [82]. During the years 1991–1998, at least 1,230 cases of TBE were reported in Germany, with a mean incidence in Baden-Württemberg of 1.2 per 100,000 inhabitants per year and a case fatality rate of 1% [81]. In a highly endemic area in Baden-Württemberg, a seroprevalence of 9% was found [83]. Also, there has been a recent diffusion of TBEV into southern European countries coming from Euro-Asiatic forests, and in part from the Danube basin [84]. The Far Eastern subtype, responsible for severer infections and also known as Russian spring-summer encephalitis, is dispersed across Russia, the Czech Republic, Austria, Poland, Hungary and the former Yugoslavia. The European subtype, responsible for a milder form called central European encephalitis, is scattered across this geographic area, but has also spread to regions bordering Austria (Italy and former Yugoslavia) [85].

In recent years, the virus has reached some Italian regions, e.g. northeast and central Italy, and has also been reported in Piedmont (northwest region). Moreover, TBEV (strain Neudörfl) has been reported in Denmark [86], Scandinavia [87] and Greece [88]. TBEV, in addition to tick bites, is also transmitted by unpasteurized milk and infected aerosols [85]. Its incubation period ranges from 1 to 2 weeks [85]. In Poland, during 1993–2002, 1,996 cases of TBE were reported [89], and in Russia, over 10,000 cases a year are recorded; about 3,000 cases per year are possible in the rest of Europe [90].

Signs and Symptoms

TBE typically takes a biphasic course. After an incubation period, usually between 7 and 14 days, the prodromal symptoms (uncharacteristic influenza-like illness with fever, headache, malaise and myalgia) are followed by CNS involvement. After an afebrile interval of approximately 1 week the second stage develops. TBE may manifest as isolated meningitis, meningoencephalitis or meningoencephalomyelitis [91]; data on the clinical course and outcome of large series of patients with TBE are sparse. The mortality was about 1%, but a higher percentage of neurologic sequelae were signaled [92]. The Russian-type disease (spring-summer encephalitis) is severer, with mortality also above 20% in patients with neurologic complications [85, 93]. In Germany, from 1991–2000, 1,500 patients were diagnosed with symptomatic infection of TBEV; neurologic manifestations were described in 47% of the cases (42% with meningoencephalitis and 11% with meningoencephalomyelitis) [94].

Diagnosis

Diagnosis of TBE can be performed by viral isolation and neutralization tests (with biohazards) or by using classical serologic tests, including complement fixation and enzyme immunoassay for IgM research [95], and more recently by more specific rE-D3 enzyme-linked immunosorbent assay (rE-D3 ELISA) and Western blot tests. The rE-D3 ELISA permits a differential diagnosis with respect to other tick-borne zoonoses [96]. Also, in recent years, real-time RT-PCR for detection and quantitation of TBEV RNA that also permits strain differentiation has been used [97].

Treatment and Prevention

There is no specific treatment for TBE. Two vaccines that prevent infection are available. Although these have a good protection rate and good efficacy, there are few data on long-term immunity. The inactivated vaccine manufactured by the Baxter Company in Austria has been extensively used in large-scale programs, which have demonstrated a significant decrease in the number of TBE cases in Austria and Germany [97].

Tick-Borne Babesiosis

Introduction

Babesiosis is an intraerythrocytic parasitic infection caused by protozoa of the genus *Babesia* and transmitted through the bite of the *Ixodes* tick, the same vector responsible for transmission of Lyme disease. The first description of *Babesia* was given by Babès in 1888 in his evaluation of the cause of febrile hemoglobinuria in cattle in Romania [98–100]. While most cases are tick-borne, transfusion and transplacental transmissions have been reported.

Babesiosis is a zoonotic disease maintained by the interaction of tick vectors, transport hosts and animal reservoirs. The primary vectors of the parasite are ticks of the genus *Ixodes*. In Europe, *I. ricinus* appears to be the primary tick vector. In each location, the *Ixodes* tick vector for *Babesia* is the same vector that locally transmits *B. burgdorferi*, the agent implicated in Lyme disease. The primary animal reservoir is cattle.

Ticks ingest *Babesia* while feeding of the host, and the parasite multiplies within the tick's gut wall. The parasites then spread to the tick's salivary glands. Inoculation into a vertebrate host occurs by a larva, nymph or adult tick [99, 100]. Infection in humans usually occurs from late spring to early fall.

After an infectious tick bite, the parasites invade red blood cells and a trophozoite differentiates, replicating asexually by budding with the formation of 2–4 merozoites; these disrupt the red blood cells and go on to invade other red blood cells. This leads to hemolytic anemia, thrombocytopenia and atypical lymphocyte formation. Alterations in red blood cell membranes cause decreased conformability and increased red blood cell adherence, which can lead to development of acute respiratory distress syndrome among those severely affected.

Epidemiology

The first case of human babesiosis was reported in 1957 from Yugoslavia in an asplenic farmer [101]. Approximately 40 cases have been reported since then, mostly in Ireland, the UK and France; 23 of these cases were caused by *B. divergens* [102, 103].

Babesiosis affects all age groups with similar frequency; however, patients older than 50 years are at increased risk of severe infection and death. Patients report traveling to an endemic area between the months of May and September; however, most do not recall the tick bite. The incubation period is between 1 and 4 weeks. The signs and symptoms mimic malaria, and range in severity from asymptomatic to septic shock.

Signs and Symptoms

Most of the patients described in Europe were asplenic, presented with acute febrile hemolytic disease, and their clinical courses have almost always been fatal [99, 100].

Symptoms include high fever (up to 40°C), chills, diaphoresis, weakness, fatigue, anorexia and headache. Later in the course of the illness, the patient may develop jaundice and dark urine. Physical examination may reveal hepatomegaly and splenomegaly or evidence of shock. Rash is an uncommon symptom in babesiosis [98–100, 104]. Signs of CNS involvement include headache, photophobia, neck and back stiffness, altered sensorium and emotional lability [100, 104, 105].

Diagnosis

A Wright- or Giemsa-stained peripheral blood smear is most commonly used to demonstrate the presence of intraerythrocytic parasites. The organisms are intraerythrocytic ring forms closely resembling *Plasmodium*. Serologic evaluation is performed by an indirect immunofluorescent antibody test with the use of *B. microti* antigen.

Inoculation of susceptible animals with whole blood from a suspected case is another diagnostic technique. Classically, hamsters are used to isolate *B. microti* [106]. Inoculation of the animal requires monitoring via blood smear examination for up to 6 weeks [107]. Thus, although this system is fairly sensitive (300 organisms per ml of blood for *B. microti* [106]), it is time-consuming and expensive. This methodology is more useful for a retrospective diagnosis, especially when a rapid diagnosis is essential.

DNA amplification by PCR has been proposed as an even more sensitive method to detect *Babesia* infection, particularly when these infections are subclinical or parasitemias are low [108]. The 18S rRNA gene is targeted because there are multiple copies present in each organism, the sequence is phylogenetically informative, and there are conserved regions that allow for the development of general primers to identify previously under-described *Babesia* parasites.

The immunofluorescent-antibody test remains the serodiagnostic test of choice for detection of antibodies against babesial parasites. The antigens of *B. divergens* also cross-react with several *Plasmodium* and *Babesia* spp. [102]. Alternatives, such as an ELISA using recombinant antigens, are being developed [109, 110], and may provide a tool for rapid screening of a large number of samples. Soluble whole parasite antigen has been used for ELISA tests for *B. divergens* for screening of cattle, and was found useful for the detection of recent infections only in these hosts [111].

Treatment

Treatment of *B. divergens* must be rapid and aggressive. A massive blood exchange transfusion (2–3 times blood volume), followed by 10 days of intravenous clindamycin (600 mg, 3–4 times per day) is recommended [111]. The current treatment recommendation for human infection with *B. microti* is combined oral quinine (650 mg, 3 times per day) and oral clindamycin (1,200 mg, twice per day) for 7 days [107].

Tick-Borne Rickettsiosis

The genus *Rickettsia* includes bacteria of the order Rickettsiales in the α-subdivision of Proteobacteria. They are Gram-negative coccobacilli bacteria in obligatory association with eukaryote cells. The spotted fever group (SFG) includes 21 valid species, mostly vectored by ticks and causing different types of spotted fever in different parts of the world. Several already described SFG species are considered to be of unknown pathogenicity because their reports have been restricted to invertebrate hosts, mostly ticks [112–114]. *Ixodid* ticks (hard ticks) are bloodsucking arthropods throughout all of their developmental stages. The percentage of infected eggs obtained from females of the same tick species infected with the same rickettsial strain may vary, depending on factors that have yet to be elucidated.

In this section, we will describe the *Rickettsia conorii* complex, including *R. conorii* subsp. *conorii* (the agent of Mediterranean spotted fever; MSF), *R. conorii israelensis* (Israeli spotted fever rickettsia; ISFR), *R. conorii caspia* (Astrakhan spotted fever rickettsia), *R. sibirica mongolitimonae* (lymphangitis-associated rickettsioses), *R. slovaca* (tick-borne lymphadenopathy or *Dermacentor*-borne necrosis erythema lymphadenopathy), *R. aeschlimannii*, *R. massiliae* and *R. raoultii.*

Rickettsia conorii *Complex*

The classification within Rickettsiales is continually modified as new data become available. Polyphasic taxonomy, which integrates phenotypic and phylogenic data, seems to be particularly useful for rickettsial taxonomy. However, experts in the field of rickettsiology frequently disagree over species definitions. Until 2005, *Rickettsia* of the so-called *R. conorii* complex, including the *R. conorii* strain Malish (MSF), *R. conorii israelensis* (ISFR) and *R. conorii caspia* (Astrakhan spotted fever rickettsia), were considered to be members of the same species. Phylogenetically, these rickettsiae constitute a homogeneous cluster supported by a significant bootstrap value and are distinct from other *Rickettsia* species. Zhu et al. [115] proposed a nomenclature of the *R. conorii* species, with the creation of the following subspecies: *R. conorii* subsp. *conorii* subsp. nov. (type strain Malish, ATCC VR-613), *R. conorii* subsp. *caspia* subsp. nov. (type strain A-167, formerly Astrakhan fever rickettsia) and *R. conorii* subsp. *israelensis* subsp. nov. (type ISTT CDC1, formerly ISFR).

Rickettsia conorii *subsp.* conorii

This *Rickettsia* was first reported in Tunisia in 1910 by Conor and Bruch. In the 1930s, the role of *Rhipicephalus sanguineus* and the causative agent, subsequently named *R. conorii,* were described. Three strains of *R. conorii* subsp. *conorii* include (1) Seven or Malish, (2) Kenya and (3) Moroccan (which is apparently a unique isolate). In 2001, the genome of *R. conorii* strain Seven was fully sequenced, and revealed several unique characteristics among bacteria genomes.

Rickettsia conorii is transmitted by *R. sanguineus*, the brown dog tick. This bacterium does not normally infect humans during its natural cycle between its arthropod host and vertebrate one, the dog. *R. sanguineus* probably has the most widespread distribution of all *Ixodid* ticks. Despite this, its distribution is patchy in that it is confined to localities within urban, suburban, periurban and rural areas in which there are both domestic dogs and human dwellings or man-made structures. *R. sanguineus* lives in peridomestic environments shared with dogs, but has relatively low affinity for humans.

MSF is endemic in the Mediterranean area, including northern Africa and southern Europe. Cases continue to be identified in new locations within this region, as some cases were recently described in Turkey, Malta, Cyprus, Slovenia, Croatia, Greece and Bulgaria. In Italy, the national incidence rate is 1.6 cases per 100,000 persons; however, when considering the Sicilian region, this incidence is much higher (10 cases per 100,000 persons). MSF is a reportable disease in Portugal, where the annual incidence rate of 9.8 cases per 100,000 persons was highest of the rates of all Mediterranean countries in the 1990s. In Spain, estimated incidence was 23–45 cases per 100,000 persons in 1983–1985. Sporadic cases in nonendemic countries are also frequently observed as a consequence of tourism, and, in North America, MSF is one of the most frequently imported rickettsioses with African tick-bite fever. Some cases have been sporadically reported in northern and Central Europe, including Belgium, Switzerland and northern France, where *R. sanguineus* can be imported with dogs and survive in peridomestic environments providing there are acceptable microclimatic conditions.

After an asymptomatic incubation of 6 days, the onset of MSF is abrupt, and typical cases present with high fever (39°C), flu-like symptoms and a black eschar (tache noire) at the site of the tick bite. In a few cases, the inoculation occurred through conjunctivae, and patients presented with conjunctivitis. One to 7 days (median, 4 days) following the onset of fever, a generalized maculopapular rash that often involves the palms and soles, but spares the face, develops. However, severe forms, including major homological manifestations and multiorgan involvement may occur in 5–6% of the cases. The mortality rate is usually estimated as around 2.5% among diagnosed cases. Classic risk factors for severe forms include advanced age, immunocompromised situations, chronic alcoholism and glucose-6-phosphate dehydrogenase deficiency.

Rickettsia conorii *subsp.* israelensis *(Israeli Spotted Fever)*

The first case of rickettsia spotted fever in Israel was reported in the late 1940s [114]. In 1971, the agent of ISFR was isolated from a patient. Two other antigenically identical agents were isolated from *R. sanguineus* ticks collected on the dogs of 2 patients with serologically documented ISFR. These 3 isolates were rickettsiae closely related to, but slightly different from, *R. conorii* isolates obtained from patients with MSF. This observation has been confirmed by recent molecular studies [115].

Rickettsia conorii subsp. *israelensis* outside of Israel was isolated from 3 patients living in semirural areas along the River Tejo in Portugal in 1999. Recently, de Sousa et al. [116] reported the clinical data of 44 patients infected with *R. conorii* subsp. *israelensis* in Portugal between 1999 and 2004, and in ticks collected in Bragança, Montesinho Natural Park, and Portalegre City. Cases were confirmed by isolation of the *Rickettsia* from blood or a PCR on skin biopsy specimens. A clinical retrospective analysis in western Sicily, from 1987 to 2001, identified by molecular-sequence-based techniques 5 out 24 patients infected with *R. conorii* subsp. *israelensis*. Recently, *R. conorii* subsp. *israelensis* was detected in Sicilian *R. sanguineus* ticks [117]. The eschar at the inoculation site is absent in 90% of cases, whereas splenomegaly and hepatomegaly are seen in 30–35% of patients.

Rickettsia conorii *subsp.* caspia *(Astrakhan Fever)*

In Astrakhan, a region of Russia located by the Caspian Sea, where cases of febrile exanthema were observed in patients in rural areas during the 1970s, most of the patients had dogs and reported having contact with *R. sanguineus* dog ticks. The agent, a member of the *R. conorii* complex, was described in 1991, and the suspected vector of this eruptive summer disease is the dog tick *R. sanguineus pumilio* [118]. The name *R. conorii* ssp. *caspia* ssp. nov. has been proposed for the agent of Astrakhan spotted fever [115]. The disease seemed to be transmitted by *R. sanguineus*, with 8% of ticks shown to be infected by the hemolymph test.

Astrakhan fever was detected in 321 cases from prospective surveillance during 1983–1988; most patients were adults (94%), specifically males (61%). The disease was similar to MSF. During the summer of 2001, French United Nations troops in Kosovo collected ticks on asymptomatic soldiers and dogs in the Morina region. By molecular methods, *R. conorii* subsp. *caspia* was detected in four *R. sanguineus* organisms, comprising 3 collected on dogs and 1 taken from an asymptomatic soldier [112].

R. conorii subsp. *caspia* (Astrakhan fever) is a similar disease to MSF, including fever associated with a maculopapular rash in 94% of the cases. However, the presence of a tache noire was reported in only 23% of the patients. Conjunctivitis was seen in 32% of the cases. No fatal cases were reported.

Rickettsia sibirica *subsp.* mongolitimonae

In 1991, a rickettsia was isolated from *Hyalomma asiaticum* ticks collected in Inner Mongolia in China. The isolate HA-91 differed antigenically and genotypically from other SFG rickettsiae. In 1996, the first case of human infection with '*R. mongolitimonae*' was documented by culture and PCR, a genetically indistinguishable isolate was obtained from the blood and the skin of a 63-year-old patient in southern France. This patient was a resident of Marseille and had no travel history; however, the patient had collected compost from a garden where migratory birds were resting. A second human case of infection with *R. sibirica* subsp. *mongolitimonae* was diagnosed in 1998 in an HIV patient who had gardened in a rural area of Marseille. That is why the initial hypothesis was that the rickettsiae were transmitted by ticks occasionally carried by birds from Asia. The name *'Rickettsia mongolitimonae'* was then first proposed for this rickettsia, referring the disparate sources of the isolates (i.e. Mongolia and La Timone Hospital in Marseille). Using gene-sequence-based criteria to define *Rickettsia* species [118, 119], *R. mongolitimonae* was identified as a member of the *R. sibirica* species complex. Nevertheless, all strains of *R. mongolitimonae* group together in phylogenetic clusters separated from other strains of *R. sibirica*.

Specific vectors and reservoirs of *R. sibirica mongolitimonae* have yet to be described, particularly in southern France. It has been hypothesized that ticks from migratory birds may have bitten French patients. The detection of *R. sibirica mongolitimonae* in *Hyalomma* spp. in Mongolia and Niger suggests a possible association of this rickettsia with ticks of this genus that are also prevalent in southern France. More arguments for this hypothesis were provided recently, when 2 cases of *R. sibirica mongolitimonae* were documented in Crete, Greece. In 1 patient, this rickettsia was simultaneously detected on a *H. anatolicum excavatum* tick that had fed on him. Recently in Portugal, *R. sibirica mongolitimonae* has been identified in one *R. pusillus* tick collected on a dead Egyptian mongoose. It now seems that the distribution area of *R. sibirica mongolitimonae* coincides with or at least corresponds to the distribution of *Hyalomma* spp. ticks worldwide.

From January 2000 to June 2004, a total of 7 culture- or PCR-proven cases of infection due to *R. sibirica mongolitimonae* were documented in southern France, 1 of them having returned from a trip in northern Africa, suggesting that this disease is likely to be more widespread than originally expected. In 3 patients, the bacterium was cultivated from the inoculation eschar. The other 4 patients were diagnosed with use of PCR of samples obtained from the eschar (2 patients) or blood (2 patients), plus specific Western blotting before (2 patients) and after (2 patients) cross-adsorption [120]. On the basis of evaluation of these 9 cases, *R. sibirica mongolitimonae* infection differs from other tick-borne rickettsioses in the Mediterranean area. More recently, 1 case was documented in a patient returning to France after a trip to Algeria. She presented with fever and 2 inoculation eschars. She had been in contact with camels, which are highly parasitized by ticks. Another European case has been recently reported. An isolate was recovered in 2004 from a 73-year-old Portuguese woman who suffered from acute febrile illness with a maculopapular rash over the body. *R. sibirica* subsp. *mongolitimonae* infection was presented clinically by fever, headache, an eschar, lymphangitis and painful satellite lymphadenopathy.

Rickettsia slovaca *(The Agent of Tick-Borne Lymphadenopathy and Dermacentor-Borne Necrosis Erythema Lymphadenopathy)*

A novel SFG rickettsia was isolated in 1968 from *D. marginatus* ticks in Czechoslovakia [121]. Based on serological studies and C+G content, 2 strains were found to be close but not identical to *R. sibirica* and *R. conorii*. Thorough studies revealed that these strains differed from all prototype strains known at that time, and a new species of SFG rickettsia, *R. slovaca*, was proposed. Subsequently, it has been detected or isolated from ticks in all European countries where *D. marginatus* and *D. reticulatus* have been evaluated for rickettsiae.

R. slovaca is an example of a human-disease-causing rickettsia that was considered as a 'nonpathogenic rickettsia' for more than 20 years following its discovery. In 1997, the first documented case of human infection with *R. slovaca* was reported in a woman who presented with a single eschar of the scalp and enlarged cervical lymph nodes following the bite of *Dermacentor* sp. ticks in France [118]. Clinically similar but undocumented cases had been seen previously in France, Slovakia and Hungary. This rickettsiosis is called tick-borne lymphadenopathy because the most pronounced sign is lymph node enlargement. In Spain, the same condition is called *Dermacentor*-borne necrosis erythema lymphadenopathy (for tick-borne lymphadenopathy) [122]. From January 1996 through April 2000, the role of *R. slovaca* infection in this syndrome was evaluated in 67 patients from France and Hungary presenting with tick-borne lymphadenopathy. Infections were most likely to occur in children and in patients who were bitten during the colder months of the year. Cases have also been reported in Bulgaria and Spain. More recently, 14 new patients were reported with tick-borne lymphadenopathy from southern France, who sought treatment between January 2004 and May 2005, and the features of these patients were compared with those in whom MSF was diagnosed during the same period [122].

Rickettsia aeschlimannii

R. aeschlimannii was first isolated from *H. marginatum marginatum* ticks in Morocco in 1992, and then characterized as a new SFG rickettsia in 1997 [123]. The first human infection caused by *R. aeschlimannii* was reported in a patient returning from Morocco to France. This patient presented with typical clinical signs of spotted fever.

R. aeschlimannii was detected in *H. m. rufipes* in southern Europe and North and sub-Saharan Africa. In Europe, it has been recently identified in *H. m. marginatum* in Croatia, from 6 tick species in Spain, including *H. m. marginatum*, and from *H. m. marginatum* in Cephalonia, the largest Ionian island of Greece. This *Rickettsia* was recently isolated from *H. m. rufipes* collected on migratory birds coming from Africa and collected in Croatia. *R. aeschlimannii* was shown to be transstadially and transovarially transmitted in ticks, indicating that *Hyalomma* ticks may be not only vectors but also reservoirs of *R. aeschlimannii.*

The first cases of human infection by *R. aeschlimannii* were reported in 2002 in a patient who was returning to France from Morocco, and also a South African patient who, on returning from a hunting and fishing trip, discovered a *Rhipicephalus appendiculatus* tick attached to his right thigh and an eschar around the attachment site. The patient was aware of the risk of tick-transmitted disease; after removing the tick, he immediately self-prescribed doxycycline [124]. Other cases were described in Algeria (unpublished data). *R. aeschlimannii* was clinically presented by eschar fever and a maculopapular rash.

Rickettsia massiliae

R. massiliae was isolated from *Rhipicephalus* ticks collected near Marseille in 1992. In Europe, this rickettsia has been detected by molecular methods in *R. sanguineus* in Greece and *R. turanicus* in Portugal. In 1996, a variant strain of *R. massiliae (Bar 29)* was isolated in *R. sanguineus* ticks from Catalonia, Spain. The first documented human infection with *R. massiliae* occurred in 2005.

In Europe, this *Rickettsia* has also been detected by molecular methods in *R. sanguineus* in Greece and *R. turanicus* in Portugal. In 1996, a variant strain of *R. massiliae* (*Bar 29*) was isolated in an *R. sanguineus* tick from Catalonia and identified in ticks removed from humans in Castilla, Spain. The transstadial and transovarial transmission of *R. massiliae Bar 29* occurs in ticks of the *R. sanguineus* group, which may also be considered to be reservoirs [112]. *R. massiliae* was isolated in 1985 from the blood of a 45-year-old man hospitalized in Palermo, Italy, with fever, a necrotic eschar, a maculopapular rash involving the palms and soles, and mild hepatomegaly. Twenty years after, the isolate was recognized as *R. massiliae,* when human infection occurred in 2005 [112]. Thus, *R. massiliae* was described in 2 patients who clinically presented with fever, necrotic eschar, a maculopapular rash involving the palms and soles, and mild hepatomegaly.

Rickettsia helvetica

R. helvetica, first isolated in *I. ricinus* ticks in Switzerland in 1979, was considered a nonpathogenic rickettsia for approximately 20 years after its discovery. In 2000, seroconversion to *R. helvetica* was described for a French patient with a nonspecific febrile illness [125]. One patient from France and 3 patients from Italy were also diagnosed using serological criteria. All 4 reported tick bites and 1 developed an eschar [126]. In 1999, *R. helvetica* was implicated in fatal perimyocarditis in several patients in Sweden. Infection was documented by electron microscopy, PCR and serology [127]. In 2003, serological findings in patients with tick bites from Switzerland were suggestive of acute or past *R. helvetica* infection. Five cases of SFG rickettsiosis, possibly caused by *R. helvetica,* were reported in patients living at the central Thai-Myanmar border. Two patients reported a tick bite, 1 presented with an eschar and another patient presented with rash. Infection were documented by microimmunofluorescence and Western blot assays. Three more cases, in patients from eastern Thailand with undifferentiated febrile illness, were serologically documented. Additional evaluation and isolation of the bacterium from clinical samples are, however, needed to confirm the pathogenicity of *R. helvetica.*

The transstadial and transovarial transmission of *R. helvetica* has been demonstrated in *I. ricinus*; this tick represents both a potential vector and a natural reservoir of *R. helvetica*. This *Rickettsia* has been identified in *I. ricinus* ticks in many European countries, including France, Sweden, Slovenia, Spain, Portugal, Italy and Bulgaria where the average infection rate is approximately 10%.

Rickettsia raoultii
This *Rickettsia* has been known for a long time as a novel genotype identified in *Ixodid* ticks collected in Russia using amplification and sequencing of *rrs* (16S rDNA), *gltA*, and *ompA*. *Rickettsia* sp. provisionally called 'genotype DnS14', was initially detected from the *D. nuttalli* tick collected in Sibirica, whereas 'genotype RpA4' was detected from *R. pumilio* ticks from the Astrakhan region. Due to their phylogenetic homogeneity, it was suggested that *Rickettsia* sp. genotype DnS14 and RpA4 belonged to the same new species.

The pathogenicity of *R. raoultii* was suggested by the amplification of its DNA from the blood of patients with a clinical picture of *R. slovaca*-like infection.

Several years later, the isolates of this *Rickettsia* were obtained using cell culture from *D. silvarum* ticks collected in Far-Eastern Russia and Sibirica and *D. reticulatus* and *D. marginatus* ticks from France and Russia. A recent study demonstrated that *Dermacento*r ticks naturally infected with *R. raoultii*, and that transovarial and transstadial transmissions occurred [128].

Treatments

The treatment of rickettsioses is based around doxycycline. Currently, it is recommended for adults (200 mg/day) and children [112]. The putative risk of tooth staining has not been established for doxycycline, and the risk of the disease is sufficient to prescribe doxycycline in children. The duration of the treatment has not been established; however, studies have shown that single-day treatment is efficient. In any case, treatment prolonged for 24 h after the obtention of apyrexia has proved to be efficient. New macrolides have been proposed in children and chloramphenicol has been widely used in the past for the treatment of rickettsioses.

References

1 Centers for Disease Control: Lyme disease – United States, 1987 and 1988. MMWR Morb Mortal Wkly Rep 1989;38:668–672.

2 Spach DH, Liles WC, Campbell GL, et al: Tick-borne diseases in the US. N Engl J Med 1993;329: 936–947.

3 Myers SA, Sexton DJ: Dermatologic manifestations of arthropod-borne diseases. Infect Dis Clin North Am 1994;8:689–712.

4 Cary NRB, Fox B, Wright DJM, et al: Fatal Lyme carditis and endodermal heterotopia of the atrioventricular node. Postgrad Med J 1990;66:134–136.

5 Paddock CD, Sumner JW, Shore GM, et al: Isolation and characterization of *Ehrlichia chaffeensis* strains from patients with fatal ehrlichiosis. J Clin Microbiol 1997;10:2496–2502.

6 Hardalo CJ, Quagliarello V, Dumler JS: Human granulocytic ehrlichiosis in Connecticut: report of a fatal case. Clin Infect Dis 1995;4:910–914.
7 Kirsch M, Ruben FL, Steere AC, et al: Fatal adult respiratory distress syndrome in a patient with Lyme disease. JAMA 1988;259:2737–2739.
8 Berglund J, Eitrem R, Ornstein K, et al: An epidemiologic study of Lyme disease in southern Sweden. N Engl J Med 1995;333:1319–1327.
9 Sonenshine DE, Azad AF: Ticks and mites in disease transmission; in Strickland GT (ed): Hunter's Tropical Medicine, ed 7. Philadelphia, WB Saunders, 1991, pp 971–981.
10 Peavy CA, Lane RS, Kleinjan JE: Role of small mammals in the ecology of *B. burgdorferi* in a peri-urban park in north coastal California. Exp Appl Acarol 1997;21:569-584.
11 Fritz CL, Kjemtrup AM, Conrad PA, et al: Seroepidemiology of emerging tick-borne infectious diseases in a northern Californian community. J Infect Dis 1997;175:1432–1439.
12 Middleton DB: Tick-borne infections: what starts as a tiny bite may have a serious outcome. Postgrad Med J 1994;5:131–139.
13 Oksi J, Viljanen MK, Kalimo H, et al: Fatal encephalitis caused by concomitant infection with tick-borne encephalitis virus and *Borrelia burgdorferi*. Clin Infect Dis 1993;16:392–396.
14 Strle F, Maraspin V, Lotric-Furlan S, et al: Epidemiologic study of a cohort of adult patients with erythema migrans registered in Slovenia in 1993. Eur J Epidemiol 1996;5:503–507.
15 Santos AS, Bacellar F, Dumler JS: Human Exposure to *Anaplasma phagocytophilum* in Portugal. Ann NY Acad Sci 2006;1078:100–105.
16 Naranjo V, Ruiz-Fons F, Höfle U, Fernandez de Mera IG, Villanua D, Almazan C, et al: Molecular epidemiology of human and bovine anaplasmosis in southern Europe. Ann NY Acad Sci 2006;1078: 95–99.
17 Inokuma H: Vectors and reservoir hosts of Anaplasmataceae; in Raoult D, Parola P (eds): Rickettsial Diseases, ed 1. New York, Informa Healthcare, 2007.
18 Brouqui P, Matsumoto K: Bacteriology and phylogeny of Anaplasmataceae; in Raoult D, Parola P (eds): Rickettsial Diseases, ed 1. New York, Informa Healthcare, 2007.
19 Barlough JE, Madigan JE, Kramer VL, Clover JR, Hui LT, Vredevoe LK: *Ehrlichia phagocytophila* genogroup rickettsiae in ixodid ticks from California collected in 1995 and 1996. J Clin Microbiol 1997;35:2018–2021.
20 Dumler JS, Madigan JE, Pusterla N, Bakken JS: Ehrlichiosis in humans: epidemiology, clinical presentation, diagnosis, and treatment. Clin Infect Dis 2007;45:45–51.
21 Chen S, Dumler JS, Bakken JS, Walker DH: Identification of a granulocytotropic *Ehrlichia* species as the etiologic agent of human disease. J Clin Microbiol 1994;32:589–595.
22 Petrovec M, Lotric Furlan S, Avsic Zupanc T, Strle F, Brouqui P, Roux V, et al: Human disease in Europe caused by a granulocytic *Ehrlichia* species. J Clin Microbiol 1997;35:1556–1559.
23 Cinco M, Padovan D, Murgia R, Heldtander M, Engvall EO: Detection of HGE agent-like *Ehrlichia* in *Ixodes ricinus* ticks in northern Italy by PCR. Wien Klin Wochenschr 1998;110:898–900.
24 Nuti M, Serafini DA, Bassetti D, Ghionni A, Russino F, Rombola P, et al: *Ehrlichia* infection in Italy. Emerg Infect Dis 1998;4:663–665.
25 Blanco JR, Oteo JA: Human granulocytic ehrlichiosis in Europe. Clin Microbiol Infect 2002;8:763–772.
26 Arnez M, Petrovec M, Lotric-Furlan S, Zupanc AT, Strle F: First European pediatric case of human granulocytic ehrlichiosis. J Clin Microbiol 2001;39: 4591–4592.
27 Lotric-Furlan S, Petrovec M, Zupanc T, Nicholson W, Summer J, Childs J, et al: Human granulocytic ehrlichiosis in Europe: clinical and laboratory findings for four patients from Slovenia. Clin Infect Dis 1998;27:424–428.
28 van Dobbenburgh A, van Dam AP, Fikrig E: Human granulocytic ehrlichiosis in western Europe. New Engl J Med 1999;340:1214–1216.
29 Oteo JA, Blanco JR, Martinez de Artola V: First report of human granulocytic ehrlichiosis from southern Europe (Spain). Emerg Infect Dis 2000;6: 430–432.
30 Bjoersdorff A, Wittesjö B, Berglund J, Massung RF, Eliasson I: Human granulocytic ehrlichiosis as a common cause of tick-associated fever in southeast Sweden: report from a prospective clinical study. Scand J Infect Dis 2002;34:187–191.
31 Misic-Majerus LJ, Bujic N, Madjaric V, Janes-Poje V: First description of the human granulocytic ehrlichiosis in Croatia. Clin Microbiol Infect 2000;25: 194–195.
32 Tylewska-Wierzbanowska S, Chmielewski T, Kondrusik M, Hermanowska-Szpakowicz T, Sawiki W, Sulek K: First cases of acute human granulocytic ehrlichiosis in Poland. Eur J Clin Microbiol 2001; 20:196–198.
33 Remy V, Hansmann Y, De Martino S, Christmann D, Brouqui P: Human anaplasmosis presenting as atypical pneumonitis in France. Clin Infect Dis 2003;37:846–848.
34 Olano JP, Walker DH: Human ehrlichioses. Med Clin North Am 2002;86:375–392.
35 Bakken JS, Dumler JS: Human granulocytic ehrlichiosis. Clin Infect Dis 2000;31:554–560.

36 Parola P, Davoust B, Raoult D: Tick- and flea-borne rickettsial emerging zoonoses. Vet Res 2005;36: 469–492.
37 Rikihisa Y, Stills H, Zimmerman G: Isolation and continuous culture of *Neorickettsia helminthoeca* in a macrophage cell line. J Clin Microbiol 1991;29: 1928–1933.
38 Bakken JS, Dumler JS: Clinical diagnosis and treatment of human granulotropic anaplasmosis. Ann NY Acad Sci 2006;1078:236–247.
39 Horowitz HW, Aguero-Rosenfeld ME, Mckenna DF, Holmgren D, Hsieh TC, Varde SA, et al: Clinical and laboratory spectrum of culture-proven human granulocytic ehrlichiosis: comparison with culture-negative cases. Clin Infect Dis 1998;27: 1314–1317.
40 Doyle CK, Labruna MB, Breitschwerdt EB, Tang YW, Corstvet RE, Hegarty BC, et al: Detection of medically important *Ehrlichia* by quantitative multicolor TaqMan real-time polymerase chain reaction of the *dsb* gene. J Mol Diagn 2005;7:504–510.
41 Bakken JS, Dumler JS: *Ehrlichia* and *Anaplasma* species; in Yu V, Weber R, Raoult D (eds): Antimicrobial Therapy and Vaccines, ed 2. New York, Apple Trees Productions, 2002.
42 Maurin M, Bakken JS, Dumler JS: Antibiotic susceptibilities of *Anaplasma* (*Ehrlichia*) *phagocytophilum* strains from various geographic areas in the United States. Antimicrob Agents Chemother 2003; 47:413–415.
43 Van Dam AP, van Gool T, Weststeyn JCFM, Dankert J: Tick-borne relapsing fever imported from West Africa: diagnosis by quantitative buffy coat analysis and in vitro culture of *Borrelia crocidurae*. J Clin Microbiol 1999;37:2027–2030.
44 Lecompte Y, Trape JF: La fièvre récurrente à tique d'Afrique de l'ouest. Ann Biol Clin (Paris) 2003;61: 541–548.
45 Brouqui P, Raoult D: Arthropod-borne diseases in homeless. Ann NY Acad Sci 2006;1078:223–235.
46 Rebaudet S, Parola P: Epidemiology of relapsing fever borreliosis. FEMS Immunol Med Microbiol 2006;48:11–15.
47 Cutler SJ, Browning P, Scott JC: *Ornithodoros moubata*, a soft tick vector for *Rickettsia* in east Africa? Ann NY Acad Sci 2006;1078:373–377.
48 Parola P, Raoult D: Ticks and tickborne bacterial diseases in humans: an emerging infectious threat. Clin Infect Dis 2001;32:897–928.
49 Vial L, Diatta G, Tall A, et al: Incidence of tick-borne relapsing fever in West Africa: longitudinal study. Lancet 2006;368:37–43.
50 Estrada-Pena A, Jongejan F: Ticks feeding on humans: a review of records on human-biting Ixodoidea with special reference to pathogen transmission. Exp Appl Acarol 1999;23:685–715.
51 Wplosz B, Mihaila-Amrouche L, Baixenh MT, et al: Imported tick-borne relapsing fever, France. Emerg Infect Dis 2005;11:1801–1803.
52 Felsenfeld O: Borreliae, human relapsing fever, and parasite-vector-host relationships. Bacteriol Rev 1965;29:46–74.
53 Anda P, Sanchez-Yebra W, del Mar Vitutia M, et al: A new *Borrelia* species isolated from patients with relapsing fever in Spain. Lancet 1996;348:162–165.
54 Cutler SJ: Possibilities for relapsing fever re-emergence. Emerg Infect Dis 2006;12:369–374.
55 Johnson WD: *Borrelia* species (relapsing fever); in Mandell GL, Bennett JE, Dolin R (eds): Principles and Practice of Infectious Diseases, ed 4. New York, Churchill Livingstone, 1995, pp 1816–1819.
56 Johnson WD, Golightly LM: *Borrelia* species (relapsing fever); in Mandell GL, Bennett JE, Dolin R (eds): Mandell, Douglas, and Bennett's Principles and Practice of Infectious Diseases, ed 5. New York, Churchill Livingstone, 2000.
57 Dupont HT, La Scola B, Williams R, Raoult D: A focus of tick-borne relapsing fever in Southern Zaire. Clin Infect Dis 1997;25:139–144.
58 Bratton RL, Corey GR: Tick-borne disease. Am Family Physician 2005:72:2323–2330.
59 Cutler SJ, Akintunde COK, Moss J, et al: Successful in vitro cultivation of *Borrelia duttonii* and its comparison with *Borrelia recurrentis*. Int J Syst Bacteriol 1999;49:1793–1799.
60 Cutler SJ, Fekade D, Hussein K, et al: Successful in-vitro cultivation of *Borrelia recurrentis*. Lancet 1994;343:242.
61 Marti Ras N, La Scola B, Postic D, et al: Phylogenesis of relapsing fever *Borrelia* spp. Int J Syst Bact 1996;46:859–865.
62 Cadavid D, Barbour AG: Neuroborreliosis during relapsing fever: review of the clinical manifestations, pathology, and treatment of infections in humans and experimental animals. Clin Infect Dis 1998;26:151–164.
63 Müller W, Bocklish H, Schüler G, Hotzel H, Neubauer H, Otto P: Detection of *Francisella tularensis* subsp. *holarctica* in a European brown hare (*Lepus europaeus*) in Thuringia, Germany. Vet Microbiol 2007;123:225–229.
64 Jiang J, Parker CE, Fuller JR, Kawula TH, Borchers CH: An immunoaffinity tandem mass spectrometry (iMALDI) assay for detection of *Francisella*. Anal Chim Acta 2007;605:70–79.
65 Chaudhui RR, Reu CP, Desmond L, et al: Genome sequencing shows that European isotopes of *Francisella tularensis subspecies tularensis* are almost identical to US laboratory strain Schu S4. PloS ONE 2007;2:e352.
66 Gurycova D: First isolation of *Francisella tularensis* subsp. *tularensis* in Europe. Eur J Epidemiol 1998; 14:797–802.

67 Eliasson H, Lindbäck J, Nuorti J, Arneborn M, Giesecke J, Tegnell A: The 2000 tularemia outbreak: a case-control study of risk factors in disease-endemic and emergent areas, Sweden. Emerg Infect Dis 2002;8:956–960.
68 Reintjes R, Dedushaj I, Gjini A, et al: Tularemia outbreak investigation in Kosovo: case control and environmental studies. Emerg Infect Dis 2002;8:969–973.
69 Johansson A, Forsman M, Sjöstedt A: The development of tools for diagnosis of tularemia and typing of *Francisella tularensis*. APMIS 2004;112:898–907.
70 De Cavalho IL, Escudero R, Garcia-Amil C, Falcao H, Anda P, Nuncio MS: *Francisella tularensis*, Portugal. Emerg Infect Dis 2007;13:666–667.
71 Bratton RL, Corey GR: Tick-borne disease. Am Fam Phys 2005;71:2323–2330.
72 Dennis DT, Inglesby TV, Henderson DA, et al: Tularemia as a biological weapon: medical and Public Health Management. JAMA 2001;285:2763–2773.
73 Evans M, Gregory D, Schaffner W, McGee ZA: Tularemia: a 30-year experience with 88 cases. Medicine (Baltimore) 1985;64:251–269.
74 Bossi P, Tegnell A, Baka A, et al: Bichat guidelines for the clinical management of tularaemia and bioterrorism-related tularaemia. Euro Surveill 2004;9: E9–E10.
75 Miller RP, Bates JH: Pleuropulmonary tularemia: a review of 29 patients. Am Rev Respir Dis 1969;99: 31–41.
76 Rubin SA: Radiographic spectrum of pleuropulmonary tularemia. AJR Am J Roentgenol 1978;131: 277–281.
77 Forsman M, Kuoppa K, Sjöstedt A, Tärnvik A: Use of RNA hybridization in the diagnosis of a case of ulceroglandular tularemia. Eur J Clin Microbiol Infect Dis 1990;9:784–785.
78 Ellis J, Oyston PC, Green M, Titball RW: Tularemia. Clin Microbiol Rev 2002;15:631–646.
79 Beers MH, Berkow R: The Merck Manual of Diagnosis and Therapy, ed 17. Whitehouse Station, Merck Research Laboratories, 1999.
80 Rizzoli A, Rosa R, Mantelli B, et al: *Ixodes ricinus*, transmitted diseases and reservoirs (in Italian). Parassitologia 2004;46:119–122.
81 Kaiser R: The clinical and epidemiological profile of tick-borne encephalitis in southern Germany 1994–1998: a prospective study of 656 patients. Brain 1999;122:2067–2078.
82 Kaiser R, Kern A, Kampa D, Neumannhaefelin D: Prevalence of antibodies to *Borrelia burgdorferi* and tick-borne encephalitis virus in an endemic region in southern Germany. Zentralbl Bakteriol 1997;286:534–541.
83 Pugliesse A, Beltramo T, Torre D: Seroprevalence study of tick-borne encephalitis, *Borrelia burgdorferi*, dengue and Toscana virus in Turin province. Cell Biochem Funct 2007;25:185–188.
84 Skarphedinsson S, Jensen PM, Kristiansen K: Survey of tick-borne infections in Denmark. Emerg Infect Dis 2005;11:1055–1061.
85 Haglund M, Vene S, Forsgren M, et al: Characterization of human tick-borne encephalitis virus from Sweden. J Med Virol 2003;71:610–621.
86 Jaussaud R, Magy N, Strady A, Dupond JL, Deville JF: Tick-borne encephalitis. Rev Med Interne 2001; 22:542–548.
87 Charrel RN, Attoui H, Butenko AM, et al: Tick-borne virus diseases of human interest in Europe. Clin Microbiol Infect 2004;10:1040–1055.
88 Kondrusik M, Biedzinska T, Pancewicz S, et al: Tick-borne encephalitis (TBE) cases in Bialostocki and Podlaski regions in years 1993–2002. Przegl Epidemiol 2004;58:273–280.
89 Gritsun TS, Nuttall PA, Gould EA: Tick-borne flaviviruses. Adv Virus Res 2003;61:317–371.
90 Ackermann R, Krüger K, Roggendorf M, et al: Spread of early summer meningoencephalitis in the Federal Republic of Germany. Dtsch Med Wochenschr 1986;111:927–933.
91 Kaiser R: Tick-borne encephalitis (TBE) in Germany and clinical course of the disease. Int J Med Microbiol 2002;291(suppl 33):58–61.
92 Seligman SJ, Gould EA: Life flavivirus vaccines: reasons for caution. Lancet 2004;363:2073–2075.
93 Pugliesse A, Beltramo T, Torre D: Emerging and re-emerging viral infections in Europe. Cell Biochem Funct 2007;25:1–13.
94 Sambri V, Marangoni A, Storni E, et al: Tick-borne zoonosis: selected clinical and diagnostic aspects. Parassitologia 2004;46:109–113.
95 Holbrook MR, Shope RE, Barrett ADT: Use of recombinant E protein domain III-based enzyme-linked immunosorbent assays for differentiation of tick-borne encephalitis serocomplex flaviviruses from mosquito-borne flaviviruses. J Clin Microbiol 2004;42:4101–4110.
96 Schwaiger M, Cassinotti P: Development of a quantitative real-time RT-PCR assay with internal control for the laboratory detection of tick-borne encephalitis virus (TBEV) RNA. J Clin Virol 2003; 27:136–145.
97 Kunz C: TBE vaccination and the Austrian experience. Vaccine 2003;21:S50–S55.
98 Gefland JA: Babesia; in Mandell GL, Bennett JE, Dolin R (eds): Principles and Practice of Infectious Diseases, ed 4. New York, Churchill Livingstone, 1995, pp 2497–2499.
99 Boustani MR, Gelfand JA: Babesiosis. Clin Infect Dis 1996;22:611–615.
100 Pruthi RK, Marshall WF, Wiltsie JC, Persing DH: Human babesiosis. Mayo Clin Proc 1995;70:853–862.
101 Skrabalo Z, Deanovic Z: Piroplasmosis in man. Doc Med Geogr Trop 1957;9:11–16.

102 Gorenflot AK, Moubri AK, Precigout E, Carcy B, Schetters TP: Human babesiosis. Ann Trop Med Parasit 1998;92:489–500.

103 Denes E, Rogez JP, Dardé ML, Weinbreack P: Management of *Babesia divergens* babesiosis without a complete course of quinine treatment. Eur J Clin Microbiol Infect Dis 1999;18:672–673.

104 Spach DH, Liles W, Campbell G, Quick R, Anderson D, Fritsche T: Tick-borne diseases in the United States. N Engl J Med 1993;329:936–947.

105 Ruebush TK, Cassaday PB, Marsh HJ, et al: Human babesiosis on Nantucket Island: clinical features. Ann Intern Med 1977;86:6–9.

106 Etkind P, Piesman J, Ruebush TK 2nd, Spielman A, Juranek DD: Methods for detecting *Babesia microti* infection in wild rodents. J Parasitol 1980;66: 107–110.

107 Telford SR 3rd, Spielman A: Babesiosis of humans; in Collier L, Balows A, Sussman M, Kreier JP (eds): Topley and Wilson's Microbiology and Microbial Infections, ed 9. London, Edward Arnold, 1997.

108 Persing DH, Mathiesen D, Marshall WF, et al: Detection of *Babesia microti* by polymerase chain reaction. J Clin Microbiol 1992;30:2097–2103.

109 Homer MJ, Aguilar-Delfin I, Telford SR 3rd, Kranse PJ, Persing DH: Babesiosis. Clin Microbiol Rev 2000;13:451–469.

110 Lodes MJ, Houghton RL, Bruinsma ES, et al: Serological expression cloning of novel immunoreactive antigens of *Babesia microti*. Infect Immun 2000;68:2783–2790.

111 Chauvin A, L'Hotis M, Valentin A, et al: *Babesia divergens*: an ELISA with soluble parasite antigen for monitoring the epidemiology of bovine babesiosis. Parasite 1995;2:257–262.

112 Parola P, Paddock CD, Raoult D: Tick-borne rickettsioses around the world: emerging diseases challenging old concepts. Clin Microbiol Rev 2005;18:719–756.

113 Brouqui P, Matsumoto K: Bacteriology and phylogeny of Anaplasmataceae; in Raoult D, Parola P (eds): Rickettsial Diseases, ed 1. New York, Informa Healthcare, 2007.

114 Valero A: Rocky Mountain spotted fever in Palestine. Harefuah 1949;36:99–101.

115 Zhu Y, Fournier PE, Eremeeva M, Raoult D: Proposal to create subspecies of *Rickettsia conorii* based on multi-locus sequence typing and an emended description of *Rickettsia conorii*. BMC Microbiol 2005;5:11.

116 de Sousa R, Santos-Silva M, Santos AS, et al: *Rickettsia conorii* Israeli tick typhus strain isolated from *Rhipicephalus sanguineus* ticks in Portugal. Vector Borne Zoonotic Dis 2007;7:444–447.

117 Giammanco GM, Vitale G, Mansueto S, Capra G, Caleca MP, Ammatuna P: Presence of *R. conorii* subsp. *israelensis*, the causative agent of Israeli spotted fever, in Sicily, Italy, ascertained in a retrospective study. J Clin Microbiol 2005;43:6027–6031.

118 Raoult D, Roux V: Rickettsioses as paradigms of new or emerging infectious diseases. Clin Microbiol Rev 1997;10:694–719.

119 Fournier PE, Dumler JS, Greub G, Zhang JZ, Wu YM, Raoult D: Gene sequence-based criteria for identification of new *Rickettsia* isolates and description of *Rickettsia heilongjiangensis* sp. nov. J Clin Microbiol 2003;41:5456–5465.

120 Fournier PE, Gouriet F, Brouqui P, Lucht F, Raoult D: Lymphangitis-associated rickettsiosis, a new rickettsiosis caused by *Rickettsia sibirica mongolotimonae*: seven new cases and review of the literature. Clin Infect Dis 2005;40:1435–1444.

121 Rehacek J: *Rickettsia slovaca*, the organism and its ecology. Acta Sci Nat Brno 1984;18:1–50.

122 Gouriet F, Rolain JM, Raoult D: Rickettsia slovaca infection, France. Emerg Infect Dis 2006;12:521–523.

123 Beati L, Meskini M, Thiers B, Raoult D: *Rickettsia aeschlimannii* sp. nov., a new spotted fever group rickettsia associated with *Hyalomma marginatum* ticks. Int J Syst Bacteriol 1997;47:548–554.

124 Pretorius AM, Birtles RJ: *Rickettsia aeschlimannii*: a new pathogenetic spotted fever group Rickettsia, South Africa. Emerg Infect Dis 2002;8:874.

125 Fournier PE, Gunnenberger F, Jaulhac B, Gastinger G, Raoult D: Evidence of *Rickettsia helvetica* infection in humans, Eastern France. Emerg Infect Dis 2000;6:389–392.

126 Fournier PE, Allombert C, Supputamongkol Y, Caruso G, Brouqui P, Raoult D: Aneruptive fever associated with antibodies to *Rickettsia helvetica* in Europe and Thailand. J Clin Microbiol 2004;42: 816–818.

127 Nilsson K, Lindquist O, Pahlson C: Association of *Rickettsia helvetica* with chronic perimyocarditis in sudden cardiac death. Lancet 1999;354:1169–1173.

128 Mediannikov O, Parola P, Raoult D: Other tick-borne rickettsioses; in Raoult D, Parola P (eds): Rickettsial Diseases. New York, Informa Healthcare, 2007, pp 139–162.

Didier Raoult
Unité des Rickettsies CNRS-IRD UMR 6236
Faculté de Médecine, Université de la Méditerranée
27, Bd Jean Moulin, FR–13385 Marseille Cedex 5 (France)
Tel. +33 4 91 32 43 75, Fax +33 4 91 38 77 72, E-Mail didier.raoult@gmail.com

Lipsker D, Jaulhac B (eds): Lyme Borreliosis.
Curr Probl Dermatol. Basel, Karger, 2009, vol 37, pp 155–166

What Should One Do in Case of a Tick Bite?

Elisabeth Aberer

Department of Dermatology, Medical University of Graz, Graz, Austria

Abstract

Ixodes ricinus is the commonest tick species in Europe, and transmits Lyme borreliosis, tick-borne encephalitis, ehrlichiosis, tularemia, rickettsiosis, and babesiosis. The risk of *Borrelia burgdorferi* infection increases with the time of tick engorgement, but not every infection necessarily causes erythema migrans or Lyme borreliosis. Therefore, the finding of *B. burgdorferi* DNA in a tick does not prove that the patient will subsequently develop Lyme borreliosis. Ticks should be removed as early as possible with fine tweezers, taking the tick's head with the forceps. Antibiotic prophylactic therapy after a tick bite is not generally recommended. Tick bites can potentially be prevented by covering the body as much as possible or by applying repellents to the body and permethrin to clothes. Tick bite areas should be inspected for 1 month. *Lyme borreliosis* should be suspected when an erythema at the tick bite site or a febrile illness develop.

Tick Vectors in Europe

More than 800 tick species have been reported worldwide, although only about 30 ticks feed on humans; among these is *Ixodes ricinus,* which is the commonest tick species in most European countries [1]. Besides *I. ricinus, I. persulcatus* was reported in the eastern part of Latvia [2]. Other ticks that feed on humans have also been reported, e.g. in Spain: besides *I. ricinus* (12.4%), *Dermacentor marginatus* (55.7%) and *Rhipicephalus bursa* (11.9%) [3]; in Slovakia, *D. marginatus* and *D. reticulatus* [4]; and in Hungary, *Dermacentor* spp. [5]. More than 300 animal species have been reported as natural hosts for *I. ricinus,* and 50 vertebrate species have been identified as reservoir hosts for *Borrelia burgdorferi.* The tick density in some areas can be about 300 ticks/100 m^2 [1]. In a forestry area in England, the average density of nymphs collected from the vegetation was 14.1/10 m^2. Children have tick bites on the head, neck and axillary region much more frequently than adults (48 vs. 10%), whereas adults are more often bitten on the lower legs [6].

Diseases Transmitted by Ticks

The spectrum of transmitted diseases comprises infections by the tick-borne encephalitis (TBE) virus, *B. burgdorferi* [7], *Francisella tularensis* [8], and *Ehrlichia (Anaplasma) phagocytophilum* [9]. Furthermore, 85.1% of *D. marginatus* ticks in Spain were *Rickettsia*-infected; 26.7% of positives were infected by *Rickettsia slovaca*, the causative agent of tick-borne lymphadenopathy [10]. Lakos [5] described tick-borne lymphadenopathy in 86 patients following tick bites caused by *R. slovaca* in Hungary.

The reported data show that the risk of tick bites depends on the geographic area, climatic factors, temperature and humidity, gender [11], the investigation method, and the infected vectors or samples (ticks, tissue of reservoir animals or their sera, human sera, or record of diseases). Thus, different rates of infections have been identified by different researchers in various countries [2, 12]. On the outskirts of Berlin, Germany, 47% of investigated *I. ricinus* nymphs showed microbial pathogenic DNA. *B. afzelii* was the commonest pathogen, followed by *Rickettsia helvetica* [13]. In northwest Poland, 1,414 *I. ricinus* ticks were investigated by PCR, and 8.9% were found to be infected with *B. burgdorferi* s.l; *B. burgdorferi* s.s. was most prevalent (96%), followed by *B. garinii* (1.3%) [14]. In altitudes between 789 m and 1,350 m in Styria, Austria, the overall positivity rate for *B. burgdorferi* in ticks was 10.9%, as investigated by dark-field microscopy, culture and by real-time PCR. Ten specimens yielded *B. afzelii* and 5 showed *B. garinii* by culture or PCR [15]. In the area around Bonn, western Germany, 17.9% of 1,394 investigated ticks were infected with *B. burgdorferi* [16]. Using genospecies-specific oligonucleotide probes, *Borrelia* infections could be assigned to *B. afzelii* in 39.5% of ticks, *B. garinii* in 27.9 %, *B. burgdorferi* s.s. in 15.7%, and *B. valaisiana* in 8.6% by DNA hybridization. In a forested area in England, infection rates were 5.2–17.0%, determined by PCR and immunofluorescence, and the genospecies *B. valaisiana* and *B. garinii* were detected [6].

Risk of Tick Bites

In southeastern Sweden, patient records focusing on exposure to tick bites, epidemiology, gender, and the clinical picture of Lyme borreliosis (LB) were analyzed retrospectively and prospectively. Women aged 40 years and older had a 48% higher risk of attracting tick bites than men of the same age group. The annual incidence rate of erythema migrans (EM) in women was 506 and in men 423 cases per 100,000 inhabitants [17]. In a study from the Aland Islands, the incidence of tick bites, with possible implications concerning the spread of LB, was recorded from 519 individuals [18]: 441 persons (85%) had been bitten by ticks, 146 of these more than 10 times. Fourteen persons had EM, and 73 had other rashes around the tick bite. In The Netherlands, all general practitioners were asked to record the number of cases of tick bites and EM in 2001 [19]. They reported seeing approximately 61,000 patients with tick bites and 12,000 patients with EM in 1 year. So, the incidence of EM was estimated at 73 cases per 100,000 habitants. The number of patients with tick bites and EM had doubled between 1994 and 2001.

B. burgdorferi – *Seropositivity in Healthy Individuals*

The seroprevalence of antibodies to *B. burgdorferi* was investigated in blood samples of 4,368 forestry workers in southwestern Germany, and ranged from 18 to 52%. Antibodies to the TBE virus were present in 0–42%, and antibodies for *Ehrlichia* spp. in 5–16% [20]. In France, 15.2% of forestry workers were seropositive for antibodies to *B. burgdorferi* [21], and 70% of them reported tick bites. No active LB was reported; thus, asymptomatic infections are predominant.

The prevalence of antibodies to *B. burgdorferi* was investigated in hunters in Burgenland, a part of eastern Austria. Blood samples of 1,214 men and 39 women were tested, and their history of tick bites was obtained by questionnaire [22]. A total of 673 (54%) sera tested positive for IgG antibodies (55% of men and 26% of women). Seropositivity was 33% among persons younger than 29 years, and 83% in those older than 70 years. The increase in seroprevalence with age and duration of hunting reflects repeated tick exposure. The seroprevalence of *B. burgdorferi* and *A. phagocytophilum* was also investigated in workers in 4 Italian regions. From a total of 712 serum samples, 387 were from workers at risk of tick bites and 325 were from individuals not considered at risk (the control group) [23]. Antibodies to *B. burgdorferi* were found in 7.5% of subjects at risk and 1.2% of the control group. Antibodies to both *B. burgdorferi* and *A. phagocytophilum* were detected in 1.6%. The prevalence of antibodies to *B. burgdorferi* was investigated in blood donors in southern Germany [24], and found to be 5.5% (hemagglutination test). The results were confirmed by immunoblotting, showing 2.7% with *B. burgdorferi*-specific antibodies. No seroconversion was observed in the recipients of blood transfusions.

Transmission of LB by Ticks

Epidemiology: Probability of Transmission

In most of Europe, the transmission risk of LB after a tick bite is low to moderate within the first 24 h of feeding, but increases to >70% after only 36 h [25]. Since the exact time of tick attachment cannot always be given, a scutal index can be determined (the ratio between tick abdominal length and scutum width) as a good measure of the level of tick engorgement; in 85–93% of people, this gives a good indication of the time of attachment.

The time of feeding and method of tick removal, potentially crucial for *B. burgdorferi* transmission, was studied in gerbils by Kahl et al. [26]. All gerbils with ticks removed after more than 47 h were infected. After 16.7 and 28.9 h of tick feeding, approximately 50% of gerbils were infected. Ticks were pulled out with forceps, or after 3 min of intensive squeezing, or after applying nail polish to the ticks 1.1 h before removal. The tick removal method had no significant effect on *B. burgdorferi* infection. The time of attachment was also studied in relation to the engorgement index [27]. Between 0 and 24 h of attachment, no detectable change was seen; only after 24 h, all engorgement indices continuously increased. So, the inspection of ticks is helpful in indicating the time of engorgement, and thus the probability of infection.

In a study in southwestern Germany, ticks were collected from 730 patients and examined by PCR for *B. burgdorferi* [28]. Patients were clinically and serologically examined after tick removal. Eighty-four ticks (11.3%) were PCR positive, and a total transmission rate of 2.6% (19 patients) was observed. The authors recommend examination of ticks, and antibiotic prophylaxis in cases of positivity.

Heininger et al. [29] reported that every fifth tick is infected. Transmission does not occur with every bite, and infection does not always lead to disease. Therefore, the risk of infection after tick bite was investigated in the area of Erlangen, Germany. In 69 patients, initially seronegative, seroconversion was detected in 4 instances, 2 of whom were asymptomatic, 1 had unspecific symptoms and 1 lymphocytoma. The conclusion was that antibiotic treatment after a tick bite cannot be recommended.

Antibodies to *B. burgdorferi* were investigated in a population living in an endemic area in Sweden, and detected in 25.7% of people [30]. Subjects were tested over a 2-year period. In the first year, 4.6% developed LB, and in the second year 3.2%. An earlier episode of LB or an elevated antibody titer did not seem to protect subjects from reinfections.

In New York State, *B. burgdorferi* was cultured from skin biopsies at tick bite sites in 2/48 samples with tick attachment for 24 h [31]. In a Polish study of 131 residents who had suffered from Lyme disease in the past, arthritis sufferers recorded a significantly higher frequency of tick bites and significantly reduced EM [32]. The authors concluded that multiple exposures to *B. burgdorferi* promote manifestation of the disease in the form of arthritis and less frequently result in EM.

Risk of EM or Other Symptoms of LB

To evaluate the risk of LB after a tick bite in Switzerland, paired serum samples of people who had been bitten very recently were investigated for seroconversion. Seroconversion was observed in 4.5% of the 376 subjects [33], which can be broken down into 3.4% of 266 patients without clinical manifestations and 7.2% of 110 patients with a local skin reaction. EM developed in 3 subjects who seroconverted and 5 subjects without seroconversion. Ticks from 160 patients were available. *Borrelia* detection in ticks did not correlate significantly with the risk of LB.

In a prospective study, patients with a tick-borne febrile illness within 6 weeks after the tick bite were analyzed [7]. Cases of TBE in 27%, LB in 7.7%, *Ehrlichia* infection in 3.1%, and infection by multiple organisms in 14.6% were identified. In another Slovenian study on 86 febrile children with a history of a tick bite within 6 weeks previously, tick-borne illness was diagnosed in 53% [34]. The most common diagnosis was TBE in 64%, followed by LB in 46%, of acute and convalescent serum samples. In 21%, there was evidence of infection with more than 1 tick-borne agent. In Poland, paired sera of 68 patients who had fever 4 weeks after tick bite were investigated. TBE was detected in 49 patients, this was concurrent in 3 patients with EM or LB, in 5 patients with possible LB, and in 2 patients with *A. phagocytophilum* infection; a further 16 patients had LB [35]. In Switzerland, 75 patients with fever within 3 weeks of a tick bite were studied [36]. Tick-borne infections were confirmed or possible in 48% of the cases; 9% had EM and 8% other specific manifestations of LB, 8% LB presenting as a nonspecific febrile illness, 11% TBE, and 10% granulocytic ehrlichiosis.

Local Reactions after Tick Bites

Nonspecific local skin reactions and itching frequently occur after a tick bite. Red macules and papules usually disappear within 1 week. In the USA, a case definition for EM specifies that the erythema should have a size of at least 5 cm for a diagnosis of acute LB [37]. In Europe, the lesions of EM can be smaller according to the definition of the European Union Concerted Action on LB [38]. In cases of erythema after a tick bite persisting for more than 1 week, a 'mini'-EM should be suspected and antibiotic treatment should be considered [37]. A definite diagnosis of a *Borrelia* infection in this case can only be proven by *Borrelia* culture or positive PCR for *B. burgdorferi* DNA. A persistent atypical lymphocytic proliferation was noted on a tick bite area of a 6-year-old girl that lasted for more than 1 year [39].

In another report, 15 skin biopsies of tick bite areas were investigated histopathologically [40]. The capillaries and postcapillary venules of the superficial and deep vascular plexus adherent to the attachment site were filled with thrombi potentially related to secretory products of the tick's saliva during inoculation.

The inserted hypostome of an *I. scapularis* female adult was investigated by electron microscopy [41]. A homogenous cement-like substance was observed under scanning electron microscopy on the dorsal hypostome, which continued into the dermis. After tick removal, no tick parts were seen in the patient's skin with a magnifying glass. Scanning microscopy of the removed tick hypostome showed some chipped and missing denticles. Two months later, the skin area which the tick had been attached to was investigated, and showed a perivascular und periadnexal infiltrate consisting of plasma cells and lymphocytes with some foreign body cells containing yellowish-brown particles.

Hypersensitivity was observed in 2 forest workers who had skin reactions following tick bites. Both patients had specific IgE antibodies to wood ticks, and 1 patient had immediate positive reactions to a skin prick test and an intradermal test [42].

Removal of Ticks

Handling of Patients after Tick Bite

Several tick removal methods have been tested, but none using controlled prospective studies. Ticks are best removed as soon as possible because the risk of disease transmission increases significantly after 24 h of attachment [43]. Stressed ticks have been suspected to salivate or regurgitate into the host.

In over 40 reports, the application of various chemical and physical methods, including petrolatum jelly, isopropyl alcohol, nail polish, hot matches, Vaseline, olive oil, vinegar, gasoline, and adhesive tape, have been recommended to aid tick removal [44]. The chemical treatments failed to induce self-detachment of the ticks within 30 min [43]; while the occlusive techniques may guarantee the removal of an intact tick, they unnecessarily extend the duration of attachment and are therefore redundant [44, 45].

The crushing of ticks during forceps extraction has been thought to increase the risk of transmission of tick-borne infections. Two methods of mechanical removal of the ticks were compared: (1) pulling them straight out with a blunt forceps, and (2) rotation of the tick around its body axis [46]. Pulling frequently resulted in the complete removal of the tick, but quite often large fragments of the mouthparts remained in the skin. When removing the tick with rotation without pulling, the tip of the hypostome usually broke off. The use of a blunt, medium-tipped, angled forceps offered the best results [43]. The tick bite should then be inspected carefully for any retained mouthparts, which the authors recommend should be excised. The area should then be cleaned with antiseptic solution, and the patient instructed to monitor for signs of local or systemic illness. Routine antibiotic prophylaxis following tick removal is not generally indicated. Removal of ticks by using disposable razors has been reported. This method instantly cuts off the tick vector's body; thus, keeping the risk of *B. burgdorferi* infection to a minimum [47]. Another removal method has been described in the article *Ticks in Australia* [48]. Here, a local anesthetic was infiltrated into the tick implantation site, which immobilized the tick and led to the eversion of mouthparts. Slow vertical traction with forceps could then be used to remove the tick with ease. Despite careful attempts, removal of ticks frequently led to breakage, and left the mouthparts (hypostomes) in the skin. The risk of transmission of LB or spotted fever was evaluated when different methods for the removal of arthropods were used [49]. The removal of ticks by pulling with fine tweezers and later disinfecting the area gave significant protection from the development of complications and infections.

Antibiotic Therapy after Tick Bite

In 1992, a double-blind placebo-controlled trial was performed in Connecticut on 387 subjects to assess the risk of infection with *B. burgdorferi* after tick bite and the efficacy of prophylactic antimicrobial treatment [50]. Amoxicillin or placebo was given for 10 days. Two persons in the placebo group developed EM, compared to none in the amoxicillin group. There was no asymptomatic seroconversion. Fifteen percent of ticks were infected. A prophylaxis with single-dose doxycycline was performed in 482 subjects who had removed ticks within 72 h [51]. EM developed in 1/235 subjects in the doxycycline group and 8/247 in the placebo group. The efficacy of treatment was 87%. No asymptomatic seroconversion occurred. As a result of these publications, a long discussion process has started on whether antimicrobial prophylaxis should be given or not. Currently, the Center for Disease Control and Prevention does not recommend antibiotics routinely [52]. Nevertheless, this treatment may be beneficial for some persons, and health care providers must determine whether the advantages of prescribing antibiotics after a tick bite outweigh the disadvantages. In Connecticut, 267 physicians were asked how they treat tick bites and EM [53]. Seventy (26%) prescribe antibiotic prophylaxis for patients with tick bites; serology was ordered by 31% of physicians for patients with tick bites and by 49% for patients with EM.

Prophylactic antibiotic treatment is not generally recommended for European patients, and different antibiotics registered for LB have been prescribed after tick bites for several reasons. In one study, 7 of 5,056 patients (0.14%) developed EM after having received antibiotic treatment [54]. From this study, it was assumed that antibiotic prophylaxis for LB after a tick bite, at least in Europe, is not entirely effective. Stanek and Kahl [55] therefore recommend a 'wait and watch' policy for European patients. One author from France also could not recommend antimicrobial prophylaxis, as the risk of transmission of LB after a tick bite is only 4% [56] and the currently available data seem to be insufficient to make a strong case for systematic antibiotic prophylaxis [57]. Most cases of LB result from unrecognized tick bites, since the great majority of attached ticks that are recognized are removed within 48 h of the time they began to feed, before they are likely to transmit infection [58, 59]. Checking carefully for ticks and removing them promptly may be the most effective strategy for preventing LB [60].

Analysis of Removed Ticks

To analyze the infection in ticks and to give further therapeutic advice, 185 tick specimens were collected from 179 Spanish patients: 26 ticks carried DNA from *Rickettsia* spp., 2 from *B. burgdorferi* and 7 from *A. phagocytophilum* [3]. It is cumbersome and expensive to analyze removed ticks, which can only be performed in special laboratories. Proof of a tick infection does not necessarily predict that the patient will actually become infected. Further, seroconversion does not always mean concomitant disease, as can be seen by the high seropositivity rate of healthy persons in endemic areas.

Prevention of Tick Bites

Strategies for the prevention of LB are to reduce the populations of ticks or host mammals, which are expensive and need to be repeated annually [56]. The primary method could be personal preventive measures, such as reducing the amount of exposed skin, wearing light-colored clothing for easy identification of crawling ticks, wearing protective garments and closed shoes, and frequently checking for ticks [61]. Further, tick repellents can be applied to the skin or to the clothing, including N,N-diethyl-m-toluamide (DEET), 2-ethyl-1,3-hexanediol, and dimethylphthalate. A study was performed upon an at-risk population in Switzerland to assess the effectiveness of a commercially available repellent spray containing both DEET and ethyl-butyl-acetyl-aminopropionate (EBAAP) [62]. The average number of tick bites per hour of exposure differed significantly between individuals receiving the placebo or the repellent. Total repellent effectiveness against tick attachment was 41.1%, and 66% on the arms. The authors concluded that an easily applied repellent is moderately effective in reducing the risk of tick bites. Permethrin is the most effective clothing repellent. DEET plus a permethrin-containing clothing repellent offers the best overall protection [61]. Rapid tick removal with fine tweezers or specials forceps followed by disinfection of the bite site appears to be the best technique. Patient education has a great influence on their behavior and leads to a reduction in tick-borne diseases. This was shown in a controlled study where there was a lower rate of tick-borne illnesses in educated participants, who were significantly more likely to take precautions as a result [63].

Conclusion – What to Do in Case of a Tick Bite

I. ricinus is the commonest tick species in Europe, and transmits LB, TBE, ehrlichiosis, tularemia, rickettsiosis, and babesiosis. In eastern Europe and in Spain, ticks of the *Dermacentor* species have been reported, which transmit *Rickettsia* infections.

The risk of tick bites and their infection rates with *B. burgdorferi* vary across different geographical areas. *B. burgdorferi* transmission increases with the time of tick engorgement. Reported data are hardly comparable since different study concepts and the investigation methods used provide different data. The seropositivity rate of healthy individuals is dependent on the amount and kind of outdoor activities, the age, and the infection rate of ticks.

Even when the tick is infected, a tick bite does not necessarily cause EM or LB. So finding *B. burgdorferi* DNA in ticks does not prove that the patient will develop LB. Seropositivity does not prevent another *B. burgdorferi* infection. When seroconversion occurs, serologic follow-up can only tell individuals that they have acquired a *B. burgdorferi* infection, with or without manifested disease. Ticks should be removed as early as possible with fine tweezers, taking the tick's head with the forceps. Any remaining mouthparts do not harm the patient. Tick granulomas and atypical lymphomatoid reactions are rare; therefore, mouthparts should not be excised or biopsied. Mouthparts cannot be completely removed by needle manipulation, so unnecessary trauma should be avoided. Antibiotic prophylactic therapy after a tick bite is not generally recommended. The same procedures should also be used in pregnant and breastfeeding women and in children. Small babies should be protected from contact with grass in areas with high tick populations, and they should not be placed on unfolded blankets in the grass.

Tick bites can be partially prevented by applying repellents to the body and permethrin to clothes. Repellents should be handled in children by carefully following the instructions. Furthermore, covering the body as much as possible with light-colored garments can also prevent tick contact, and allows identification of ticks on the clothes. Moreover, regularly checking all body sites once a day for ticks and taking a shower with soap after outdoor activities can help to identify ticks within 24 h. Ticks should be removed as soon as possible. The tick bite area should be inspected regularly for about 1 month. Unspecific papules at the tick bite site should decrease in size and vanish within about 1 week. In case of persistent erythema for longer than 1 week, the erythema should be seen by a dermatologist since *Borrelia* infection cannot be excluded. Furthermore, the patient should be aware of any febrile illness within 6 weeks of the tick bite, which is a sign of possible disseminated LB.

Tick bites should be seen as a natural occurrence for individuals participating in outdoor activities. LB is a treatable disease, in contrast to TBE where vaccination provides protection against infection. The fear of getting LB after a tick bite is exaggerated, and can be diminished or even abolished with adequate information.

References

1 Gern L: The biology of the *Ixodes ricinus* tick (in German). Ther Umsch 2005;62:707–712.

2 Bormane A, Lucenko I, Duks A, Mavtchoutko V, Ranka R, Salmina K, Baumanis V: Vectors of tick-borne diseases and epidemiological situation in Latvia in 1993–2002. Int J Med Microbiol 2004; 293:(suppl 37):36–47.

3 Merino FJ, Nebreda T, Serrano JL, Fernandez-Soto P, Encinas A, Perez-Sanchez R: Tick species and tick-borne infections identified in population from a rural area of Spain. Epidemiol Infect 2005;133: 943–949.

4 Smetanova K, Schwarzova K, Kocianova E: Detection of *Anaplasma phagocytophilum*, *Coxiella burnetii*, *Rickettsia* spp., and *Borrelia burgdorferi* s.l. in ticks, and wild-living animals in western and middle Slovakia. Ann NY Acad Sci 2006;1078:312–315.

5 Lakos A: Tick-borne lymphadenopathy (TIBOLA). Wien Klin Wochenschr 2002;114:648–654.

6 Robertson JN, Gray JS, Stewart P: Tick bite and Lyme borreliosis risk at a recreational site in England. Eur J Epidemiol 2000;16:647–652.

7 Lotric-Furlan S, Petrovec M, Avsic-Zupanc T, Nicholson WL, Sumner JW, Childs JE, Strle F: Prospective assessment of the etiology of acute febrile illness after a tick bite in Slovenia. Clin Infect Dis 2001;33:503–510.

8 Golubic D, Zember S: Dual infection: Tularemia and Lyme borreliosis acquired by single tick bite in northwest Croatia. Acta Med Croatica 2001;55: 207–209.

9 Strle F: Human granulocytic ehrlichiosis in Europe. Int J Med Microbiol 2004;293(suppl 37):27–35.

10 Marquez FJ, Rojas A, Ibarra V, Cantero A, Rojas J, Oteo JA, Muniain MA: Prevalence data of *Rickettsia slovaca* and other SFG Rickettsiae species in *Dermacentor marginatus* in the southeastern Iberian peninsula. Ann NY Acad Sci 2006;1078:328–330.

11 Bennet L, Halling A, Berglund J: Increased incidence of Lyme borreliosis in southern Sweden following mild winters and during warm, humid summers. Eur J Clin Microbiol Infect Dis 2006;25: 426–432.

12 Rizzoli A, Rosa R, Mantelli B, Pecchioli E, Hauffe H, Tagliapietra V, Beninati T, Neteler M, Genchi C: *Ixodes ricinus*, transmitted diseases and reservoirs (in Italian). Parassitologia 2004;46:119–122.

13 Pichon B, Kahl O, Hammer B, Gray JS: Pathogens and host DNA in *Ixodes ricinus* nymphal ticks from a German forest. Vector Borne Zoonotic Dis 2006; 6:382–387.

14 Wodecka B, Skotarczak B: Genetic diversity of *Borrelia burgdorferi* sensu lato in *Ixodes ricinus* ticks collected in north-west Poland (in Polish). Wiad Parazytol 2000;46:475–485.

15 Stunzner D, Hubalek Z, Halouzka J, Wendelin I, Sixl W, Marth E: Prevalence of *Borrelia burgdorferi* sensu lato in the tick *Ixodes ricinus* in the Styrian mountains of Austria. Wien Klin Wochenschr 2006;118:682–685.

16 Maetzel D, Maier WA, Kampen H: *Borrelia burgdorferi* infection prevalences in questing *Ixodes ricinus* ticks (Acari: Ixodidae) in urban and suburban Bonn, western Germany. Parasitol Res 2005;95:5–12.

17 Bennet L, Stjernberg L, Berglund J: Effect of gender on clinical and epidemiologic features of Lyme borreliosis. Vector Borne Zoonotic Dis 2007;7:34–41.

18 Wahlberg P: Incidence of tick-bite in man in Aland islands: reference to the spread of Lyme borreliosis. Scand J Infect Dis 1990;22:59–62.

19 den Boon S, Schellekens JF, Schouls LM, Suijkerbuijk AW, Docters van Leeuwen B, van Pelt W: Doubling of the number of cases of tick bites and Lyme borreliosis seen by general practitioners in the Netherlands (in Dutch). Ned Tijdschr Geneeskd 2004;148:665–670.

20 Oehme R, Hartelt K, Backe H, Brockmann S, Kimmig P: Foci of tick-borne diseases in southwest Germany. Int J Med Microbiol 2002;291(suppl 33):22–29.

21 Zhioua E, Rodhain F, Binet P, Perez-Eid C: Prevalence of antibodies to *Borrelia burgdorferi* in forestry workers of Ile de France, France. Eur J Epidemiol 1997;13:959–962.

22 Cetin E, Sotoudeh M, Auer H, Stanek G: Paradigm Burgenland: risk of *Borrelia burgdorferi* sensu lato infection indicated by variable seroprevalence rates in hunters. Wien Klin Wochenschr 2006;118:677–681.

23 Santino I, Cammarata E, Franco S, Galdiero F, Oliva B, Sessa R, Cipriani P, Tempera G, Del Piano M: Multicentric study of seroprevalence of *Borrelia burgdorferi* and *Anaplasma phagocytophila* in high-risk groups in regions of central and southern Italy. Int J Immunopathol Pharmacol 2004;17:219–223.

24 Bohme M, Schembra J, Bocklage H, Schwenecke S, Fuchs E, Karch H, Wiebecke D: Infections with *Borrelia burgdorferi* in Wurzburg blood donors: antibody prevalence, clinical aspects and pathogen detection in antibody positive donors (in German). Beitr Infusionsther 1992;30:96–99.

25 Meiners T, Hammer B, Gobel UB, Kahl O: Determining the tick scutal index allows assessment of tick feeding duration and estimation of infection risk with *Borrelia burgdorferi* sensu lato in a person bitten by an *Ixodes ricinus* nymph. Int J Med Microbiol 2006;296(suppl 40):103–107.
26 Kahl O, Janetzki-Mittmann C, Gray JS, Jonas R, Stein J, de Boer R: Risk of infection with *Borrelia burgdorferi* sensu lato for a host in relation to the duration of nymphal *Ixodes ricinus* feeding and the method of tick removal. Zentralbl Bakteriol 1998; 287:41–52.
27 Yeh MT, Bak JM, Hu R, Nicholson MC, Kelly C, Mather TN: Determining the duration of *Ixodes scapularis* (Acari: Ixodidae) attachment to tick-bite victims. J Med Entomol 1995;32:853–858.
28 Maiwald M, Oehme R, March O, Petney TN, Kimmig P, Naser K, Zappe HA, Hassler D, von Knebel Doeberitz M: Transmission risk of *Borrelia burgdorferi* sensu lato from *Ixodes ricinus* ticks to humans in southwest Germany. Epidemiol Infect 1998;121:103–108.
29 Heininger U, Zimmermann T, Schoerner C, Brade V, Stehr K: Tick bite and Lyme borreliosis: an epidemiologic study in the Erlangen area (in German). Monatsschr Kinderheilkd 1993;141:874–877.
30 Gustafson R, Svenungsson B, Forsgren M, Gardulf A, Granstrom M: Two-year survey of the incidence of Lyme borreliosis and tick-borne encephalitis in a high-risk population in Sweden. Eur J Clin Microbiol Infect Dis 1992;11:894–900.
31 Berger BW, Johnson RC, Kodner C, Coleman L: Cultivation of *Borrelia burgdorferi* from human tick bite sites: a guide to the risk of infection. J Am Acad Dermatol 1995;32:184–187.
32 Zalezny W, Flisiak R, Prokopowicz D: Effect of exposure to tick-bites on the course of Lyme borreliosis in Bialowieza residents (in Polish). Przegl Epidemiol 2002;56:419–424.
33 Nahimana I, Gern L, Blanc DS, Praz G, Francioli P, Peter O: Risk of *Borrelia burgdorferi* infection in western Switzerland following a tick bite. Eur J Clin Microbiol Infect Dis 2004;23:603–608.
34 Arnez M, Luznik-Bufon T, Avsic-Zupanc T, Ruzic-Sabljic E, Petrovec M, Lotric-Furlan S, Strle F: Causes of febrile illnesses after a tick bite in Slovenian children. Pediatr Infect Dis J 2003;22:1078–1083.
35 Grzeszczuk A, Ziarko S, Kovalchuk O, Stanczak J: Etiology of tick-borne febrile illnesses in adult residents of north-eastern Poland: report from a prospective clinical study. Int J Med Microbiol 2006; 296(suppl 40):242–249.
36 Baumann D, Pusterla N, Peter O, Grimm F, Fournier PE, Schar G, Bossart W, Lutz H, Weber R: Fever after a tick bite: clinical manifestations and diagnosis of acute tick bite-associated infections in northeastern Switzerland (in German). Dtsch Med Wochenschr 2003;128:1042–1047.
37 Weber K, Wilske B: Mini erythema migrans – a sign of early Lyme borreliosis. Dermatology 2006;212: 113–116.
38 Stanek G, O'Connell S, Cimmino M, Aberer E, Kristoferitsch W, Granstrom M, Guy E, Gray J: European Union Concerted Action on Risk Assessment in Lyme Borreliosis: clinical case definitions for Lyme borreliosis. Wien Klin Wochenschr 1996; 108:741–747.
39 Hwong H, Jones D, Prieto VG, Schulz C, Duvic M: Persistent atypical lymphocytic hyperplasia following tick bite in a child: report of a case and review of the literature. Pediatr Dermatol 2001;18:481–484.
40 Stefanato CM, Phelps RG, Goldberg LJ, Perry AE, Bhawan J: Type-I cryoglobulinemia-like histopathologic changes in tick bites: a useful clue for tissue diagnosis in the absence of tick parts. J Cutan Pathol 2002;29:101–106.
41 Aoki K, Kamata H, Iida T, Suzuki H: Tick bite: two cases studied by scanning electron microscopy. Br J Dermatol 1984;110:233–240.
42 Beaudouin E, Kanny G, Guerin B, Guerin L, Plenat F, Moneret-Vautrin DA: Unusual manifestations of hypersensitivity after a tick bite: report of two cases. Ann Allergy Asthma Immunol 1997;79:43–46.
43 Gammons M, Salam G: Tick removal. Am Fam Physician 2002;66:643–645.
44 Lanschuetzer CM, Wieser M, Laimer M, Emberger M, Hintner H: Improving the removal of intact ticks. Australas J Dermatol 2003;44:301.
45 Fingerle V, Wilske B: Ticks, tick bites and how best to remove the tick (in German). MMW Fortschr Med 2006;148:30–32.
46 De Boer R, van den Bogaard AE: Removal of attached nymphs and adults of *Ixodes ricinus* (Acari: Ixodidae). J Med Entomol 1993;30:748–752.
47 Moehrle M, Rassner G: How to remove ticks? Dermatology 2002;204:303–304.
48 Storer E, Sheridan AT, Warren L, Wayte J: Ticks in Australia. Australas J Dermatol 2003;44:83–89.
49 Oteo JA, Martinez de Artola V, Gomez-Cadinanos R, Casas JM, Blanco JR, Rosel L: Evaluation of methods of tick removal in human ixodidiasis. Rev Clin Esp 1996;196:584–587.
50 Shapiro ED, Gerber MA, Holabird NB, Berg AT, Feder HM Jr, Bell GL, Rys PN, Persing DH: A controlled trial of antimicrobial prophylaxis for Lyme disease after deer-tick bites. N Engl J Med 1992;327: 1769–1773.

51 Nadelman RB, Nowakowski J, Fish D, Falco RC, Freeman K, McKenna D, Welch P, Marcus R, Aguero-Rosenfeld ME, Dennis DT, Wormser GP: Prophylaxis with single-dose doxycycline for the prevention of Lyme disease after an *Ixodes scapularis* tick bite. N Engl J Med 2001;345:79–84.
52 www.cdc.gov/ncidod/dvbid/lyme/Prevention/ld_Prevention_Antibiotics.htm.
53 Murray T, Feder HM Jr: Management of tick bites and early Lyme disease: a survey of Connecticut physicians. Pediatrics 2001;108:1367–1370.
54 Maraspin V, Lotric-Furlan S, Strle F: Development of erythema migrans in spite of treatment with antibiotics after a tick bite. Wien Klin Wochenschr 2002;114:616–619.
55 Stanek G, Kahl O: Chemoprophylaxis for Lyme borreliosis? Zentralbl Bakteriol 1999;289:655–665.
56 Guy N: Lyme disease: Basis for treatment strategy, primary preventive care and secondary preventive care (in French). Med Mal Infect 2007;37:381–393.
57 Patey O: Lyme disease: prophylaxis after tick bite (in French). Med Mal Infect 2007;37:446–455.
58 Shapiro ED: Doxycycline for tick bites – not for everyone. N Engl J Med 2001;345:133–134.
59 Falco RC, Fish D, Piesman J: Duration of tick bites in a Lyme disease-endemic area. Am J Epidemiol 1996;143:187–192.
60 des Vignes F, Piesman J, Heffernan R, Schulze TL, Stafford KC 3rd, Fish D: Effect of tick removal on transmission of *Borrelia burgdorferi* and *Ehrlichia phagocytophila* by *Ixodes scapularis* nymphs. J Infect Dis 2001;183:773–778.
61 Couch P, Johnson CE: Prevention of Lyme disease. Am J Hosp Pharm 1992;49:1164–1173.
62 Staub D, Debrunner M, Amsler L, Steffen R: Effectiveness of a repellent containing DEET and EBAAP for preventing tick bites. Wilderness Environ Med 2002;13:12–20.
63 Daltroy LH, Phillips C, Lew R, Wright E, Shadick NA, Liang MH: A controlled trial of a novel primary prevention program for Lyme disease and other tick-borne illnesses. Health Educ Behav 2007;34:531–542.

Prof. Elisabeth Aberer, MD
Department of Dermatology, Medical University of Graz, Austria
Auenbrugger Platz 8
AT–8036 Graz (Austria)
Tel. +43 316 385 80317, Fax +43 316 385 2466, E-Mail elisabeth.aberer@medunigraz.at

Lipsker D, Jaulhac B (eds): Lyme Borreliosis.
Curr Probl Dermatol. Basel, Karger, 2009, vol 37, pp 167–177

When Is the Best Time to Order a Western Blot and How Should It Be Interpreted?

K.-P. Hunfeld · P. Kraiczy

Institute of Medical Microbiology and Infection Control, Hospital of the Johann Wolfgang Goethe-University Frankfurt, Frankfurt am Main, Germany

Abstract

Despite significant progress in the diagnostics of Lyme borreliosis, including molecular methods, the detection of a specific antibody response remains the mainstay in the laboratory diagnosis of the disease. Current guidelines propose the combination of highly sensitive screening assays, such as ELISAs, with very specific confirmatory tests, such as immunoblots, to guarantee a cost-effective, sensitive and specific diagnostic approach. For a correct interpretation of the serological findings, the investigator must always consider a whole series of clinical and laboratory facts. Here, we summarize current laboratory algorithms in the diagnosis of Lyme borreliosis, with a special emphasis on when to order a Western blot and how to interpret it correctly in the context of additional clinical and laboratory information.

Despite the substantial advancements in our knowledge of the biological properties of *Borrelia burgdorferi* and the introduction of molecular detection methods, the detection of antibodies still remains the mainstay in the laboratory diagnosis of Lyme borreliosis mainly because specimen collection is simple and convenient [1–3]. In this context, the introduction of immunoblot assays using constantly improving panels of whole cell and/or recombinant antigen preparations led to a very diverse armamentarium of tests, which are usually employed as part of 2-tier testing protocols (fig. 1) in the serodiagnosis of Lyme borreliosis [1, 2, 4–8].

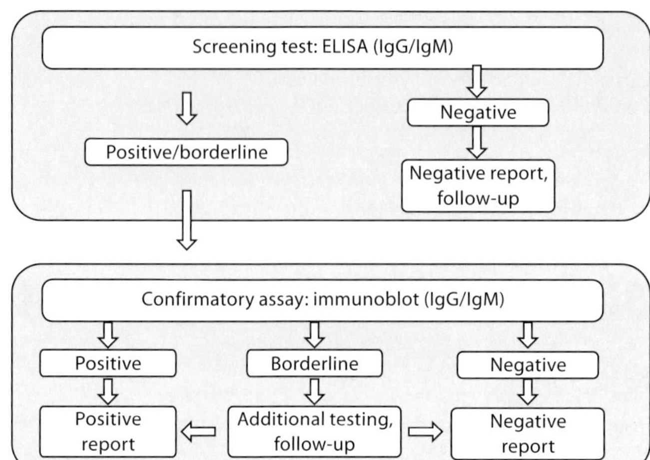

Fig. 1. Laboratory diagnosis of Lyme borreliosis: rational stepwise serological testing.

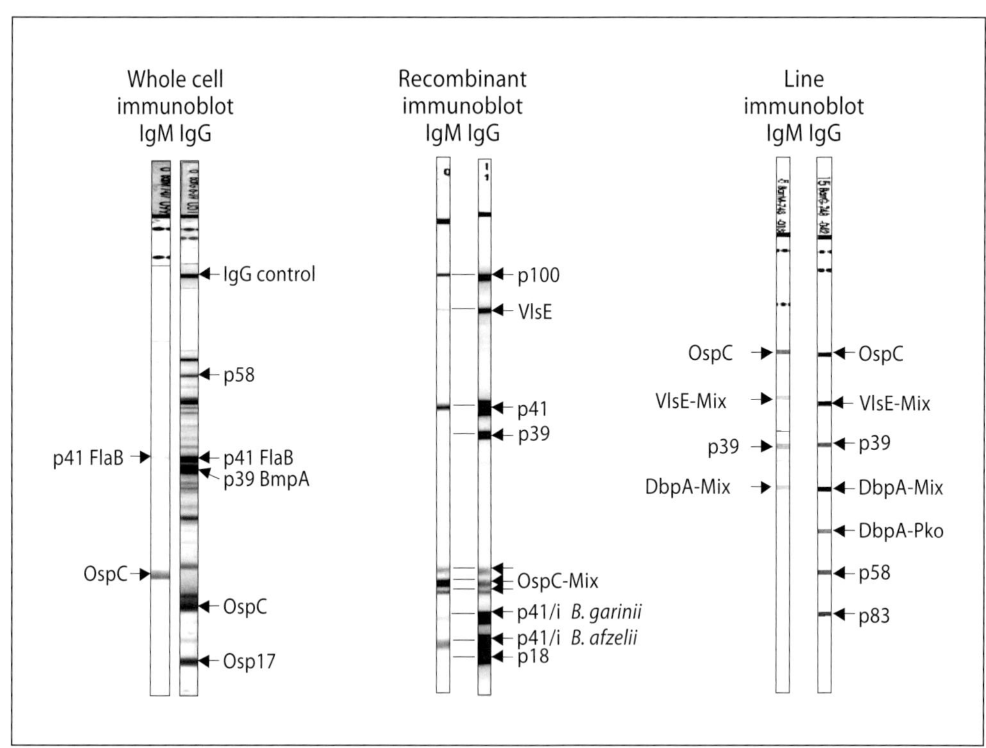

Fig. 2. Examples of the variable antigen preparations and diagnostic formats of currently available immunoblot assays.

Table 1. Immunodominant antigens of *B. burgdorferi* s.l. according to their occurrence in the course of infection (early or late) with a special notion on specificity and cross-reactivities (modified from [1])

Protein	Phase in which antigen expressed	Specificity	Cross-reactivity
p83/100	late	high	infrequent
p58	early/late	fair	infrequent
p43	early/late	fair	infrequent
p41 (flagellin)	early/late	low	common
p39 (BmpA)	late	fair	infrequent
OspA	late	fair	infrequent
OspC	early/late	high	infrequent
Osp17/p18 (DbpA)	late	fair	infrequent
VlsE	early/late	high	infrequent
p41 (flagellin, internal fragment)	early/late	fair	infrequent

Western Blot Techniques for Serological Antibody Detection in Lyme Borreliosis Diagnostics

The classical Western blot technique is based on the transfer of proteins already separated by SDS polyacrylamide gel electrophoresis (SDS-PAGE) to a nitrocellulose or polyvinyl difluoride (PVDF) membrane. Line immunoblots represent a modification of conventional immunoblots, where various recombinant antigens of proven diagnostic value are produced, purified and directly sprayed onto the membrane without previous denaturation through electrophoretic separation [4, 9, 10]. In both approaches, proteins remain fixed to the membrane due to hydrophobic interactions, and such prepared membranes can easily be stored for longer time periods. The number and kind of antigens used (native or recombinant) for such tests are essential for diagnostic quality. Although immunoblots are mainly used as confirmatory tests, in general, such assays offer both high sensitivity and specificity [1, 2, 4]. In contrast to the qualitative and quantitative test results of ELISA, the immunoblot provides a qualitative result. One particular advantage of this technique, however, is that it can provide both reliable information on the class and antigen specificities of the immune response for a large number of *Borrelia*-specific antigens (fig. 2; table 1). In general, an immunoblot is carried out by incubating antigen-loaded blot strips with the patient's serum. Specific antibodies then bind to the proteins and can be identified/visualized as marked bands after specific staining with enzyme-labeled anti-human immunoglobulins, similar to the sandwich principle used in ELISA. Each band then specifically corresponds to an antigen-antibody reaction with the underlying fraction of proteins. However, unlike the ELISA technique, this method does not just detect the presence of antibodies but, instead, the nature and number of detected bands in an immunoblot (fig. 1; table 1), and therefore permits additional analysis of the individual class- and antigen-specific antibody patterns expressed by the patient [1, 2]. In regard to the currently available diagnostic tests, 3 different assay types have to be distinguished: whole cell antigen immunoblots, recombinant immunoblots, and the so-called line immunoblots that have been more recently developed.

Whole Cell Antigen Immunoblot

Borrelia whole cell extracts of a defined borrelial strain obtained during the exponential growth phase provide the starting material for the classical immunoblot (fig. 2). The advantage of this method is that all the naturally occurring antigens of a defined strain are available for antibody detection. In addition to highly specific immunodominant antigens, numerous less specific or non-specific cross-reactive antigens are present for blot testing [1, 2]. Because both highly specific and less specific antigens can react with antibodies from the patient (IgM and/or IgG) such tests need a high level of test standardization and expertise of the investigator to avoid false-positive test results. In addition, reliable identification and correct evaluation of the bands are decisive for the quality of the diagnosis. To improve handling and specificity of such tests, the Centers of Disease Control and Prevention and the German Society for Hygiene and Medical Microbiology (DGHM) developed standard criteria (table 2) for the laboratory evaluation of immunoblot test results [1, 2, 11, 12]. A set of interpretation rules has also been defined on the basis of a multicentric European study [14]. Because of a general lack of standardization and the highly variable format and antigen composition of the currently available commercial assays, however, the diagnostic assessment of a given test has to be performed according to the evaluation criteria of the individual manufacturer. Although the assay evaluation depends greatly on the individual diagnostic algorithm of the test manufacturer, in general, the detection of specific IgM antibodies by whole cell antigen immunoblot is regarded as reliable and specific if at least 2 of the following 3 bands are detected: OspC, p39 (BmpA) and p41 (flagellin). Similarly, the presence of several of the following bands is regarded as particularly important for the reliable and specific detection of specific IgG antibodies: Osp17/p18 (DbpA), OspC, OspA, p58, p39 (BmpA), p41 (flagellin), p66 (Oms66), VlsE and p83/100.

Another diagnostic difficulty is that the immunodominant antigens of the 4 *Borrelia* species so far known to be pathogenic in humans *(B. burgdorferi* s.s., *B. afzelii, B. garinii* and *B. spielmanii)* tend to show a significant amount of variability [4, 6, 9, 15, 16]. Serological studies performed in the US and Europe pertaining to this problem have demonstrated that the currently available strains are not equally suitable as an antigen source for whole cell antigen immunoblot production [2, 11, 12]. Comparative serological evaluations revealed that the antigens of *B. afzelii* isolate Pko are particularly suitable for the sensitive and specific diagnosis of specific antibodies by

Table 2. Current published interpretative criteria for recombinant and whole cell antigen immunoblots in the serodiagnosis of Lyme borreliosis in Europe and the USA

IgG	IgM
B. afzelii (strain PKo) whole cell antigen immunoblot evaluation criteria for Europe according to Hauser et al. [10]	
IgG positive: ≥2 bands	IgM positive: ≥1 bands
p100, p58, p43, p39, p30, OspC, p21, Osp17, p14	p41 (strongly positive), p39, OspC, Osp17
B. burgdorferi s.s. (strain G39/40) whole cell antigen immunoblot evaluation criteria according to the CDC recommendations for the USA only [11, 12]	
IgG positive: ≥5 bands	IgM positive: ≥2 bands
p83/100, p66, p58, p45, p41, p39, p30, p28, OspC, or p18	p39, OspC, p41
Recombinant immunoblot, according to Wilske et al. [13] and Schulte-Spechtel et al. [6]	
IgG positive: ≥2 bands	IgM positive: ≥2 bands
p100, p58, p39, VlsE, OspC, p41 internal fragment, Osp17/p18	p39, OspC, p41 internal fragment, Osp17/p18; or strong reaction against OspC only

immunoblot, at least in the European context [10, 14, 16]. This is why the users of whole cell antigen immunoblots should critically evaluate the source and preparation of antigens used for their specific assays for the diagnostic suitability in a given epidemiological setting [1, 2].

Recombinant Immunoblot

The recombinant immunoblot (fig. 2) commonly uses defined highly purified borrelial proteins produced by genetic engineering [3]. These antigens are then transferred to the blot membrane after purification and separation by SDS-PAGE [1, 10, 14]. A positive test result corresponds to the specific staining of the binding of the patient's antibodies (IgM and/or IgG) to selected highly specific immunodominant *Borrelia*-specific antigens such as p83/100, VlsE, p58, p41 (flagellin), internal fragment of p41 (p41i), p39 (BmpA), OspA, OspC and Osp17/p18 (DbpA) [2, 4, 9]. As compared to whole cell antigen immunoblots, the recombinant ones are easier to read and are generally better standardized. It is helpful to combine different antigen preparations from different *Borrelia* species on a single blot, so that antibodies to specific antigenic determinants of all 4 pathogens responsible for human Lyme borreliosis *(B. burgdorferi* s.s., *B. afzelii, B. garinii* and also *B. spielmanii)* can be detected in a single test [4, 6]. They also allow users to incorporate antigens which are expressed in vivo only (e.g. VlsE). One disadvantage of these tests, however, is their substantially higher cost. The diagnostic evaluation of the recombinant immunoblot test is based on the previously cited criteria, but depends on the given standards and precautions of the individual manufacturer and also on the particular immunoblot batch [1, 2, 4–6].

Line Immunoblot

Antigens used for the production of line immunoblots (fig. 2) are essentially the same as those applied in the regular recombinant immunoblots. The production and further processing of the antigens is mainly identical. However, no electrophoretic separation step is necessary prior to the blotting procedure. For such tests, the individual antigens are sprayed on the membranes without conventional blotting procedures. In doing so, several homologous immunodominant antigens of different borrelial strains with identical or similar molecular weights can be combined in diagnostic groups on a single strip [4]. The line immunoblot technology thus allows for a much more variable combination and application of very diverse antigen panels on individual test strips. As such, a broad spectrum of antigens derived from various different strains belonging to the diagnostically important genospecies of *B. burgdorferi* s.l. can be covered by the assay to improve diagnostic sensitivity and guarantee high specificity [4, 9]. An additional advantage of the line immunoblot is the application of non-denaturated antigens for the detection of immunoreactive antibodies directed exclusively to native structural determinants [17].

Stage-Dependent Antibody Kinetics in Lyme Borreliosis

For the critical evaluation of immunoblot results and the correct interpretation of serological findings in the context of given clinical symptoms, a good knowledge of the temporal course of the antibody response directed against the major immunodominant antigens (table 1) is essential [1, 2]. The antigenic specificities of the outer membrane proteins and flagellin from *B. burgdorferi* have been the subjects of extensive investigations. By contrast, there is still fragmentary information available on structure and immunological significance of many other potential immunodominant antigens [1, 3]. Specific antibodies directed against borrelial antigens can usually be detected by any test 3–6 weeks after the infection has taken place. The development of IgM antibodies usually precedes that of IgG antibodies, but in individual cases IgM production may be delayed or even absent [1, 2]. This remains true also in cases of reinfection, where a broad IgG antibody response without significant IgM production can be expected. Early on in the infection, the primary immune response to both classes of immunoglobulin is directed against a narrow spectrum of borrelial antigens only. Such antigens comprise, in particular, the flagellin (p41), the VlsE and the outer surface protein OspC of *B. burgdorferi*. Antibodies directed against VlsE and OspC are of particular diagnostic relevance because they are regarded as highly specific [2]. However, a substantial proportion of false-negatives should be expected in the early stages of Lyme borreliosis, as in many patients a significant antibody titer may develop very slowly after initial infection. Correspondingly, seroprevalence studies show a serologically detectable antibody response in 20–60% of European patients with localized infection (stage I: erythema migrans) mainly depending on the assay and test criteria used [1, 2, 12]. Among seropositive patients, IgM antibodies can be detected in up to 90% of cases, but a corresponding IgG response is only present in up to 70% of the cases. The number of seropositive patients increases as borrelial infection progresses to the early disseminated stage (stage II) and reaches almost 100% for IgG in late disseminated disease manifestations (stage III) [1, 2]. IgG antibodies directed against a broad spectrum of borrelial antigens are characteristic of early disseminated and late disseminated disease manifestations (stages II and III of Lyme borreliosis). Antibodies against specific antigens such as the p83/100 protein, p58, p38 (BmpA), the internal fragment of p41 (flagellin) and Osp17/p18 (DbpA) are of particularly high diagnostic significance. In contrast, antibodies against OspA, which is also specific, are rare (except at the late stage, i.e. in Lyme arthritis cases) because of a switch in antigen expression from OspA to OspC by the pathogen upon entering the mammalian host.

As with other serological tests, normal immune status and the ability of the patient to produce antibodies remains an important prerequisite for the serological detection of antibodies by immunoblotting. Seronegative Lyme borreliosis is extremely rare, except in the very early course of the disease, but should be borne in mind in patients with a short duration of the disease and clinically unambiguous symptoms. In such cases, direct detection of the pathogen should always be considered if Lyme borreliosis is strongly suspected clinically in immunocompromised patients or when unambiguous or borderline findings are repeatedly obtained by serological tests [1].

Value of Immunoblot Testing for the Laboratory Diagnosis of Lyme Borreliosis

In the serodiagnosis of many bacterial and viral pathogens, as a general principle, highly sensitive screening methods such as ELISA are best combined with very specific confirmatory tests such as immunoblots to guarantee a cost effective, sensitive and specific diagnostic approach (fig. 1) [1, 2, 18]. This is why the general application of immunoblots as first-line tests for the serodiagnosis of Lyme borreliosis is rejected by most European (DGHM, EUCALB) and American diagnostic guidelines [1, 2, 11, 12]. Using immunoblots as a first-line test will also increase the asymptomatic seroprevalence of the pathogen and decrease the clinical value of the result.

Unfortunately, diagnostic assays for Lyme borreliosis do not require peer-reviewed competent pre-market approval in the majority of countries outside the USA, and therefore a wide range of commercial and home-brewed tests with substantially different diagnostic qualities are currently being used by diagnostic laboratories [18]. As such, the level of test standardization and the diagnostic quality of serological testing for Lyme borreliosis still lags far behind when compared to syphilis diagnostics [19]. Immunoblots, especially those using recombinant antigens, represent confirmatory tests of high specificity and sensitivity when antigens included are accurately selected [1, 2, 4]. Keeping in mind the inclusion of recombinant homologues, truncated proteins or fusion proteins derived from different *Borrelia* species can broaden the diagnostic coverage of such tests in regard to the pronounced antigenic heterogeneity of the different *B. burgdorferi* s.l. isolates [4, 9]. By creating recombinant protein compositions that include conserved amino acid sequences which are recognized by antibodies to antigens from all 4 species pathogenic in humans, such 'designer' immunoblots are highly sensitive, standardized and more easily interpretable than most currently available whole cell immunoblots [1, 4]. When performed carefully, the immunoblot can fairly reliably distinguish between antibody responses to specific and non-specific proteins. Although test quality has steadily increased during recent years, it should be mentioned that immunoblot testing for diagnosing of *Borrelia* infection in individual cases can be significantly influenced by 3 major factors: (1) the kind of strain infecting the individual patient, (2) the kind of antigens and type of assay used for serological testing, and (3) the individual course and duration of the infection. Moreover, the evaluation and interpretation of test results depends largely on the individual diagnostic expertise of the investigator.

When to Order a Western Blot and How to Interpret Serological Findings

Combinations of Tests for Standard Diagnostics

In recent years, there have been many studies dealing with the improvement and standardization of serological diagnostics in Lyme borreliosis [1, 3, 5, 10, 14, 18, 20]. In truth, it is almost impossible for serological test methods to combine absolute specificity with best possible sensitivity [1, 2, 18]. To come close to this objective, therefore, a combination of very sensitive screening tests with highly specific confirmatory tests is commonly used to provide serological diagnostics which are both reliable and economic. The improved selection of specific antigens has made possible the replacement of earlier diagnostic protocols by means of 3 steps (IHAT, IFA/ELISA, immunoblot) by 2-tier testing protocols using ELISA and immunoblot (fig. 1). Our own experience also shows that a combination of a screening test (ELISA) with a confirmatory test (whole cell antigen immunoblot, recombinant immunoblot or line immunoblot) is in most cases sensitive and reliable for assessing Lyme borreliosis infection status [1, 2]. The use of other test combinations, or the use of ELISA or immunoblot in a single step only, is not currently recommended as it increases the risk of false-positive results by reducing test specificity [1, 2, 18].

How to Perform Rational Stepwise Diagnostics

The currently employed rational stepwise serological procedure for Lyme borreliosis is described briefly below:

- If the screening test is negative, it is usually not helpful to carry out further immunoblot testing and the Lyme borreliosis serology is reported as negative. However, it is not possible to exclude a *Borrelia* infection because seronegative courses are common in the early stages of the disease, and therefore a serological follow-up should be performed 2–3 weeks later if clinical suspicion remains.
- If, on the other hand, the screening test is positive, it is indicated to perform further investigations with confirmatory tests such as immunoblot assays. In addition to the whole cell antigen immunoblot, recombinant immunoblots and line immunoblots are now available for different *Borrelia* genospecies. In many cases, confirmatory tests, carried out to affirm an initially positive or borderline screening test result, remain negative, and from a serological point of view the presence of specific antibodies in such cases cannot be substantiated. Such findings, however, may be consistent with early stage I or II of the disease, and again carrying out a serological follow-up 3–4 weeks later can be helpful if clinical suspicion persists. If the following-up test turns out positive for antibodies (IgM and IgG) against specific antigens of *B. burgdorferi* s.l., clearly indicating seroconversion, an infection with the pathogen is regarded as having been established [1, 2].
- If, however, a borderline or positive screening test is supported by specific immunoblot testing according to the previously mentioned rules of interpretation, the criteria for a positive *Borrelia* serology are fulfilled. The resulting laboratory report should clearly state the number and kind of *Borrelia*-specific antigens (bands) as recognized by corresponding antibodies in the patient's serum [1, 2]. This is the only way to allow for comparison with the findings from follow-up samples and to permit the clinician to answer the question of whether or not the serological findings comply with the clinical picture, i.e. with early- or late-stage manifestations of the disease.

Rational Interpretation of Serological Findings

For a correct interpretation of the serological findings, the investigator must consider a whole series of questions and facts in the evaluation of immunoblot results. The first point to establish is whether the findings provide sufficient evidence to support the fact that borrelial infection did occur. If specific antibodies have been detected, it is necessary to clarify whether the findings obtained are suspicious of a more recent infection or whether they may reflect a long-lasting or past infection [1, 2]. Most importantly, the findings concerning the subclass of specific antibodies (IgM, IgG) and the pattern of detected antigens must fit into the clinical context of the patient (erythema migrans, neuroborreliosis, acrodermatitis chronica atrophicans, arthritis, etc.). For example, on the one hand, solely IgM-positive immunoblot findings and a narrow pattern of antigens such as flagellin (p41), and its internal fragment (p41i), and OspC clearly exclude clinical suspicion of late-stage disease manifestations, but are consistent with a recent infection. In the latter case, seroconversion can be demonstrated upon serological follow-up, such findings are a clear proof of a very recent time point of infection. On the other hand, a predominant IgG response and a broad pattern of positive antigens in the immunoblot [p83/100, VlsE, p58, Oms66/p66, OspA, p39 (BmpA), Osp17/p18 (DbpA)] are clearly consistent with late-stage disease manifestations or past infection (table 1) but, with the exception of re-infection, clearly argue against a recent time point of infection [1, 2].

References

1 Hunfeld KP, Oschmann P, Kaiser R, Schulze J, Brade V: Diagnostics; in Oschmann P, Kraiczy P, Halperin J, Brade V (eds): Lyme-Borreliosis and Tick-Borne Encephalitis. Bremen, Unimed, 1999, pp 80–108.

2 Wilske B, Fingerle V, Schulte-Spechtel U: Microbiological and serological diagnosis of Lyme borreliosis. FEMS Immunol Med Microbiol 2007;49:13–21.

3 Hunfeld KP, Ernst M, Zachary P, Jaulhac B, Sonneborn HH, Brade V: Development and laboratory evaluation of a new recombinant ELISA for the serodiagnosis of Lyme disease. Wien Klin Wochenschr 2002;114:580–585.

4 Goettner G, Schulte-Spechtel U, Hillermann R, Liegl G, Wilske B, Fingerle V: Improvement of Lyme borreliosis serodiagnosis by a newly developed recombinant immunoglobulin G (IgG) and IgM line immunoblot assay and addition of VlsE and DbpA homologues. J Clin Microbiol 2005;43: 3602–3609.

5 Magnarelli LA, Fikrig E, Padula SJ, Anderson JF, Flavell RA: Use of recombinant antigens of *Borrelia burgdorferi* in serologic tests for diagnosis of Lyme borreliosis. J Clin Microbiol 1996;34:237–240.

6 Schulte-Spechtel U, Lehnert G, Liegl G, Fingerle V, Heimerl C, Johnson BJ, Wilske B: Significant improvement of the recombinant Borrelia-specific immunoglobulin G immunoblot test by addition of VlsE and a DbpA homologue derived from *Borrelia garinii* for diagnosis of early neuroborreliosis. J Clin Microbiol 2003;41:1299–1303.

7 Wilske B, Fingerle V, Herzer P, Hofmann A, Lehnert G, Peters H, Pfister HW, Preac-Mursic V, Soutschek E, Weber K: Recombinant immunoblot in the serodiagnosis of Lyme borreliosis: comparison with indirect immunofluorescence and enzyme-linked immunosorbent assay. Med Microbiol Immunol 1993;182:255–270.

8 Wilske B, Fingerle V, Preac-Mursic V, Jauris-Heipke S, Hofmann A, Loy H, Pfister HW, Rössler D, Soutschek E: Immunoblot using recombinant antigens derived from different genospecies of *Borrelia burgdorferi* sensu lato. Med Microbiol Immunol 1994; 183:43–59.

9 Schulte-Spechtel U, Fingerle V, Goettner G, Rogge S, Wilske B: Molecular analysis of decorin-binding protein A (DbpA) reveals five major groups among European *Borrelia burgdorferi* sensu lato strains with impact for the development of serological assays and indicates lateral gene transfer of the *dbpA* gene. Int J Med Microbiol 2006;296(suppl 40):250–266.

10 Hauser U, Lehnert G, Lobentanzer R, Wilske B: Interpretation criteria for standardized Western blots for three European species of *Borrelia burgdorferi* sensu lato. J Clin Microbiol 1997;35:1433–1444.

11 Recommendations for test performance and interpretation from the Second National Conference on Serologic Diagnosis of Lyme Disease. MMWR Morb Mortal Wkly Rep 1995;44:590–591.

12 Aguero-Rosenfeld ME, Wang G, Schwartz I, Wormser GP: Diagnosis of Lyme borreliosis. Clin Microbiol Rev 2005;18:484–509.

13 Wilske B, Habermann C, Fingerle V, Hillenbrand B, Jauris-Heipke S, Lehnert G, Pradel I, Rössler D, Schulte-Spechtel U: An improved recombinant IgG immunoblot for serodiagnosis of Lyme borreliosis. Med Microbiol Immunol 1999;188:139–144.

14 Robertson J, Guy E, Andrews N, Wilske B, Anda P, Granström M, Hauser U, Moosmann Y, Sambri V, Schellekens J, Stanek G, Gray J: A European multicenter study of immunoblotting in serodiagnosis of Lyme borreliosis. J Clin Microbiol 2000;38:2097–2102.

15 Hauser U, Krahl H, Peters H, Fingerle V, Wilske B: Impact of strain heterogeneity on Lyme disease serology in Europe: comparison of enzyme-linked immunosorbent assays using different species of *Borrelia burgdorferi* sensu lato. J Clin Microbiol 1998;36:427–436.

16 Wilske B, Hauser U, Lehnert G, Jauris-Heipke S: Genospecies and their influence on immunoblot results. Wien Klin Wochenschr 1998;110:882–885.
17 Rossmann E, Kitiratschky V, Hofmann H, Kraiczy P, Simon MM, Wallich R: *Borrelia burgdorferi* complement regulator-acquiring surface protein 1 of the Lyme disease spirochetes is expressed in humans and induces antibody responses restricted to nondenaturated structural determinants. Infect Immun 2006;74:7024–7028.
18 Hunfeld KP, Stanek G, Straube E, Hagedorn HJ, Schörner C, Mühlschlegel F, Brade V: Quality of Lyme disease serology: lessons from the German Proficiency Testing Program 1999–2001. A preliminary report. Wien Klin Wochenschr 2002;114: 591–600.
19 Muller I, Brade V, Hagedorn HJ, Straube E, Schörner C, Frosch M, Hlobil H, Stanek G, Hunfeld KP: Is serological testing a reliable tool in laboratory diagnosis of syphilis? Meta-analysis of eight external quality control surveys performed by the German Infection Serology Proficiency Testing Program. J Clin Microbiol 2006;44:1335–1341.
20 Ledue TB, Collins MF, Craig WY: New laboratory guidelines for serologic diagnosis of Lyme disease: evaluation of the two-test protocol. J Clin Microbiol 1996;34:2343–2350.

K.-P. Hunfeld, MD, MPH
Institute of Medical Microbiology and Infection Control
Hospital of the Johann Wolfgang Goethe-University Frankfurt
Paul-Ehrlich-Strasse 40
DE–60596 Frankfurt am Main (Germany)
Tel. +49 69 6301 6441, Fax +49 69 6301 5767, E-Mail k.hunfeld@em.uni-frankfurt.de

Lipsker D, Jaulhac B (eds): Lyme Borreliosis.
Curr Probl Dermatol. Basel, Karger, 2009, vol 37, pp 178–182

Is Serological Follow-Up Useful for Patients with Cutaneous Lyme Borreliosis?

R.R. Müllegger[a] · M. Glatz[b]

[a]Department of Dermatology, State Hospital Wiener Neustadt, Wiener Neustadt, and
[b]Department of Dermatology, Medical University Graz, Graz, Austria

Abstract

Serologic follow-up examinations are frequently performed in patients with erythema migrans, borrelial lymphocytoma, and acrodermatitis chronica atrophicans (the 3 dermatoborrelioses) to evaluate treatment efficacy. There is, however, substantial proof in the literature that antibody titer development after therapy is unpredictable and variable, and moreover it is largely uncorrelated with the clinical course and mode of antibiotic treatment. For example, persistent positive IgG and/or IgM antibody titers do not indicate treatment failure. Thus, repeated serologic testing is of very limited value for assessing therapy efficacy, and therefore not recommended in the follow-up of dermatoborrelioses patients. Since cultivation of the etiologic agent, *Borrelia burgdorferi* sensu lato, and polymerase chain reaction are also inadequate for this purpose, the assessment of patients with cutaneous manifestations of Lyme borreliosis in the follow-up rests primarily on the clinical picture.

The typical cutaneous manifestations of Lyme borreliosis (LB), a multisystem infectious disease caused by *Borrelia burgdorferi* sensu lato (*B. burgdorferi* s.l.), are erythema migrans (EM), borrelial lymphocytoma (BL), and acrodermatitis chronica atrophicans (ACA) [1]. The extrapolated incidence of these 3 entities is about 200/100,000 people per year. EM, the hallmark of early LB, is clinically defined as an expanding round to oval, sharply demarcated, red to bluish-red skin lesion of at least 5 cm in diameter, sometimes disseminated and/or accompanied by extracutaneous signs and symptoms. BL, a B cell pseudolymphoma, represents a subacute lesion and predominantly affects children. Clinically, it is a sharply demarcated, soft bluish-red nodule or plaque of 1–5 cm, typically on the ear, breast, or scrotum, rarely with extracutaneous symptoms. ACA is the characteristic cutaneous manifestation of late-stage LB. It mostly affects elderly woman and typically develops on the extensor surfaces of the distal extremities. It slowly (weeks to months) progresses from an early inflammatory stage with bluish-red discoloration and doughy swelling to a chronic persistent stage with thinning and wrinkling of the skin.

Antibiotic therapy is obligatory in every case of cutaneous LB to eliminate *B. burgdorferi* s.l., resolve skin changes, and prevent extracutaneous complications. Response to appropriate therapy (usually doxycycline, amoxicillin or cefuroxime) is generally excellent for cutaneous and extracutaneous features in EM and BL, although delayed by weeks to months in the latter [1]. However, major complications (including meningitis) or minor symptoms over a period of several months to 1 year after therapy persist or newly develop in a small percentage of patients, particularly after EM. In ACA, inflammatory changes (erythema and swelling) gradually subside over a period of 1 year after treatment, whereas atrophy, telangiectases, and pseudo-sclerodermatous changes are usually not influenced by antimicrobials. Peripheral neuropathy, which is associated with ACA in about two thirds of patients, improves very slowly, if at all. True therapy failures (persistence or recurrence of cutaneous or associated signs and symptoms and/or survival of *B. burgdorferi* s.l.) have to be retreated, whereas sustained subjective symptoms, such as fatigue, musculoskeletal pain, and cognitive dysfunction ('post-Lyme disease syndrome'), which are not caused by *B. burgdorferi* s.l. persistence, do not respond to repeated antimicrobial treatment. Thus, laboratory tests would be desirable to prove the efficacy of treatment. To date, great uncertainty exists about the application and interpretation of such tests, particularly regarding serologic follow-up examinations. Analyses of skin biopsy samples for the presence of *B. burgdorferi* s.l. (-specific DNA) from the site of infection by cultivation or (quantitative) polymerase chain reaction (PCR) are very specific, but their sensitivity is insufficient, and they are available only in specialized laboratories [2, 3]. PCR is a quick method, but cultivation of *B. burgdorferi* s.l. is laborious and does not yield timely results. Also, both procedures are invasive and do not provide any evidence about possible (residual) *B. burgdorferi* s.l. infection of organs other than the skin. Culture or PCR testing of other clinical samples (e.g. blood or urine) is even far less valuable [2, 3]. In 2 post-treatment studies, PCR analyses of previous dermatoborrelioses sites proved to be a reliable method for demonstrating eradication of the spirochete [4, 5]. Molecular analyses were consistent with clinical response in most cases; in 2% of patients, PCR results were positive, but they were asymptomatic clinically [4].

So far, analyses of serum anti-*B. burgdorferi* s.l. antibodies have been frequently used because of the misconception that serologic follow-up examinations could support the assessment of the clinical course after treatment. They are convenient to use and generally available, although not cheap. However, interpretation of serologic results is difficult due to several possibilities of false-positive (e.g. seroprevalence, immunologic cross-reactions) or false-negative (e.g. lack of seroconversion early in the infection) outcomes [1, 6]. Also, results from different assays and laboratories are not comparable because of missing standardization. Serology is most reliable in substantiating the clinical diagnosis of ACA (100% positive) and BL (about 90% positive), but without value for EM [1, 6]. In the convalescent phase, up to 1 month after therapy in EM, seroconversion (increase in antibody titers) is found in at least two thirds of patients [1, 6]. Thus, analyses of sequential serum samples may ironically be diagnostically helpful instead of indicating successful therapy. On the other hand, about half of EM patients remain seronegative during their whole disease course, including on follow-up examinations [6–9]. This may be due to antibiotic abrogation [6] or that EM (in Europe) may represent a localized infection without systemic immune response. IgG and/or IgM antibodies can persist in 10–60% of EM patients for (many) years after adequate therapy [6, 7, 10–12]. It could be speculated that persistence of the antibody response is associated with the survival of spirochetes due to treatment failure. It has been proven, however, by PCR from skin lesions before and after therapy that antibiotic treatment leads to bacterial eradication in most cases [5]. It is instead plausible that the persistence of antibody response results from unspecific polyclonal activation of memory B cells [12, 13]. Several studies [6–8, 11], including a large investigation of more than 100 patients with serial serologic analyses [6] over a follow-up period of a minimum of 1 year, found no correlation between development of serologic titers and type of therapy or post-treatment clinical course. In a recent study, immunoblot analyses confirmed the missing correlation between antibody kinetics to specific *B. burgdorferi* s.l. antigens and clinical outcome in EM patients [14]. It was initially thought that serologic follow-up using a novel ELISA test based on C6 (part of VlsE, variable major protein-like sequence, expressed) is a better indicator of therapy efficacy (fast decrease of IgG antibody titers after antibiotic therapy), but serology was not put into statistical correlation with clinical characteristics [15, 16]. In contrast, other studies found a persistent IgG antibody response to C6 in clinically successfully treated EM patients [17]. Consequently, retreatment of EM patients solely based on a positive antibody titer after treatment without persistent or newly developed specific symptoms is not indicated, although everyday practice shows that less experienced physicians tend to reapply antibiotics in such cases, often driven by demanding patients. For BL patients who test positive for anti-*B. burgdorferi* s.l. IgG and/or IgM antibodies before therapy (70–95%) [1], only 1 study provides data on serologic development after therapy. One quarter to half of patients remain seropositive during a follow-up of 2 months. Seropositivity seems to be independent from type of therapy or disease course after therapy, although this aspect was not specifically looked into [18]. Several studies, in which ACA patients were followed up after therapy, have demonstrated a (clear) decline in the serologic response to *B. burgdorferi* s.l. over 1 to several years, although IgG titers (the predominant antibody class in ACA) remain positive in the great majority of patients [8–11, 19]. It was assumed that the observed serologic decline is due to effective therapy, but the course of seroreactivity and the type of treatment or clinical outcome were not correlated [8, 11, 19]. In accordance, we found essentially unchanged antibody titers during an average observation period of 18 months after treatment in 82 ACA patients, irrespective of the kind of therapy or time to clinical resolution of the skin lesion [unpublished data]. Thus, persistent antibody titers do not necessarily indicate a treatment failure, but rather represent a serologic scar after a chronic spirochetosis that is without clinical relevance.

In conclusion, anti-*B. burgdorferi* s.l. antibody titers after therapy develop differently in the 3 dermatoborrelioses. Antibody kinetics are unpredictable and variable, but generally independent of the clinical outcome and duration and type of antibiotic treatment. Importantly, persistent positive IgG and/or IgM antibody titers do not indicate treatment failure. Therefore, repeated serologic testing is of very limited value for the evaluation of therapy efficacy, and not recommended in the follow-up of dermatoborrelioses patients. To date, the key assessment parameter in follow-up examinations of patients with cutaneous manifestations of LB is the clinical picture.

References

1 Müllegger RR: Dermatological manifestations of Lyme borreliosis. Eur J Dermatol 2004;14:296–309.

2 Dumler JS: Molecular diagnosis of Lyme disease: review and meta-analysis. Mol Diagn 2001;6:1–11.

3 Lebech AM, Hansen K, Bandrup F, Clemmensen O, Halkier-Sorensen L: Diagnostic value of PCR for detection of *Borrelia burgdorferi* DNA in clinical specimens from patients with erythema migrans and Lyme neuroborreliosis. Mol Diagn 2000;5:139–150.

4 Hunfeld KP, Ruzic-Sabljic E, Norris DE, Kraiczy P, Strle F: In vitro susceptibility testing of *Borrelia burgdorferi* sensu lato isolates cultured from patients with erythema migrans before and after antimicrobial chemotherapy. Antimicrob Agents Chemother 2005;49:1294–1301.

5 Müllegger RR, Zöchling N, Schlüpen EM, Soyer HP, Hödl S, Kerl H, Volkenandt M: Polymerase chain reaction control of antibiotic treatment in dermatoborreliosis. Infection 1996;24:76–79.

6 Glatz M, Golestani M, Kerl H, Müllegger RR: Clinical relevance of different IgG and IgM serum antibody responses to *Borrelia burgdorferi* after antibiotic therapy for erythema migrans: long-term follow-up study of 113 patients. Arch Dermatol 2006;142:862–868.

7 Feder HM Jr, Gerber MA, Luger SW, Ryan RW: Persistence of serum antibodies to *Borrelia burgdorferi* in patients treated for Lyme disease. Clin Infect Dis 1992;15:788–793.

8 Hulshof MM, Vandenbroucke JP, Nohlmans LM, Spanjaard L, Bavnick JN, Dijkmans BA: Long-term prognosis in patients treated for erythema chronicum migrans and acrodermatitis chronica atrophicans. Arch Dermatol 1997;133:33–37.

9 Lomholt H, Lebech AM, Hansen K, Bandrup F, Halkier-Sorensen L: Long-term serological follow-up of patients treated for chronic cutaneous borreliosis or culture-positive erythema migrans. Acta Derm Venereol 2000;80:362–366.

10 Asbrink E, Hovmark A, Hederstedt B: Serologic studies of erythema chronicum migrans Afzelius and acrodermatitis chronica atrophicans with indirect immunofluorescence and enzyme-linked immunosorbent assays. Acta Derm Venereol 1985;65:509–514.

11 Hammers-Berggren S, Lebech AM, Karlsson M, Svenungsson B, Hansen K, Stiernstedt G: Serological follow-up after treatment of patients with erythema migrans and neuroborreliosis. J Clin Microbiol 1994;32:1519–1525.

12 Kalish RA, McHugh G, Granquist J, Shea B, Ruthazer R, Steere AC: Persistence of immunoglobulin M or immunoglobulin G antibody responses to *Borrelia burgdorferi* 10–20 years after active Lyme disease. Clin Infect Dis 2001;33:780–785.

13 Bernasconi NL, Traggiai E, Lanzavecchia A: Maintenance of serological memory by polyclonal activation of human memory B-cells. Science 2002;298:2199–2202.

14 Glatz M, Fingerle V, Wilske B, Ambros-Rudolph C, Kerl H, Müllegger RR: Immunoblot analysis of the seroreactivity to recombinant *Borrelia burgdorferi* sensu lato antigens, including VlsE, in the long-term course of treated patients with erythema migrans. Dermatology 2008;216:93–103.

15 Marangoni A, Sambri V, Accardo S, Cavrini F, Mondardini V, Moroni A, Storni E, Cevenini R: A decrease in the immunoglobulin G antibody response against the VlsE protein of *Borrelia burgdorferi* sensu lato correlates with the resolution of clinical signs in antibiotic-treated patients with early Lyme disease. Clin Vaccine Immunol 2006;13:525–529.

16 Philipp MT, Wormser GP, Marques AR, Bittker S, Martin DS, Nowakowski J, Dally LG: A decline in C6 antibody titer occurs in successfully treated patients with culture-confirmed early localized or early disseminated Lyme borreliosis. Clin Diagn Lab Immunol 2005;12:1069–1074.

17 Peltomaa M, McHugh G, Steere AC: Persistence of the antibody response to the sixth invariant region (IR6) peptide of *Borrelia burgdorferi* after successful antibiotic treatment of Lyme disease. J Infect Dis 2003;187:1178–1186.

18 Maraspin V, Cimperman J, Lotric-Furlan S, Ruzic-Sabljic E, Jurca T, Picken R, Strle F: Solitary borrelial lymphocytoma in adult patients. Wien Klin Wochenschr 2002;114:515–523.

19 Olsson I, Asbrink E, von-Stedingk M, von-Stedingk LV: Changes in *Borrelia burgdorferi*-specific serum IgG antibody levels in patients treated for acrodermatitis chronica atrophicans. Acta Derm Venereol (Stockh) 1994;74:424–428.

Prof. Dr. Robert Müllegger
Department of Dermatology, State Hospital Wiener Neustadt
Corvinusring 3–5
AT–2700 Wiener Neustadt (Austria)
Tel. +43 2622 321 4901, Fax +43 2622 321 4905, E-Mail robert.muellegger@wienerneustadt.lknoe.at

Lipsker D, Jaulhac B (eds): Lyme Borreliosis.
Curr Probl Dermatol. Basel, Karger, 2009, vol 37, pp 183–190

How Do I Manage Tick Bites and Lyme Borreliosis in Pregnant Women?

Vera Maraspin · Franc Strle

Department of Infectious Diseases, University Medical Center Ljubljana, Ljubljana, Slovenia

Abstract

In this report, we present basic data pertinent to the current understanding of borrelial infection in pregnancy, and propose a rationale for the management of Lyme borreliosis in pregnant women. We advocate early detection of attached ticks and their prompt removal. We do not recommend the use of prophylactic antibiotics in pregnant women but support the 'wait and watch' strategy, including early treatment with antibiotics if signs/symptoms of the disease arise. We encourage the approach that antibiotic treatment of pregnant patients is restricted to those having a reliable clinical diagnosis of Lyme borreliosis, and propose intravenous antibiotic treatment with penicillin, or preferably ceftriaxone 2 g daily for 14 days, not only for patients with early disseminated disease but also for those with solitary erythema migrans.

The objectives of this report are to present basic data pertinent to the current understanding of borrelial infection in pregnancy, and to propose a rationale for the management of Lyme borreliosis in pregnant women.

Management of pregnancy encompasses management of the woman herself and of her fetus. Although this distinction is usually somewhat artificial, it is useful for appreciation of the suggestions presented here for management of tick bites in pregnant women and for treatment of Lyme borreliosis during pregnancy, both of which are based on rather elusive evidence.

There are no precise data on the natural course and outcome of Lyme borreliosis during pregnancy, but there is a general belief that there are no substantial differences between pregnant and nonpregnant individuals with Lyme borreliosis, and that pregnant women treated for Lyme borreliosis have an outcome similar to those of the corresponding adult population. However, to our best knowledge there has been no direct comparison of the outcome of treatment for individual clinical manifestations of Lyme borreliosis in pregnant and non-pregnant women of comparable age.

Information on the influence of borrelial infection on the fetus is also incomplete. In general, circumstances in which an infection of a pregnant woman may have detrimental influence on the fetus include: (1) severe illness of the mother, associated with circulatory instability and/or other harmful effects that subsequently damage her fetus, (2) induction of immunological mechanisms and/or (3) production of toxins that damage the fetus directly or indirectly through impairment of the placenta, and/or (4) damage of the fetus by the microorganisms causing the illness in the pregnant woman either directly or indirectly through damage of the placenta. The prerequisite for the latter outcome is (hematogenous) dissemination of the causative agent to the placenta and eventually to the fetus.

With the possible exception of complete atrioventricular block (which is a fairly rare clinical manifestation), Lyme borreliosis in adults is not an acute life-threatening illness causing circulatory instability [1, 2]. It has also never been known to induce severe immune reactions or production of toxins, and thus does not detrimentally influence the fetus in this mode [1, 2]. However, it is recognized that in Lyme borreliosis patients, borreliae do enter the blood [1–7], although it is less well established precisely when in the course of the illness the dissemination begins, what the duration of this dissemination is, whether it is continuous or intermittent, and if it occurs only during the initial illness or also later in the course of the disease.

The majority of patients with Lyme borreliosis present with erythema migrans, an early clinical manifestation of the disease. Erythema migrans usually develops at the site of a tick bite and consequent inoculation of the causative agent (*Borrelia burgdorferi* sensu lato) into the skin. In some patients not (properly) treated for their erythema migrans, days to months later skin, neurologic, cardiac, joint and/or ocular manifestations of Lyme borreliosis may appear; these are interpreted as the result of hematogenous dissemination of borreliae from the infected skin to other tissues or organs [1, 2]. According to current information, the presence of *B. burgdorferi* sensu lato in blood, as determined by culture, has been reported nearly exclusively in the course of early Lyme borreliosis, i.e. in patients with solitary or multiple erythema migrans, but – with a few exceptions indicated by individual case reports – not in other manifestations of Lyme borreliosis [3–6]. In patients with erythema migrans, blood-borne borreliae have been found more often (in up to 44%) [6] in the USA, where the only known causative agent of Lyme borreliosis in humans is *B. burgdorferi* sensu stricto [1, 2], than in Europe (in 9% children and in 1.2% adults), where the predominant agent associated with erythema migrans is *B. afzelii* [1, 2, 4, 5]. Nevertheless, because of methodological dissimilarities, including the precise volume of blood cultured for the presence of borreliae, the differences are not completely reliable and should be interpreted with caution. Whereas the majority (up to 89%) of American patients with erythema migrans and borreliae present in their blood had systemic symptoms such as fatigue, arthralgia, myalgia, headache, fever and/or stiff neck [7], the proportion of corresponding adult European patients with systemic symptoms was much lower (7/35, 20%) [4]. Thus, at least in Europe, in a patient with solitary erythema migrans, no reliable simple surrogate clinical indicator of the presence of borreliae in blood is available. We were not able to find any systematic analysis on the presence of blood-borne *B. burgdorferi* sensu lato in manifestations of Lyme borreliosis other than in solitary and multiple erythema migrans. Thus, although the absence of spirochetemia later in the course of Lyme borreliosis seems logical and is generally acknowledged, it is based on assumptions and is not supported by facts.

Although it is well known that *B. burgdorferi* sensu lato may be present in the blood early in the course of Lyme borreliosis, the consequences of this for the fetus are not clear cut. It is recognized that in spirochetal diseases, such as syphilis, relapsing fever and leptospirosis, the causative agents can pass transplacentally from the infected mother to the offspring and cause an adverse outcome [8]. In Lyme borreliosis, in utero transmission of *B. burgdorferi* sensu lato during pregnancy, resulting in fetal involvement, has been reported in humans [9–12] and in animals such as cows, horses, dogs and mice [13–15]. Nevertheless, several reports of fetal involvement in humans are limited to the description of single cases, and in some articles the proof of borrelial infection is rather vague by present standards.

Suggested Measures after a Tick Bite in a Pregnant Woman

Early Detection of the Attached Tick and its Prompt Removal

After returning from outdoor activities, pregnant women should make careful inspection of their entire body for attached ticks, and in Lyme borreliosis endemic areas routine daily checking is warranted [16].

The risk of transmission of borreliae increases with the duration of attachment; therefore, prompt removal of the attached ticks is important in preventing the disease [1, 2, 16]. The tick should be grasped with fine (sharply pointed) forceps as close as possible to the point of attachment and pulled out with a steady motion directed away from the skin. Local disinfection is required [1, 2, 16].

Testing Ticks for the Presence of B. burgdorferi *sensu lato*

Testing ticks for tick-borne infectious agents is not recommended, except in research studies [16].

Chemoprophylaxis with Antibiotics after a Tick Bite

Chemoprophylaxis after a tick bite has most probably been used extensively in everyday clinical practice in several European countries and in the USA, in spite of the absence of official general recommendations for such an approach. The prophylaxis is most probably based on the belief that antimicrobial agents, given within a short period after a tick bite, could eradicate an incubating borrelial infection and prevent the illness. Data on the effectiveness of this measure are limited and mainly restricted to information from the USA. In several studies, the efficacy of prophylactic antibiotics, such as phenoxymethylpenicillin [17, 18], doxycycline [19] or amoxicillin [20], was not ascertained (theoretically, at least partly because the studies were statistically underpowered). However, a single dose of 200 mg doxycycline given within 72 h after tick detachment has been shown to prevent Lyme borreliosis in 87% (95% CI: 25–98%) of individuals [21]. An expert panel of the Infectious Diseases Society of America (IDSA) recently updated guidelines on the management of Lyme disease (American Lyme borreliosis) [16]. According to IDSA, the routine use of prophylaxis with antibiotics is not recommended, but a single dose of doxycycline 'may be offered when all of the following circumstances exist: (1) the attached tick can be reliably identified as an adult or nymphal *Ixodes scapularis* tick that is estimated to have been attached for ≥36 h on the basis of the degree of engorgement of the tick with blood or of certainty about the time of exposure to the tick; (2) prophylaxis can be started within 72 h of the time that the tick was removed; (3) ecologic information indicates that the local rate of infection of these ticks with *B. burgdorferi* is ≥20%; (4) doxycycline treatment is not contraindicated'. Because doxycycline is known to have several adverse effects, including slowed bone growth, enamel hypoplasia, permanent yellowing of the teeth and increased susceptibility to cavities in offspring, and occasionally induces liver failure in pregnant women, it is contraindicated during pregnancy. The panel 'does not believe that amoxicillin should be substituted for doxycycline in persons for whom doxycycline prophylaxis is contraindicated because of the absence of data on an effective short-course regimen for prophylaxis, the likely need for a multi-day regimen (and its associated side effects), the excellent efficacy of antibiotic treatment of Lyme disease if infection were to develop, and the extremely low risk that a person with a recognized bite will develop a serious complication of Lyme disease' [16]. The reported findings on the effectiveness of prophylaxis with doxycycline are valid for *I. scapularis* ticks and *B. burgdorferi* sensu stricto, and might not be the same for other *Ixodes* or *Borrelia* species. The value of antibiotic prophylaxis is also restricted by potential side effects, and by the danger of inducing antimicrobial resistance as a consequence of antibiotic overuse [2]. We therefore do not recommend antibiotic prophylaxis in a pregnant woman after a tick bite.

Other Measures

The skin should be carefully observed for eventual development of erythema migrans for at least a month after removal of a tick. If signs and symptoms of Lyme borreliosis appear, prompt antibiotic treatment is warranted [1, 2, 22].

Suggested Treatment of Lyme Borreliosis in Pregnant Women

Treatment with antibiotics is beneficial in all stages of Lyme borreliosis; however, its effectiveness is highest in early disease [1, 2, 22]. Antibiotic therapy not only reduces the duration of erythema migrans and alleviates and shortens associated symptoms, but is also reasonably effective in preventing further progression of the illness. Through early recognition and prompt treatment of erythema migrans, later manifestations of Lyme borreliosis can be effectively prevented [1, 2, 22].

From the standpoint of the health of pregnant women, approaches for treatment of Lyme borreliosis could be the same as those for nonpregnant women. However, because of potential harmful effects on the fetus of some of the recommended antibiotics there are several restrictions, and it is probable that somewhat different approaches are warranted to ensure effective prevention and treatment of potential *Borrelia* infection of the placenta and/or the fetus.

In general, pregnant women, even more so than for other patients, should not be given antibiotics without strong evidence of a bacterial infection. Use of any antibiotic during pregnancy should be based on whether benefits outweigh risk, which may vary by trimester. The chosen antibiotic has to be effective in the treatment of infection, and safe for both the mother and the developing fetus. All antimicrobial agents cross the placenta to some degree, enabling not only the possibility of effective antibiotic treatment, but also exposure of the fetus to the potentially adverse effect of the drug. Taking into account the level of risk the drug poses to the fetus, the Food and Drug Administration (FDA) has assigned drugs into categories A, B, C, D and X. Currently, there are no completely safe antibiotics for treatment in pregnancy (category A – studies in pregnant women show no risk). Several antibiotics, including penicillins, cephalosporins, erythromycin and some other macrolides, metronidazole, monobactams and the majority of carbapenems, are classified as category B. These drugs are thought to be relatively safe (animal studies show no risk, but human data are insufficient; or animal studies show toxicity, but human data show no risk) and are an appropriate choice for treatment in pregnancy. Among the less safe antimicrobial drugs belonging to FDA group C (animal studies show toxicity, human data are insufficient, but clinical benefit may exceed risk) are antibiotics such as fluoroquinolones, some aminoglycosides, linezolid, telithromycin and teicoplanin. For use, risk and benefits must be carefully evaluated. Among drugs that should be avoided (FDA group D – there is evidence of human risk, but clinical benefits may outweigh the risk), unless necessary for serious or life-threatening infections during pregnancy, are tetracyclines, tigecycline, and some aminoglycosides.

However, for antibiotics that cross the placenta, not only their safety but also their effectiveness must be considered. Dosages of drugs often need to be adjusted (usually increased) to accommodate changes deriving from physiologic alterations in pregnancy.

For the treatment of Lyme borreliosis, antibiotics such as tetracyclines (usually doxycycline), penicillins (including amoxicillin, penicillin V and penicillin G), second-generation cephalosporins (cefuroxime axetil), third-generation cephalosporins (ceftriaxone, cefotaxime) and some macrolides (predominantly for patients allergic to β-lactam antibiotics) are usually recommended [1, 2, 16, 22]. Patients with (solitary) erythema migrans are normally treated with oral antibiotics, whereas the main indication for intravenous treatment is (potential) nervous system involvement [1, 2, 16, 22]. Recommendations for the treatment of gestational Lyme borreliosis are diverse. There is consensus that tetracyclines should be avoided during pregnancy and that the antibiotics of choice are penicillins and cephalosporins, but there are disagreements on several other issues. Some clinicians recommend treatment of gestational Lyme borreliosis with penicillins or cephalosporins determined by clinical manifestation and severity of the infection. This usually consists of oral antibiotic treatment for early localized Lyme borreliosis and intravenous treatment for early disseminated and late disease, because of their impression that the actual risk of development of congenital Lyme borreliosis is exceedingly low and that there is no need for more aggressive treatment of gestational Lyme borreliosis [16]. Other clinicians, concerned about (potential) transplacental spread of borreliae, recommend longer [23] or more aggressive therapy such as intravenous antibiotic treatment for (all cases of) gestational Lyme borreliosis [22, 23]. No investigation comparing the efficacy of these 3 approaches (i.e. an approach similar to that used in the general population, prolonged treatment, or more aggressive treatment) has been published. There are also no reliable studies on the outcome of Lyme borreliosis after treatment with the approach as used in the nonpregnant population, or with longer treatment using identical antibiotics, dosages and mode of application as used for the nonpregnant population. The only published prospective study on treatment of Lyme borreliosis during pregnancy is a report on 58 consecutively enrolled patients treated for gestational erythema migrans with ceftriaxone 2 g daily for 14 days [24] and its extension with the addition of 47 further patients [25]. According to these 2 reports, none of the 105 consecutive pregnant women so treated for erythema migrans developed any subsequent manifestation of Lyme borreliosis. The majority of them (93/105, 88.6%) gave birth at term to healthy babies with normal later psychomotor development. The other 12 (11.4%) pregnancies ended with abortion in 2 cases (1 missed abortion at 9 weeks, 1 spontaneous abortion at 10 weeks), preterm delivery in 6 cases (2 of these 6 babies died, 1 was established as having heart abnormality) and congenital abnormalities in 4 babies delivered at term (urinary tract abnormalities in 3, syndactylia in 1). A causative relationship with borrelial infection was not established in any of these 12 cases, and in several of them acceptable alternative explanations for the unfavorable outcomes were found [24, 25].

Based on the encouraging results of these studies and in the absence of reliable information on the efficacy of other therapeutic approaches, we propose intravenous antibiotic therapy, preferably with ceftriaxone 2 g daily for 14 days, for all gestational

Lyme borreliosis. This suggestion is offered because case reports, although rare, have suggested that Lyme borreliosis during pregnancy may be associated with adverse outcomes for the fetus [9–12], and out of concern that neither the occurrence of transplacental dissemination nor the timing of such an occurrence during the acute infection can be accurately assessed.

Lactating patients may be treated in the same way as nonlactating patients with the same disease manifestations, except that doxycycline should be avoided [16].

Conclusions

We advocate early detection of attached ticks and their prompt removal. We do not recommend the use of prophylactic antibiotics in pregnant women but support the 'wait and watch' strategy, including early treatment with antibiotics if signs/symptoms of the disease arise.

We encourage the approach that antibiotic treatment of pregnant patients is restricted to those having a reliable clinical diagnosis of Lyme borreliosis, and propose intravenous antibiotic treatment with penicillin, or preferably ceftriaxone 2 g daily for 14 days, not only for patients with early disseminated disease but also for those with solitary erythema migrans.

Lactating patients may be treated in the same way as nonlactating patients with the same disease manifestations, except that doxycycline should be avoided.

References

1 Steere AC: Lyme disease. N Engl J Med 2001;345: 115–125.

2 Stanek G, Strle F: Lyme borreliosis. Lancet 2003; 362:1639–1647.

3 Nadelman RB, Pavia CS, Magnarelli LA, Wormser GP: Isolation of *Borrelia burgdorferi* from the blood of seven patients with Lyme disease. Am J Med 1990;88:21–26.

4 Maraspin V, Ružić-Sabljić E, Cimperman J, Lotrič-Furlan S, Jurca T, Picken RN, Strle F: Isolation of *Borrelia burgdorferi* sensu lato from blood of patients with erythema migrans. Infection 2001;29: 65–70.

5 Arnez M, Ružić-Sabljić E, Ahcan J, Radsel-Medvescek A, Pleterski-Rigler D, Strle: Isolation of *Borrelia burgdorferi* sensu lato from blood of children with solitary erythema migrans. Pediatr Infect Dis J 2001;20:251–255.

6 Wormser GP, Bittker S, Cooper D, Nowakowsky J, Nadelman RB, Pavia C: Yield of large-volume blood cultures in patients with early Lyme disease. J Infect Dis 2001;184:1070–1072.

7 Wormser GP, McKenna D, Carlin J, Nadelman RB, Cavaliere LF, Holmgren D, Byrne DW, Nowakowski J: Hematogenous dissemination in early Lyme disease. Ann Intern Med 2005;142:751–755.

8 Taber LH, Feigin RD: Spirochetal infections. Pediatr Clin North Am 1979;26:377–413.

9 Schlesinger PA, Duray PH, Burke SA, Steere AC, Stillman MT: Maternal-fetal transmission of the Lyme disease spirochete, *Borrelia burgdorferi*. Ann Intern Med 1985;103:67–68.

10 Markowitz LE, Steere AC, Benach JL, Slade JD, Broome CV: Lyme disease during pregnancy. JAMA 1986;255:3394–3396.

11 MacDonald AB, Benach JL, Burgdorfer W: Stillbirth following maternal Lyme disease. NY State J Med 1987;87:615–616.

12 Weber K, Bratzke HJ, Neubert U, Wilske B, Duray PH: *Borrelia burgdorferi* in a newborn despite oral penicillin for Lyme borreliosis during pregnancy. Pediatr Infect Dis J 1988;7:286–289.
13 Burgess EC: *Borrelia burgdorferi* infection in Wisconsin horses and cows. Ann NY Acad Sci 1988; 539:235–243.
14 Gustafson J, Burges EC, Wachal MD, Steinberg H: Intrauterine transmission of *B. burgdorferi* in dogs. Am J Vet Res 1993;54:882–890.
15 Silver R, Yang L, Daynes RA, Branch DW, Salafia CM, Weis JJ: Fetal outcome in murine Lyme disease. Infect Immun 1995;63:66–72.
16 Wormser GP, Dattwyler RJ, Shapiro ED, Halperin JJ, Steere AC, Klempner MS, Krause PJ, Bakken JS, Strle F, Stanek G, Bockenstedt L, Fish D, Dumler S, Nadelman R: The clinical assessment, treatment, and prevention of Lyme disease, human granulocytic anaplasmosis, and babesiosis: clinical practice guidelines by the Infectious Diseases Society of America. Clin Infect Dis 2006;43:1089–1134.
17 Costello CM, Steere AC, Pinkerton RJ, Feder HM Jr: A prospective study of tick bites in an endemic area for Lyme disease. J Infect Dis 1989;159:136–139.
18 Agre F, Schwartz R: The value of early treatment of deer tick bites for the prevention of Lyme disease. Am J Dis Child 1993;147:945–947.
19 Korenberg EI, Vorobyeva NN, Moskvitina HG, Ya Gorban L: Prevention of borreliosis in persons bitten by infected ticks. Infection 1996;24:187–189.
20 Shapiro ED, Gerber MA, Holabird ND, Berg AT, Feder HM Jr, Bell GL, Rys PN, Persing DH: A controlled trial of antimicrobial prophylaxis for Lyme disease after deer-tick bites. N Engl J Med 1992;327: 1769–1773.
21 Nadelman RB, Nowakowski J, Fish D, Falco RC, Freeman K, McKenna D, Welch P, Marcus R, Aguero-Rosenfeld ME, Dennis DT, Wormser GP: Prophylaxis with single-dose doxycycline for the prevention of Lyme disease after an *Ixodes scapularis* tick bite. N Engl J Med 2001;345:79–84.
22 Strle F: Principles of the diagnosis and antibiotic treatment of Lyme borreliosis. Wien Klin Wochenschr 1999;111:911–915.
23 Gardner T: Lyme disease; in Remington JS, Klein JO (eds): Infectious Diseases of the Fetus and Newborn Infant. Philadelphia, WB Saunders, 2001, pp 519–641.
24 Maraspin V, Cimperman J, Lotric-Furlan S, Pleterski-Rigler D, Strle F: Treatment of erythema migrans in pregnancy. Clin Infect Dis 1996;22:788–793.
25 Maraspin V, Cimperman J, Lotric-Furlan S, Pleterski-Rigler D, Strle F: Erythema migrans in pregnancy. Wien Klin Wochenschr 1999;111:933–940.

Vera Maraspin, MD, PhD
Department of Infectious Diseases, University Medical Center Ljubljana
Japljeva 2
SI–1525 Ljubljana (Slovenia)
Tel. +386 1 522 2110, Fax +386 1 522 2456, E-Mail vera.maraspin@kclj.si

Lipsker D, Jaulhac B (eds): Lyme Borreliosis.
Curr Probl Dermatol. Basel, Karger, 2009, vol 37, pp 191–199

What Should Be Done in Case of Persistent Symptoms after Adequate Antibiotic Treatment for Lyme Disease?

Xavier Puéchal[a] · Jean Sibilia[b]

[a]Service de Rhumatologie, Centre Hospitalier du Mans, Le Mans, et [b]Service de Rhumatologie, Hôpital de Hautepierre, Hôpitaux Universitaires de Strasbourg, Strasbourg, France

Abstract

The most common cause of treatment failure is incorrect diagnosis. Most patients cured of Lyme disease remain seropositive for long periods, and no laboratory test allows one to differentiate between cured and active infection. The first step is to check that the patient fulfils the diagnostic criteria for Lyme disease and that the antibiotic regimen has been administered according to the current recommendations. In the case of persistent arthritis after a first course of antibiotics, it is generally recommended to give a second course of treatment with a different drug. Ceftriaxone should be administered intravenously for arthritis that did not respond to previous oral therapy with doxycycline or amoxicillin. Despite resolution of the objective manifestations of Lyme disease after antibiotic treatment, a small proportion of patients still complain of subjective musculoskeletal pain, fatigue, difficulties with concentration or short-term memory, or all these symptoms. Given the risk of serious adverse events and the lack of efficacy, a consensus has emerged that repeated courses of antibiotic therapy are not indicated for persistent subjective symptoms following Lyme disease. The patient should be thoroughly examined for medical conditions that could explain the symptoms. If a diagnosis is made for which no specific treatment can be proposed, emotional support and management of pain, fatigue and other symptoms is required.

The persistence of complaints in a patient with a prior diagnosis of Lyme disease raises a number of issues [1]: (1) The most common cause of treatment failure is incorrect diagnosis. Thus, in patients with chronic objective complaints, a lack of response to therapy suggests above all the possibility of initial misdiagnosis and the need for prompt reassessment rather than retreatment. (2) True persistent infection is a rare situation, and persistence or progression of the disease has only been documented with the use of lower-dose or shorter-duration antibiotic therapy than is now recommended. The most likely explanation is that the initial regimen was inappropriate due to insufficient tissue penetration or concentration of the antibiotic. Many such patients can be cured by a longer duration or higher dose of antibiotics [2]. (3) Another possible explanation in some situations is the long time lapse before achieving a complete cure. (4) Irreversible tissue damage exists in some clinical situations, and can be misinterpreted in some patients as evolving Lyme disease. (5) Local immune reactivity to poorly degraded antigens or evolution towards a 'reactive' or autoimmune process can explain persistent arthritis in certain patients. (6) Although some patients relapse with objective symptoms despite an appropriate antibiotic regimen, very few with persisting complaints fall into this category. It is generally recommended that a different drug, a longer duration and/or a higher dose of a previous antibiotic be given for a second course of treatment. There may have been inadequate penetration of the first drug to privileged sites where the spirochetes reside, 'resistance', intracellular survival of the organism [1] or reinfection [3]. (7) Finally, in some individuals who have had Lyme disease, there have been reports of subjective musculoskeletal complaints, fatigue and disorders of sleep. The management of such patients will be discussed in the final section of this chapter.

The management of a patient with persistent symptoms of Lyme disease requires this type of structured reasoning, bearing in mind that no laboratory test currently available allows differentiation between cured and active infection and that most patients with cured Lyme disease remain seropositive for long periods. Specialist advice is often necessary to explain the absence of a need for further antibiotic treatment potentially involving significant side effects and costs.

After having checked that the patient fulfils the international diagnostic criteria for Lyme disease and that the antibiotic regimen has been administered according to the actual recommendations, the management of these patients varies according to the clinical features.

Persistent Cutaneous Manifestations of Early Lyme Disease

Natural Evolution of Erythema Migrans

The cutaneous symptoms of the early manifestations of Lyme borreliosis may last several weeks after the end of an appropriate antibiotic regimen. This delay should not be interpreted as a treatment failure.

Management

In this clinical setting, there is no need to extend the duration of antibiotic treatment or to give an additional antibiotics [4]. However, if lesions persist more than 3 months after the end of treatment, the diagnosis of erythema migrans should be reconsidered. A cutaneous biopsy is then indicated.

Persistent Arthritis

Natural Evolution of Arthritis

The natural evolution of Lyme arthritis has been documented in historical cohorts before the use of antibiotics [5, 6]. Lyme arthritis, which had a tendency to persist during the second and third years of the disease [7], finally healed after a few years despite the absence of antibiotic therapy [7, 8].

In patients with arthritis, clinical recovery typically coincides with antibiotic therapy. In a cost-effectiveness analysis, Magid et al. [9] found that oral doxycycline was effective in 70% of cases and intravenous ceftriaxone in 50%. Despite antibiotic treatment, joint swelling persists for some months to a few years in about 10% of adults with Lyme arthritis [5, 6, 10] and may be associated with bone and cartilaginous damage. Refractory Lyme arthritis is defined as chronic persistent arthritis sometimes with destructive changes, and with no improvement after at least a 2-month course of antibiotic therapy.

Management

In the case of persistent arthritis after a first course of antibiotics, it is generally recommended to give a second course of treatment with a different drug. Ceftriaxone should be administered intravenously for arthritis that did not respond to previous oral therapy with doxycycline or amoxicillin.

In the case of non-response despite correct diagnosis and antibiotic treatment, it is important for the clinician to document evidence of inflammation and consider other causes of arthralgia or arthritis. Non-inflammatory joint pain after Lyme disease is not Lyme arthritis. Quadriceps femoris muscle atrophy can result from Lyme arthritis and may cause mechanical patellofemoral joint dysfunction and pain. In this case, physiotherapy should restore normal quadriceps tone. Mechanical pain may also result from long-standing arthritis with subsequent cartilage damage, and analgesics or nonsteroidal anti-inflammatory drugs (NSAID) can improve the pain and function.

Polymerase Chain Reaction Analysis

At this stage, an arthrocentesis should be performed to confirm the synovial inflammation and allow synovial fluid to be studied by PCR analysis with specific primers. When possible, a synovial tissue biopsy should be analyzed since it is a more sensitive medium than synovial fluid for the PCR detection of *Borrelia burgdorferi*.

The persistence of organisms or of some of their antigens may be crucial for the perpetuation of a local inflammatory reaction. *B. burgdorferi* DNA can be detected by PCR in the synovial fluid of up to 96% of patients with Lyme arthritis having received no treatment or only short courses of oral antibiotics [11]. Its detection is less frequently successful in patients who had received previous antibiotic therapy, and even more rare in patients with chronic refractory Lyme arthritis after several courses of antibiotics. The mechanisms of treatment resistance in Lyme arthritis remain controversial. The theory of intra-articular survival of bacteria opposes that of the induction of a self-perpetuating autoreactive reaction by cross-reactivity between certain bacterial antigens and host components.

When PCR gives a positive result for *B. burgdorferi*, another course of antibiotic treatment should be given using a drug different from the one previously prescribed. Local treatment should be proposed if the PCR results are negative. This strategy generally cures the joint inflammation, although it does not always prevent cartilage damage.

Intra-Articular Corticosteroid Injections

In chronic Lyme arthritis, intra-articular corticosteroids are useful to immediately relieve a symptomatic joint effusion [8, 12, 13]. Nevertheless, since a few studies have provided weak methodological evidence of a deleterious effect, it would seem advisable not to carry out articular injections before or during antibiotic therapy. Injections are recommended for patients whose joint effusion persists after antibiotic treatment [12] or despite 2 courses of oral therapy or 1 course of IV therapy antibiotics [13]. Some authors [7, 8, 14] argue that injections should only be performed after having checked that PCR results in the joint fluid are negative.

Chemical or Radiation Synovectomy

A few isolated case reports have pointed to the efficacy of chemical (osmic acid) or radiation synovectomy (rhenium, yttrium) in refractory Lyme arthritis [15]. Radiation synovectomy may be indicated in persistent synovitis after antibiotics and before a surgical procedure. Further studies will be necessary to address its role in the local therapeutic arsenal. Chemical or radiation synovectomy is not at present mentioned in the IDSA (Infectious Diseases Society of America) recommendations [13].

Arthroscopic Synovectomy

Arthroscopic synovectomy can reduce the period of joint inflammation when persistent synovitis is associated with significant pain or limited function [8, 13]. Several authors recommend opting for this procedure only when the synovitis persists after 2 months of antibiotics and the PCR joint test is negative [7]. On the other hand, arthroscopic synovectomy remains a matter of debate in refractory Lyme arthritis given its inconstant efficacy [16] and the possibility of postoperative sequelae [17], particularly in childhood [4]. These aspects are to be considered in the light of the spontaneous favorable outcomes of most cases of Lyme arthritis after a few years, even without antibiotic therapy.

Disease Modifying Anti-Rheumatic Drugs

Hydroxychloroquine has been described to be of some benefit [8], but this has not been confirmed [12]. Disease-modifying anti-rheumatic drugs used in reactive arthritis, such as methotrexate or sulfasalazine, have not been evaluated in appropriate studies of refractory Lyme arthritis.

Systemic Corticosteroids

There are concordant experimental data showing that systemic corticosteroids are deleterious and their use is not indicated in Lyme disease.

Nonsteroidal Anti-Inflammatory Drugs

NSAID are often prescribed for their non-specific symptomatic effects [5, 10]. Symptomatic treatment with NSAID is recommended in the case of persistent arthritis [13].

In summary, after a second course of antibiotic therapy for refractory Lyme arthritis, negative PCR results for synovial fluid generally indicate removal of synovial fluid and local injection of long-term corticosteroids. Analgesics and NSAID are also useful. In the case of failure or relapse after a few weeks, another injection may be performed. On the other hand, one should give an additional course of antibiotics according to the usual recommendations [4, 13] if the PCR results are positive. In the very rare instance of relapse after this therapy, radiation or mechanical synovectomy should be discussed. The outcome is usually favorable.

Persistent Neurological Symptoms

Natural Evolution of Neuroborreliosis

In the majority of patients with early neuroborreliosis, the pain intensity diminishes markedly after 1–4 days [18]. After an average of 1–2 months and up to 12 months of treatment for early neuroborreliosis, 20% of patients still complain of intermittent radicular pain and dysesthesia. A mean period of 7–8 weeks is required for complete recovery of motor deficits [19]. Significant disabling sequelae are mainly reported in patients with central nervous system involvement, although some individuals with motor weakness may display residual deficits after treatment, such as mild seventh nerve palsy. Sensory complaints may also persist [18].

In patients with long-lasting meningitis or chronic encephalomyelitis, the onset of improvement after therapy is slower, but nevertheless marked [18].

Management

Patients whose condition does not improve after appropriate antibiotic therapy may have irreversible damage to the nervous system, particularly if the prior disease has been of long duration. There is no evidence in the literature to support additional antibiotic treatment in patients with persistent neurological symptoms after an adequate first course of antibiotics. Nevertheless, as the equivalence of tetracyclines and ceftriaxone remains to be established, a course of ceftriaxone should be administered to patients previously treated with oral drugs. In the event of relapse after a 2-week course of intravenous ceftriaxone, the most likely explanation is failure to completely eradicate the spirochete, and a 1-month course usually leads to improvement [20]. Analgesics and medications used for neuropathic pain are often useful. Systemic corticosteroids have been proposed to obtain analgesia more quickly [21], but this treatment cannot be recommended on account of the low level of supporting evidence and possible deleterious effects.

Persistent Fatigue Immediately after Treatment of Lyme Disease

Up to 10% of patients with Lyme disease in some endemic areas are coinfected with babesiosis (due to *Babesia microti*) [22]. Other tick-transmitted zoonoses such as human granulocytic ehrlichiosis (rickettsiosis due to *Anaplasma phagocytophilum*) also occur in areas where these 2 pathogens are endemic.

Patients with Lyme disease and laboratory evidence of coinfection with babesiosis are more likely to present constitutional symptoms (e.g. fatigue, headache, sweats, chills) than patients with isolated Lyme disease [22]. Persistent and debilitating fatigue is characteristic of coinfection. Persistent symptoms lasting for 3 months or more, among which fatigue is the most common, are encountered in half of coinfected patients, but are very unusual (4%) in individuals with isolated Lyme disease. Serologic testing for babesiosis should be performed in patients with fatigue persisting for more than 2 months after a history of Lyme disease. Anti-babesial therapy consists of clindamycin and quinine. It should be pointed out that coexposure to *B. burgdor-*

feri and *Babesia microti* does not worsen the long-term outcome of Lyme disease [23]. Patients examined years after coinfection do not display any differences in regard to the prevalence of constitutional, musculoskeletal or neurological complaints as compared to those affected by isolated Lyme disease. There is thus no reason to search for coinfection in patients with symptoms persisting years after Lyme disease.

A search for dual infection with the agents of Lyme borreliosis and human granulocytic ehrlichiosis cannot be recommended for persistent symptoms following Lyme disease because it remains to be determined whether this coinfection may result in more prolonged disease than infection with either agent alone [24].

Persistent Subjective Symptoms after Treatment of Lyme Disease

Despite resolution of the objective manifestations of Lyme disease after antibiotic treatment, a small proportion of patients still complain of subjective musculoskeletal pain, fatigue, difficulties with concentration or short term memory, or all these symptoms [25].

Natural Evolution of Lyme Disease

In prospective studies of patients with erythema migrans, subjective symptoms were present 1 year or more after treatment in 0.5–13.1% of cases [26]. Whether this prevalence exceeds that of such symptoms in the general population is unknown, since none of these studies included a control group [25]. Moreover, nearly 40% of these patients with subjective symptoms following Lyme disease had a positive response to placebo [27].

Several lines of evidence suggest that symptoms occurring after Lyme disease are not caused by an active occult infection of the central nervous system [4, 25]. There is no inflammation in the cerebrospinal fluid [27, 28], the results of both cultures and PCR assays for *B. burgdorferi* in the cerebrospinal fluid are negative [27], there are no structural abnormalities of the brain parenchyma, neurological function is normal and antibiotic treatment has no effect (as compared to placebo) on cognitive function [28, 29].

Management

Three double-blind randomized placebo-controlled studies have shown that there is a substantial risk, with little or no benefit, associated with additional antibiotic treatment in patients who have long-standing subjective symptoms after appropriate initial treatment of Lyme disease [27–29]. Given the risk of serious adverse events, a consensus has emerged that repeated courses of antibiotic therapy are not indicated for persistent subjective symptoms following Lyme disease, including those related to fatigue and cognitive dysfunction [28].

The patient should be thoroughly examined for medical conditions which could explain the symptoms [25]. The scientific evidence against the concept of chronic Lyme disease should be discussed, and the patient should be informed about the risk of unnecessary antibiotic therapy. If a diagnosis is made for which no specific treatment can be proposed, emotional support and management of pain, fatigue and other symptoms are required [25].

References

1 Sigal LH: Persisting complaints attributed to chronic Lyme disease: possible mechanisms and implications for management. Am J Med 1994;96:365–374.

2 Steere AC, Hutchinson GJ, Rahn DW, Sigal LH, Craft JE, DeSanna ET, et al: Treatment of the early manifestations of Lyme disease. Ann Intern Med 1983;99:22–26.

3 Krause PJ, Foley DT, Burke GS, Christianson D, Closter L, Spielman A; Tick-Borne Disease Study Group: Reinfection and relapse in early Lyme disease. Am J Trop Med Hyg 2006;75:1090–1094.

4 SPILF: 16ème conférence de consensus en thérapie anti-infectieuse. Borréliose de Lyme: démarches diagnostiques, thérapeutiques et préventives. http://www.infectiologie.com/site/medias/_documents/consensus/2006-lyme-long.pdf

5 Steere AC, Schoen RT, Taylor E: The clinical evolution of Lyme arthritis. Ann Intern Med 1987;107:725–731.

6 Szer IS, Taylor E, Steere AC: The long-term course of Lyme arthritis in children. N Engl J Med 1991;325:159–163.

7 Steere AC: Diagnosis and treatment of Lyme arthritis. Med Clin North Am 1997;81:179–194.

8 Steere AC, Levin RE, Molloy PJ, Kalish RA, Abraham JH 3rd, Liu NY, Schmid CH: Treatment of Lyme arthritis. Arthritis Rheum 1994;37:878–888.

9 Magid D, Schwartz B, Craft J, Schwartz JS: Prevention of Lyme disease after tick bites: a cost-effectiveness analysis. N Engl J Med 1992;327:534–541.

10 Steere AC, Green J, Schoen RT, Taylor E, Hutchinson GJ, Rahn DW, Malawista SE: Successful parenteral penicillin therapy of established Lyme arthritis. N Engl J Med 1985;312:869–874.

11 Nocton JJ, Dressler F, Rutledge BJ, Rys PN, Persing DH, Steere AC: Detection of Borrelia burgdorferi DNA by polymerase chain reaction in synovial fluid from patients with Lyme arthritis. N Engl J Med 1994;330:229–234.

12 Cimmino MA, Moggiana GL, Parisi M, Accardo S: Treatment of Lyme arthritis. Infection 1996;24:91–93.

13 Wormser GP, Nadelman RB, Dattwyler RJ, Dennis DT, Shapiro ED, Steere AC, Rush TJ, Rahn DW, Coyle PK, Persing DH, Fish D, Luft BJ: Practice guidelines for the treatment of Lyme disease. The Infectious Diseases Society of America. Clin Infect Dis 2000;31(suppl 1):1–14.

14 Sood SK, Ilowite NT: Lyme arthritis in children: is chronic arthritis a common complication? J Rheumatol 2000;27:1836–1838.

15 Limbach FX, Jaulhac B, Puéchal X, Monteil H, Kuntz JL, Piemont Y, Sibilia J: Treatment resistant Lyme arthritis caused by Borrelia garinii. Ann Rheum Dis 2001;60:284–286.

16 Bentas W, Karch H, Huppertz HI: Lyme arthritis in children and adolescents: outcome 12 months after initiation of antibiotic therapy. J Rheumatol 2000;27:2025–2030.

17 Steere AC, Gibofsky A, Patarroyo ME, Winchester RJ, Hardin JA, Malawista SE: Chronic Lyme arthritis: clinical and immunogenetic differentiation from rheumatoid arthritis. Ann Intern Med 1979;90:896–901.

18 Hansen K, Lebech AM: The clinical and epidemiological profile of Lyme neuroborreliosis in Denmark 1985–1990: a prospective study of 187 patients with *Borrelia burgdorferi* specific intrathecal antibody production. Brain 1992;115:399–423.

19 Pachner AR, Steere AC: The triad of neurologic manifestations of Lyme disease: meningitis, cranial neuritis, and radiculoneuritis. Neurology 1985;35:47–53.

20 Logigian EL, Kaplan Steere AC: Chronic neurologic manifestations of Lyme disease. N Engl J Med 1990;323:1438–1444.

21 Pfister HW, Einhäupl KM, Franz P, Garner C: Corticosteroids for radicular pain in Bannwarth's syndrome: a double-blind, randomized, placebo-controlled trial. Ann NY Acad Sci 1988;539:485–487.
22 Krause PJ, Telford SR 3rd, Spielman A, Sikand V, Ryan R, Christianson D, et al: Concurrent Lyme disease and babesiosis: evidence for increased severity and duration of illness. JAMA 1996;275:1657–1660.
23 Wang TJ, Liang MH, Sangha O, Phillips CB, Lew RA, Wright EA, et al: Coexposure to *Borrelia burgdorferi* and *Babesia microti* does not worsen the long-term outcome of Lyme disease. Clin Infect Dis 2000;31:1149–1154.
24 Nadelman RB, Horowitz HW, Hsieh TC, Wu JM, Aguero-Rosenfeld ME, Schwartz I, et al: Simultaneous human granulocytic ehrlichiosis and Lyme borreliosis. N Engl J Med 1997;337:27–30.
25 Feder HM Jr, Johnson BJ, O'Connell S, Shapiro ED, Steere AC, Wormser GP; Ad Hoc International Lyme Disease Group, et al: A critical appraisal of 'chronic Lyme disease'. N Engl J Med 2007;357:1422–1430.
26 Shapiro ED, Dattwyler R, Nadelman RB, Wormser GP: Response to meta-analysis of Lyme borreliosis symptoms. Int J Epidemiol 2005;34:1437–1439.
27 Klempner MS, Hu LT, Evans J, Schmid CH, Johnson GM, Trevino RP, et al: Two controlled trials of antibiotic treatment in patients with persistent symptoms and a history of Lyme disease. N Engl J Med 2001;345:85–92.
28 Krupp LB, Hyman LG, Grimson R, Coyle PK, Melville P, Ahnn S, Dattwyler R, Chandler B: Study and treatment of post Lyme disease (STOP-LD): a randomized double masked clinical trial. Neurology 2003;60:1923–1930.
29 Kaplan RF, Trevino RP, Johnson GM, Levy L, Dornbush R, Hu LT, et al: Cognitive function in post-treatment Lyme disease: do additional antibiotics help? Neurology 2003;60:1916–1922.

Xavier Puéchal, MD, PhD
Service de Rhumatologie, Centre Hospitalier du Mans
194, avenue Rubillard
FR–72037 Le Mans Cedex 9 (France)
Tel. +33 2 43 43 26 56, Fax +33 2 43 43 28 10, E-Mail xpuechal@ch-lemans.fr

Lipsker D, Jaulhac B (eds): Lyme Borreliosis.
Curr Probl Dermatol. Basel, Karger, 2009, vol 37, pp 200–206

What Are the Indications for Lumbar Puncture in Patients with Lyme Disease?

Tobias A. Rupprecht · Hans-Walter Pfister

Department of Neurology, Ludwig-Maximilians University, Munich, Germany

Abstract

Lyme neuroborreliosis (LNB) is a tick-borne disease of the nervous system, caused by the spirochete *Borrelia burgdorferi*. Having entered the host at the site of the tick bite, the spirochetes can initially cause a local inflammatory reaction, called erythema migrans. If left untreated, the *Borrelia* can disseminate in the second stage of the disease and invade the central nervous system, causing LNB. The diagnosis of LNB is based on a compatible clinical picture (meningitis, cranial neuritis or radiculoneuritis), lymphocytic pleocytosis in the cerebrospinal fluid (CSF) and intrathecal *Borrelia burgdorferi*-specific antibody production. As the clinical picture of LNB may be unspecific, a lumbar puncture to analyze the CSF is usually mandatory for confirmation of the suspected diagnosis. The indications for a lumbar puncture and the limitations of the different diagnostic procedures are the main topics of this review. In addition, a short overview of the epidemiology and the therapeutic principles of LNB is given.

Lyme borreliosis is the most common human tick-borne disease in the northern hemisphere. The prevalence is estimated to be 20–100 cases per 100,000 people in the USA and about 100–130 cases per 100,000 in Europe [1, 2]. It is caused by the spirochete *Borrelia burgdorferi* sensu lato. *B. burgdorferi* can be divided into 4 human pathogenic species: *B. burgdorferi* sensu stricto (the only human pathogenic species present in the USA), *B. afzelii*, *B. garinii* and *B. spielmanii* [3]. The infection by *B. burgdorferi* is a complex process beginning with the transition from the gut to the salivary glands of the tick during the feeding process on the host. After invasion into the skin, *B. burgdorferi* can cause a local infection called erythema migrans. During the second stage of Lyme disease, *B. burgdorferi* can spread from the site of the tick bite on the skin to various secondary organs throughout the body, including the heart, joints, and the peripheral and central nervous systems (CNS) [4].

Lyme Neuroborreliosis

Up to 10% of untreated erythema migrans patients in Europe develop a borrelial infection of the nervous system, called Lyme neuroborreliosis (LNB) [2]. The most frequent manifestation of LNB in Europe is meningoradiculitis, the so-called Garin-Bujadoux-Bannwarth's syndrome (GBBS) [5]. It is characterized by intense lancinating radicular pain especially at night, paresis of the cranial nerves (for example the facial or the abducens nerve) or the extremities, and inflammatory cerebrospinal fluid (CSF) changes. In GBBS, the most frequent species isolated from the CSF is *B. garinii* [6, 7]. In parallel, GBBS rarely occurs in the USA, where *B. burgdorferi* sensu stricto but not *B. garinii* is found, and instead meningitis is the predominant neurological manifestation, suggesting a certain organotropism of the different genospecies [8]. In contrast to its frequency in adults, GBBS is rather rare in children, occurring in less than 5% of the patients with neuroborreliosis. The most common manifestations in children with neuroborreliosis are acute facial nerve palsy (55% of patients) and lymphocytic meningitis (27%) [9]. Apart from GBBS and lymphocytic meningitis, other neurological manifestations of Lyme borreliosis during stage II are cranial neuritis, plexus neuritis, mononeuritis multiplex, and, rarely, acute encephalitis and myelitis [4, 8]. In contrast to the acute form of LNB, chronic neuroborreliosis is a rare manifestation, so far only observed months to years after infection in untreated patients. It mainly includes chronic progressive encephalomyelitis and cerebral vasculitis. Furthermore, acrodermatitis chronica atrophicans may be associated with axonal polyneuropathy in about 40% of patients [10].

Diagnosis of LNB: When Is a Lumbar Puncture Indicated?

The diagnosis of a nervous system infection with *B. burgdorferi* is based on a clinical picture compatible with LNB, lymphocytic pleocytosis in the CSF and intrathecal *B. burgdorferi*-specific antibody production (table 1) [10]. Therefore, the analysis of the CSF is mandatory for a reliable diagnosis.

However, when is a lumbar puncture indicated in patients with a borrelial infection and when should a LNB be suspected? There are several arguments to be considered:

Should Every Patient with a Local or Systemic Infection with B. burgdorferi *Undergo a Lumbar Puncture?*

Patients with a local or systemic infection with *B. burgdorferi* – either with a dermatologic manifestation, like erythema migrans, lymphocytoma or acrodermatitis chronica atrophicans, or an extracutaneous finding, like carditis or arthritis – do not

Table 1. Diagnostic criteria of LNB

Possible neuroborreliosis Typical clinical features (e.g. meningitis, meningoradiculitis, cranial nerve deficits) *B. burgdorferi*-specific IgG and/or IgM serum antibodies CSF findings not available/lumbar puncture not performed
Probable neuroborreliosis Criteria of possible neuroborreliosis plus: Inflammatory CSF changes (lymphocytic pleocytosis, elevated protein content, intrathecal IgG antibody production) Exclusion of other causes
Definite (proven) neuroborreliosis Criteria of probable neuroborreliosis plus: Intrathecal *B. burgdorferi*-specific antibody production (and/or positive culture or PCR)

need a routine lumbar puncture, as long as they do not have clinical signs of central or peripheral nervous system involvement. Only patients with neurological symptoms and signs compatible with LNB should undergo a lumbar puncture.

Are There Certain Constellations Where the Presence of Serum Antibodies Is Sufficient for the Diagnosis of LNB?

The combination of radicular signs and *B. burgdorferi*-specific antibodies in the serum is not sufficient for the definite diagnosis of LNB. Positive *B. burgdorferi*-specific antibodies can be detected in the serum of 5–25% of healthy persons [11]. Therefore, an analysis of the serum alone is insufficient, and would lead to a high rate of false-positive diagnoses. There might be the exception of a patient with characteristic GBBS, presenting with lancinating pain exacerbated at night and, for example, a facial palsy and a tick bite or even an erythema migrans in the recent history, where one has sufficient arguments for LNB. However, a lumbar puncture would be recommended even in this case, as only the CSF analysis can confirm the suspected diagnosis and exclude differential diagnoses.

Does the Detection of B. burgdorferi*-Specific IgM Antibodies Indicate an Acute Infection with* B. burgdorferi*?*

In contrast to many other microbial infections, *B. burgdorferi*-specific IgM antibodies do not necessarily indicate an acute infection. These IgM antibodies can persist for years, and even after sufficient antibiotic therapy [12]. Therefore, only an inflammatory reaction in the CSF (i.e. lymphocytic pleocytosis) documents the active infection and helps to distinguish acute infectious causes from previous neuroborreliosis (as the *B. burgdorferi*-specific antibodies might only be an indicator of an earlier, currently not active, borrelial infection) [10]. On the other hand, the lack of serum or CSF *B. burgdorferi*-specific IgM antibodies does not contradict a very recent primary infection, as IgM-antibodies might be absent in early stages of the disease and do not have to precede the production of *B. burgdorferi*-specific IgG antibodies [12]. Taken together, the presence or absence of *B. burgdorferi*-specific IgM antibodies in the serum neither proves nor excludes an acute infection. Therefore, the measurement of IgM antibodies is not a substitute for a lumbar puncture.

In conclusion, the only method to prove the diagnosis of acute LNB is the analysis of the CSF. Lumbar puncture is indicated in every patient with a clinical picture compatible with LNB and no otherwise obvious causes, even in the absence of other manifestations of borreliosis or a documented tick bite. Many tick bites may have occurred without being noticed and the involvement of organs other than the brain could have passed unrecognized. Even negative serum antibodies do not exclude a LNB in early phases of infection, as the immune reaction in the CSF might precede the production of antibodies in the blood. Up to now, no blood parameter has been found that could replace CSF analysis.

Analysis of the CSF

The CSF has to be analyzed for several factors. First, the inflammatory reaction of the CNS has to be documented. A minimal routine analysis, including the count and differentiation of the CSF leukocytes, the total amount of CSF protein and the CSF-to-serum glucose ratio, is mandatory. Patients with acute LNB generally have moderate, lymphocytic pleocytosis (30–1,000 cells/mm^3), a moderate to severely disturbed blood-brain barrier (resulting in an increased total CSF protein of up to several hundred mg/dl), and a normal CSF-to-serum glucose ratio [5]. Additional parameters are the CSF albumin-, IgM-, IgG-, and IgA-to-serum ratio and the presence of oligoclonal IgG bands. Obtaining these further data can aid in the interpretation of borderline values of the routine analysis.

The *Borrelia*-specificity of the infection can be detected in several ways. The most common method is to calculate the CSF-to-serum antibody index (AI) [5]. This *Borrelia* AI is the ratio of *B. burgdorferi*-specific CSF-to-serum antibodies and the CSF-to-serum ratio of albumin or IgG. It allows discrimination between elevated CSF *B. burgdorferi*-specific antibodies caused by a passive transfer due to a blood-CSF barrier dysfunction and those caused by intrathecal production. In contrast to this diagnostic gold standard, the cultivation of *B. burgdorferi* from the CSF is possible in only 10–15% of patients with GBBS in specialized laboratories [13]. A similar diagnostic yield can be achieved by PCR analysis to detect *B. burgdorferi* DNA in the CSF.

A promising diagnostic marker for the future might be the chemokine CXCL13, which was found to be highly elevated in the CSF of LNB patients, but not in other inflammatory and noninflammatory CNS diseases [14]. In contrast to *B. burgdorferi*-specific antibodies, which are found to be absent in 20–30% of cases in the first 2 weeks, CXCL13 was already highly elevated in early stages [15]. Finally, its concentration quickly decreases during therapy [14], making it a promising tool for differentiation between an active or an earlier infection. However, the sensitivity and specificity of CXCL13 has to be evaluated in further prospective studies, and it can therefore not yet be recommended for routine analysis.

On the other hand, there are several further laboratory methods that have not been validated in adequate clinical studies, even though they are already used by some clinicians in the diagnostic workup. Among them are antigen detection from body fluids other than the serum or CSF, PCR of serum or urine, the lymphocytic transformation test, and the so-called 'visual contrast sensitivity test' [10]. All these tests are not suitable for the diagnosis of LNB, and therefore cannot be recommended.

Differential Diagnoses

Several differential diagnoses of LNB have to be considered. The intense radicular pain of BS can be mistaken for a herniated disc or herpes zoster. While the first warrants a CT or MRI scan of the spine, the latter (apart from the typical rash) would result in moderate lymphocytic CSF pleocytosis, just as LNB but without the finding of intrathecal *B. burgdorferi*-specific antibody production. In cases with a predominant meningitis, other forms of meningeal infection or inflammation have to be excluded – among them viral meningitis, carcinomatous meningitis, neurosarcoidosis, fungal meningitis, and other spirochetal infections such as syphilis, leptospirosis and relapsing fever. These differential diagnoses have to be discriminated by microbiological and/or serological methods as the extent of the CSF pleocytosis can be similar to LNB. The facial palsy requires diagnostic differentiation from Guillain-Barré syndrome, Miller-Fisher syndrome and Bell's palsy. These entities can be distinguished from LNB by the lack of an elevated CSF cell count, while they can have similarly elevated total CSF protein resulting from a disturbance in the blood-brain barrier. Finally, chronic progressive Lyme encephalomyelitis has to be differentiated from multiple sclerosis. This can be a diagnostic challenge as the clinical picture in both diseases may be very similar, and both might lead to increased signal intensity of periventricular distribution on T_2-weighted MRI scans. However, the CSF pleocytosis is mostly higher in patients with LNB (>30 cells/μl), and the absence of intrathecal *B. burgdorferi*-specific antibody production as well as a relapsing-remitting course of the disease would exclude a chronic neuroborreliosis. Taken together, only a CSF analysis can reliably differentiate between all these diagnoses, and this further underlines the value of the lumbar puncture in the diagnostic workup of LNB.

Therapeutic Principles

In contrast to the sometimes challenging diagnostic workup, the therapy is rather straightforward. The standard treatment of LNB is ceftriaxone 2 g/day for 2–3 weeks, the latter being recommended for chronic cases [10]. Doxycycline is an alternative in early LNB especially in case of cephalosporin allergy [16]. Though there are no controlled studies comparing different dosages, 300 mg/day might be necessary in view of the low blood-brain barrier penetration of this agent.

When Is a Repeat Lumbar Puncture Indicated?

A repeat puncture is not necessary in patients who become free of symptoms within days to weeks during/after antibiotic therapy. A progression of the infection after adequate antibiotic therapy hardly ever occurs. Symptoms evolving the first time after adequate therapy are merely due to reinfection or other non-*Borrelia* associated causes, rather than representing ongoing infection. A repeat puncture is indicated in suspected treatment failures or relapses. On the one hand, it reveals the course of the inflammatory CNS response. A decrease or normalization of the CSF cell count indicates an adequate treatment response. In case of a persistent clinical syndrome, there might be either irreversible defects independent of the microbiological cure (as the radicular symptoms in LNB are not always reversible [5, 17]), or other noninflammatory reasons are responsible for the clinical picture. It is of note, however, that the normalization of the CSF cell count might take weeks to sometimes months; therefore, a regression of the CSF pleocytosis without normalization within 6 months after treatment does not necessarily indicate a treatment failure and has to be interpreted cautiously. The previously mentioned chemokine, CXCL13, as a diagnostic marker that rapidly decreases during antibiotic treatment, might be an alternative in these cases [14].

On the other hand, a repeat puncture gives the opportunity for additional microbiological testing. In addition, it allows the reanalysis of the different antibody titers, as a significant increase in a certain antibody titer would indicate an active infection with the respective causative organism, and implies a different diagnosis which should lead to treatment adaptation. However, as the diagnosis of LNB is definite in most cases, treatment failures are rare and the rapid decrease in pain in GBBS within 3–5 days after the initiation of therapy is a suitable indicator for an adequate treatment response, the necessity of a repeat puncture should be an exception.

Conclusion

In conclusion, lumbar puncture is the main tool in the diagnosis of LNB. As this infection can be effectively treated with antibiotics and lumbar puncture is a rapid and safe procedure (except, for example, in the case of bleeding abnormalities), every patient with a suspected LNB should undergo a CSF analysis. This can help us to avoid a treatment delay (with potentially irreversible deficits) in confirmed cases and non-indicated ineffective antibiotic treatments, as well as false expectations in misdiagnoses.

Acknowledgment

We thank Ms. Katie Ogston for copyediting the manuscript.

References

1 Huppertz HI, Bohme M, Standaert SM, Karch H, Plotkin SA: Incidence of Lyme borreliosis in the Wurzburg region of Germany. Eur J Clin Microbiol Infect Dis 1999;18:697–703.

2 Hengge UR, Tannapfel A, Tyring SK, Erbel R, Arendt G, Ruzicka T: Lyme borreliosis. Lancet Infect Dis 2003;3:489–500.

3 Wilske B, Fingerle V, Schulte-Spechtel U: Microbiological and serological diagnosis of Lyme borreliosis. FEMS Immunol Med Microbiol 2007;49:13–21.

4 Pfister HW, Wilske B, Weber K: Lyme borreliosis: basic science and clinical aspects. Lancet 1994;343:1013–1016.

5 Hansen K, Lebech AM: The clinical and epidemiological profile of Lyme neuroborreliosis in Denmark 1985–1990: a prospective study of 187 patients with *Borrelia burgdorferi* specific intrathecal antibody production. Brain 1992;115(part 2):399–423.

6 Wilske B, Busch U, Eiffert H, Fingerle V, Pfister HW, Rossler D, Preac-Mursic V: Diversity of OspA and OspC among cerebrospinal fluid isolates of *Borrelia burgdorferi* sensu lato from patients with neuroborreliosis in Germany. Med Microbiol Immunol (Berl) 1996;184:195–201.

7 Ornstein K, Berglund J, Nilsson I, Norrby R, Bergstrom S: Characterization of Lyme borreliosis isolates from patients with erythema migrans and neuroborreliosis in southern Sweden. J Clin Microbiol 2001;39:1294–1298.

8 Steere AC: Lyme disease. N Engl J Med 2001;345:115–125.

9 Christen HJ: Lyme neuroborreliosis in children. Ann Med 1996;28:235–240.

10 Pfister HW, Rupprecht TA: Clinical aspects of neuroborreliosis and post-Lyme disease syndrome in adult patients. Int J Med Microbiol 2006;9:11–16.

11 Kaiser R, Kern A, Kampa D, Neumann-Haefelin D: Prevalence of antibodies to *Borrelia burgdorferi* and tick-borne encephalitis virus in an endemic region in southern Germany. Zentralbl Bakteriol 1997;286:534–541.

12 Hammers-Berggren S, Hansen K, Lebech AM, Karlsson M: *Borrelia burgdorferi*-specific intrathecal antibody production in neuroborreliosis: a follow-up study. Neurology 1993;43:169–175.

13 Karlsson M, Hovind-Hougen K, Svenungsson B, Stiernstedt G: Cultivation and characterization of spirochetes from cerebrospinal fluid of patients with Lyme borreliosis. J Clin Microbiol 1990;28:473–479.

14 Rupprecht TA, Pfister HW, Angele B, Kastenbauer S, Wilske B, Koedel U: The chemokine CXCL13 (BLC): a putative diagnostic marker for neuroborreliosis. Neurology 2005;65:448–450.

15 Rupprecht TA, Koedel U, Angele B, Fingerle V, Pfister HW: Cytokine CXCL13 – a possible early CSF marker for neuroborreliosis (in German). Nervenarzt 2006;77:470–473.

16 Halperin JJ, Shapiro ED, Logigian E, Belman AL, Dotevall L, Wormser GP, Krupp L, Gronseth G, Bever CT Jr: Practice parameter: treatment of nervous system Lyme disease (an evidence-based review): report of the Quality Standards Subcommittee of the American Academy of Neurology. Neurology 2007;69:91–102.

17 Kalish RA, Kaplan RF, Taylor E, Jones-Woodward L, Workman K, Steere AC: Evaluation of study patients with Lyme disease, 10–20-year follow-up. J Infect Dis 2001;183:453–460.

Hans-Walter Pfister, MD
Department of Neurology, Klinikum Grosshadern, Ludwig-Maximilians University
Marchioninistrasse 15, DE–81377 Munich (Germany)
Tel. +49 89 7095 3676, Fax +49 89 7095 6673, E-Mail hans-walter.pfister@med.uni-muenchen.de

Author Index

Subject Index